Mosby's

Review for
Long-Term Care
Certification

for Practical and Vocational Nurses

D1569778

Mosby's

Review for
Long-Term Care
Certification

for Practical and Vocational Nurses

Mary O. Eyles, MA, RN
Director of Education
Kessler Institute for Rehabilitation, Inc.
West Orange, New Jersey

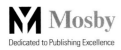

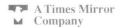

Vice President and Publisher: Nancy L. Coon
Senior Editor: Susan R. Epstein
Associate Developmental Editors: Laurie K. Muench, Jerry Schwartz
Project Manager: Deborah L. Vogel
Production Editor: Mamata Reddy
Manuscript Editor: Lavon Wirch Peters
Electronic Production Coordinator: Joan Herron
Designer: Pati Pye
Cover Art: Elizabeth Rohne Rudder
Manufacturing Manager: David Graybill

Printed in the United States of America
Composition by Mosby Electronic Production, St. Louis
Printing/Binding by R.R. Donnelley & Sons Company

National Council of State Boards of Nursing, Inc.
676 North St. Clair Street
Suite 550
Chicago, Illinois 60611-2921

International Standard Book Number 0-8151-3170-4

96 97 98 99 00 / 9 8 7 6 5 4 3 2 1

To all LPNs/LVNs in long-term care who give untiringly of themselves
to the care of those individuals in need of their skills,
commitment, dedication, and, most of all, caring.

EDITOR

Mary O. Eyles, MA, RN
Director of Education
Kessler Institute for Rehabilitation, Inc.
West Orange, New Jersey

CONTRIBUTING EDITORS

Anita A. Brooks, BA, RN
LPN Instructor (Retired)
Quality Resource Management Analyst (Retired)
Toms River, New Jersey

G. Constance Butherus, MA, RN
Director of Professional and Residential Services
Hunterdon Developmental Center
Clinton, New Jersey

Laura Hart Cole, BS
Education Coordinator
Kessler Institute for Rehabilitation, Inc.
West Orange, New Jersey

Nuha D. Hababo, BSN, CPM
Director of Nursing
Vineland Developmental Center Hospital
Vineland, New Jersey

Shirley Woerner Kallen, BS, RN,C
Director of Nursing
Crest Haven Nursing Home
Cape May Court House, New Jersey

CONSULTANT

Maria C. Dixon, LPN
Private Duty Nursing,
Long Term Care
Harleigh, Pennsylvania

M. Catherine Dulio, LNHA, LPN
Administrator
Holy Family Residence
West Paterson, New Jersey

Foreword

Congratulations! If you are an LPN/LVN and have bought this book, you have taken a major step toward the National Association for Practical Nurse Education and Service, Inc. (NAPNES) Certification in Long-Term Care (LTC). When you pass the examination and become certified, you can proudly wear the NAPNES Certified in Long-Term Care (CLTC) pin that tells your employer, your patients, and the world that your skills in long-term care are nationally recognized! You have taken the opportunity to enhance your career by skill building beyond the competence your license indicates. Passing the certification test developed by the National Council of State Boards of Nursing (the National Council) and receiving the certificate and pin issued by NAPNES sets you apart. To be sure, as an LPN/LVN, you already provide excellent care. The valuable information in this book builds on that quality because it takes you, step by step, through the process of preparing for the LTC certification examination that enhances your competence.

This book is conveniently divided into five units with a total of 24 chapters. Unit One consists of two introductory chapters that orient you to the Fundamental Practice Issues in Long-Term Care and prepare you for studying for the examination. Unit Two comprises 14 chapters that cover Physiologic Integrity. The unit starts with General Nursing Management and takes you through all of the body systems, focusing on nursing responsibilities in Long-Term Care settings. Chapters on Pharmacology, Aging, and Pediatrics highlight important concepts and special needs.

Unit Three, Psychologic Integrity, follows with chapters on the Developmental Continuum, Communication, and Cognitive and Emotional Considerations. Unit Four takes you into Specialty Practice Issues with chapters on Education Issues as well as Ethical and Legal Considerations. The last unit of this comprehensive study guide, Unit Five, brings closure to your study by concentrating on Leadership and Management. These chapters, on the Interdisciplinary Team, Leadership and Management Issues, as well as Safe and Effective Care Environment are just as pertinent and valuable as the rest of the information. Study questions at the end of each chapter and a comprehensive examination provide additional insight to the subject material and serve as check points to validate your knowledge.

The leadership, integrity and personal best of each contributing editor are reflected in every chapter. The product of their collective effort, based on years of education and experience, will have a positive impact on long-term care through the enhancement of your skills.

It is my pleasure to tell you that NAPNES, the National Council, and Mosby wish you much success in this endeavor.

Helen M. Larsen, JD, BS, LPN
President
National Association for Practical Nurse
Education and Service, Inc. (NAPNES)

Preface

Mosby's Review for Long-Term Care Certification for Practical and Vocational Nurses has been developed for nurses in long-term care settings for use as a clinical reference or review for the Certification Examination for Practical Nurses (CEPN) for Long-Term Care. This book is based on the test plan for the CEPN as developed by The National Council of State Boards of Nursing, Inc. (the National Council) in cooperation with the National Association for Practical Nurse Education and Service, Inc. (NAPNES).

An extensive outline overview of content is provided in the following areas:

- Physiologic integrity coverage includes review of all body systems.
- Chapters on Pharmacology, Aging, and Pediatrics highlight important concepts and special needs.
- Psychosocial integrity coverage includes chapters on the Developmental Continuum, Communication, and Cognitive and Emotional Considerations.
- Discussion of Specialty Practice focuses on resident education and ethical and legal issues.
- Leadership and Management issues include the practical/vocational nurse as a key part of the interdisciplinary team and the promotion of a safe and effective care environment.

Review questions are provided for each chapter, and a comprehensive examination at the end of the book parallels the CEPN. Answers for all questions include rationales that explain why the correct answer is correct and why each of the remaining options is wrong.

For the sake of clarity and consistency, the word *nurse* is used to indicate a practical/vocational nurse. The recipient of care is termed the *resident* to provide consistency as well, although we acknowledge that the term *client* or *patient* may be preferred.

The editor of and contributors to this text have the upmost respect for and recognize the LPN/LVN as a valued member of today's health care team, providing quality nursing care to long-term care residents nationwide. It is because of this respect and recognition that this text has been developed, with the hope that individuals preparing for certification in long-term care will find a dependable source with which to prepare for the examination.

As a coordinating editor, I would like to thank all those individuals who have worked so diligently in the preparation of this text. This includes all contributors and consultants, as well as all those at Mosby, especially Suzi Epstein and Laurie Muench, without whom this text would not have been possible. I would also like to extend a special note of thanks to my husband Robert, for being so supportive of our efforts during the preparation of this text.

To those who will use this text, we wish you all the best and much success. Remember that POSITIVE ATTITUDE!

Mary O. Eyles

Table of Contents

UNIT FIVE
LEADERSHIP AND MANAGEMENT

Introduction

chapter one

Preparing for the Long-Term Care Certification Examination

The purpose of this text is threefold: (1) to assist you in determining the extent of your knowledge relative to your specific strengths and weaknesses in long-term care nursing, (2) to increase your understanding of that knowledge through additional study, and (3) to increase your familiarity with and ability to respond to written test questions and corresponding clinical situations similar to those presented in the certification examination.

The National Council of State Boards of Nursing (the National Council) test plan for this examination encompasses four categories of practical/vocational nursing activities. Each category is vital to the assurance of the final intent of the examination: to recognize the expanded role of the nurse in long-term care. The four categories as given in the actual test plan, including the percent of questions allocated to each specific category on the examination are provided below.

PHYSIOLOGIC INTEGRITY—35% TO 42%

The nurse certified in long-term care meets the physiologic integrity needs of residents with the goal of promoting quality of life. The knowledge, skills, and abilities needed to meet the physiologic integrity needs of the resident include an ability to identify potential problems and ongoing changes in the resident that could affect outcomes of treatment, to respect the individuality of each resident, to identify significant early cues to prevent complications, to utilize alternate interventions, to initiate and follow through with intended actions, and to use communication and organization skills to work with others. The nursing process (assessment, analysis, planning, implementation, and evaluation) is incorporated in all aspects of meeting the physiologic integrity needs of the resident.

PSYCHOSOCIAL INTEGRITY—18% TO 22%

The nurse certified in long-term care meets the psychosocial integrity needs of residents with the goal of promoting quality of life. The knowledge, skills, and abilities needed to meet the psychosocial integrity needs of the resident include knowledge of growth, development, and family dynamics; respect for the individual resident; and the ability to communicate. The nursing process (assessment, analysis, planning, implementation, and evaluation) is inherent in all aspects of meeting residents' needs related to psychosocial integrity.

SPECIALTY PRACTICE ISSUES—13% TO 17%

The nurse certified in long-term care meets the specialty practice issues to improve the quality of life and to serve as a resource to others. The knowledge, skills, and abilities needed to meet the specialty practice issues needs of the resident include knowledge of teaching and learning concepts, nursing process, communication skills, respect for the uniqueness of the individual, and knowledge of federal and state legislation, as well as policy issues affecting long-term care residents.

LEADERSHIP AND MANAGEMENT—23% TO 27%

The nurse certified in long-term care meets the leadership and management needs required in a long-term care setting. The knowledge, skills, and abilities needed to meet these needs include utilizing the nursing process, communication, and organization skills to work with others as a team leader, as well as a team member. The nurse, because of extensive experience in the long-term care environment and current knowledge, serves as a resource to others.

Effective Study

The key to effective study and the use of this text can only be determined by you. The review is presented in a manner that is easily adaptable to various forms of study habits, in addition to affording you the opportunity to become familiar with taking timed examinations.

Each unit outlines a specific content area within the long-term care test plan followed by a set of questions relative to that particular content area. You will find the correct answers and the rationales for both the correct and incorrect responses for each unit at the end of the text.

You may want to start with the questions to determine areas in which you need more study and then return to review the outline of that particular unit. Should you feel more in-depth study is needed, you may choose to select resources from the reference list found at the end of this text.

Once you have completed review of all units and corresponding questions, you are ready to take the comprehensive examination. The comprehensive examination contains 150 questions and should take 2^1/$_2$ hours to complete. Time yourself or have someone time you.

Although the examination may be administered by computers in the future, the examination initially comprises a test booklet. You are required to indicate your answer choice for each question directly in this booklet. To help you become accustomed to this procedure, you should darken your answer choice on the unit review questions. On the comprehensive examination questions, you should indicate your response as you did on the unit review questions. Marking your answers in this manner also eliminates the need to keep your place on an answer sheet and permits you to concentrate on answering the questions.

This review book contains one full examination and simulates the certification examination in length, as well as content. Proper use of this text will not only increase your nursing knowledge but will also increase your self-confidence in your test-taking abilities.

Remember, intelligence plays a vital role in your ability to learn. However, being "smart" involves more than just intelligence. Being practical and applying common sense are also part of the learning experience.

Regardless of how you choose to study, following these simple study guides may be helpful:

1. Establish priorities and the goals by which to achieve those priorities.

2. Enhance organizational skills by developing a checklist and creating ways to improve your ability to retain information, such as index cards, which are easy to carry.
3. Enhance time-management skills by designing a study schedule that best suits your needs and by considering the following:
   - Amount of time needed
   - Amount of time available
   - "Best" time to study
   - Allowance for emergencies/free time
4. Prepare for study by considering the following:
   - Conducive environment
   - Appropriate study material
   - Planned study sessions alone or with friend/group
   - Formal review course

One word of caution: do not expect to achieve the maximum benefits of this text by cramming a few days before sitting for the examination. It does not work. Instead, organize planned study sessions, by yourself or with others, over a reasonable period of time in an environment that you find relaxing and conducive to learning.

Test-Taking Skills

By now you more than likely have been exposed to a variety of objective and subjective testing. The certification examination, however, deals only with the objective type and more precisely with the objective multiple choice form of testing. Although this form of testing may be familiar to you, let's examine how you can avoid some common test-taking errors:

1. Answer the question that is asked. To do so, you need to read, not scan, the question carefully, looking for key words or phrases. Do not read anything into the question or apply what you did in a similar situation during your clinical experiences. No one is trying to trick you. Each question contains a stem (the main intent of the question), followed by four plausible answers or alternatives that either complete a statement or answer the question presented. Only one of the alternatives is the best answer; the remaining three alternatives are known as distractors, because they are written in such a way that they could be the correct answer and may distract you to a certain degree. Your nursing knowledge will, however, lead you to the correct answer.

2. Listen to the examiner and read the written directions carefully. Failure to listen or read the directions thoroughly may lead to an incorrect answer, which could cause you considerable loss of points. Should you have any questions about the directions, ask the examiner for clarification.
3. Have confidence in your initial response to a question, because it will probably be the correct answer. If you are unable to answer immediately, eliminate the alternatives you know are incorrect and proceed from there. Remember there is a time factor involved, so don't spend an excessive amount of time on any one question. The maximum time allotted to any question should be 1 minute. If you do find it necessary to move on, make a note of the question omitted and return to it later. Not all questions will consume a full minute; some may take only 20 or 30 seconds to read and answer.
4. Taking a wild guess at an answer should be avoided at all costs; however, should you feel insecure about a question, eliminate the alternatives you feel are definitely incorrect. This will increase your chances of randomly selecting the correct answer. There is no penalty for guessing on the examination, so be sure to answer every question.
5. Above all, begin with a positive attitude about yourself, your nursing knowledge, and your test-taking abilities. A positive attitude is achieved through self-confidence gained by studying effectively. Stated simply this means (a) answering questions (assessment), (b) explore available resources (analysis), (c) organizing study time (planning), (d) reading and further study (implementation), and (e) again answering questions (evaluation).

Being emotionally prepared for an examination is also a key factor to your success; however, proper use of this text over an extended period will eliminate any mystery relative to the mechanics of the examination as well as increase your confidence about the nursing knowledge you possess. Practicing a few relaxation techniques may also prove helpful to you, especially on the day of the examination.

Before you begin your review sessions or take the licensing examination, here are some additional words of advice:

- Many times the correct answer is the longest alternative given; however, don't count on it. Individuals who prepare the examination are also aware of this fact and so attempt to avoid offering you any such "helpful hints."
- Avoid looking for an answer pattern or code. Many times four or five consecutive questions will have the same letter or number for the correct answer.
- Key words or phrases in the stem of the question, such as first, primary, early, and best, are also important. Likewise, words such as only, always, never, and all in the alternatives will often be evidence of a wrong response, as in life, there are no real absolutes in nursing. Of course, there are exceptions to every rule, so answer with care.
- Be alert for grammatical inconsistencies. If the response is intended to complete the stem (an incomplete sentence) but makes no grammatical sense to you, it can be considered to be a distractor rather than the correct answer. Great effort is expended by test developers, however, to eliminate such inconsistencies.
- Answer all questions. You have at least a 25% chance of selecting the correct answer.
- The night before the examination you may want to review some material, but then relax and get a good night's sleep. In the morning allow yourself plenty of time to dress, have breakfast, and arrive at the testing site a few minutes early. Be sure you know where to park and where the test will be given. By doing so you will reduce your stress/tension level. Remember that *positive attitude!*

Scoring

Tests are computer-scored to determine the number of correct answers (raw score). The raw score is then equated onto a scale that allows comparison with the passing standard set by the National Association for Practical Nurse Education and Service (NAPNES).

You started preparation for this certification examination the day you began working in long-term care. Every clinical experience and resident interaction has had meaning and purpose. *Mosby's Review for Long-Term Care Certification for Practical and Vocational Nurses* has been developed to assist the practitioner in the certification preparation process. It is now in your hands, for only your initiative and dedication to achieve well-deserved recognition as a long-term care clinician will be rewarded with success.

chapter two

Fundamental Practice Issues in Long-Term Care

Long-Term Care Defined

A. Refers to the type of services provided either in an institutional setting such as a nursing home or rehabilitation center, in a day-care program, or at home once the acute phase of an illness has past

B. Generally provides supportive maintenance and/or restorative interdisciplinary health intervention for individuals with chronic or long-term health problems

C. Types of long-term care settings
  1. Nursing homes
    a. Provide all degrees of skilled nursing care and related services such as medical, dietary, social services, activities, pharmacy, and rehabilitation from maintenance to restorative care
    b. Some nursing homes have a special mission to provide services to residents with a specific health problem (e.g., nursing for residents who have positive test results for the human immunodeficiency virus (HIV); whose test results are positive for HIV and who have a history of substance abuse; or who have a diagnosis of Alzheimer's disease or head trauma
    c. The Nursing Home Reform Law of 1987 has abolished the titles *skilled nursing facility* and *health-related facility* and replaced them with the title *nursing home*
  2. Adult day health care: an institutional daytime program that provides all degrees of care from skilled nursing care to personal care and from rehabilitation to social programs, depending on whether they are based on a medical, nursing, or social model; the resident is able to live at home during the evening and night, which provides an alternative to institutionalization

  3. Hospice care: emotional, physical, and supportive care to the terminally ill resident and significant others; may be provided on an inpatient or outpatient basis; provides pain control; supports quality of life; does not institute life support or other extraordinary means to prolong the life; hospice services may be in an independent institution, a unit within another setting, or in the home

  4. Rehabilitation center: institution that provides multiple services and facilities that assist a resident and family to make an adjustment to living; the resident can obtain an optimal level of health by developing personal abilities to their fullest potential and using the following resources
    a. Medical and nursing: total health assessment and planning, physical therapy, occupational therapy, and speech therapy
    b. Psychosocial: personal counseling, social service, and psychiatric service
    c. Vocational: work evaluation, vocational counseling, vocational training, trial employment in sheltered workshops, terminal employment in sheltered workshops, and job placement

5. Home care: comprehensive services for people who do not need to be hospitalized and yet require more care than an outpatient facility can provide; prevents or delays institutionalization; care is provided by both nonprofessional and professional staff (e.g., public health nurses, homemaker services, medical home care programs, and home health aides)
6. Respite care: a form of short-term health care service provided in either an institution or in the home to enable the primary care giver to rest temporarily; allows the primary care giver time to pursue personal interests, enjoy time alone with other family members, be away from the home, or go on vacation
7. Adult housing: residence in which an individual lives; meals and recreational programs may often be supplied; however, medical and nursing supervision are generally not provided on a full-time basis

The Nursing Process In Long-Term Care

A. Basis of personalized care is planned rather than relying on intuitive intervention
B. Most efficient way to accomplish this in a time of exploding knowledge and rapid social change is by the nursing process
   1. Theoretic framework used by the nurse
   2. Assists in solving or alleviating both simple and complex nursing problems
C. Changing, expanding, more responsible role demands knowledgeably planned, purposeful, and accountable action by nurses
D. Documentation of nursing care is done to:
   1. Provide comprehensive and systematic nursing care through use of the nursing process
   2. Satisfy requirements of regulatory agencies
      a. Hospitals and nursing homes are licensed by the state in which they operate; the state sets regulations that must be met
      b. The Joint Commission on Accreditation of Healthcare Organizations (JCAHO) accredits hospitals and some nursing homes; hospitals must be accredited by JCAHO for Medicare and Medicaid reimbursement

   c. Health Care Financing Administration (HCFA) certifies nursing homes; nursing homes must be certified by HCFA for Medicare and Medicaid reimbursement
   d. Documentation of care by staff is vital and it becomes a focal point of the accreditation/certification process
   3. Provide a legal document that reflects the care given to and the progress of the resident
   4. Provide a data base for continuous quality improvement programs
E. Decision making that systematically selects and uses relevant information is a requisite for individualized resident care
F. Cognitive, affective, and activity nursing components can best be integrated by the nursing process
G. Process consists of assessing, diagnosing, planning, implementing, and evaluating a resident's problem and its proposed solution through the nursing care plan; it is continuous throughout the resident's stay

STEPS IN THE NURSING PROCESS

A. Assessment
   1. Collection of personal, social, medical, and general data
      a. Sources: primary (resident and diagnostic test results) and secondary (family, colleagues, Kardex, literature)
      b. Methods
         (1) Interviewing formally (nursing health history) and informally during various nurse-resident interactions
         (2) Observation
         (3) Review of records
B. Analysis/nursing diagnosis
   1. Classification of data: screening, organizing, and grouping significant and related information
   2. Definition of resident problem: making a nursing diagnosis
      a. A nursing diagnosis is a definitive statement of the resident's actual or potential difficulties, concerns, or deficits that are amenable to nursing interventions; there are two components to the statement of a nursing diagnosis:

(1) Part I: a determination of the problem (unhealthful response of resident)

(2) Part II: identification of the etiologic (contributing) factors

(3) The two parts are joined together by the phrase "related to"

b. Development of diagnoses (see list of NANDA-approved Nursing Diagnoses, pp. 10-12).

(1) Excludes all nonnursing diagnoses (e.g., medical diagnoses or diagnostic tests)

(2) Excludes medical treatments, as well as the nurse's problems with the resident

(3) Involves inductive and deductive reasoning

(4) Includes both internal and external environmental stresses

(5) Includes data that have been clustered (grouping of related data) during assessment

C. Planning: the nursing care plan, a blueprint for action

1. Previously identified nursing diagnoses are written on the care plan

2. Planned intervention may include both independent and interdependent functions of the nurse; prescriptions made by physician or allied health professionals may be included

3. New diagnoses should be noted on the nursing care plan and progress notes as they are identified

4. Resident outcomes (goals of nursing intervention) are reflected in expected changes in the resident

a. Expected resident outcome is written next to each nursing diagnosis on nursing care plan

b. These outcomes must be objective, realistic, measurable, observable alterations in the resident's behavior, activity, or physical state; a time period should be set for achievement of the outcome

c. The outcome provides a standard of measure that can be used to determine if the goal toward which the resident

and nurse are working has been achieved

5. Nursing interventions (nursing orders) are written for each nursing diagnosis and should be specific to the stated outcome or goal; each goal may have one or more applicable interventions

D. Implementation: the actual administration of the planned nursing care

E. Evaluation/outcome and revision of nursing care plan

1. Process is ongoing throughout the resident's treatment/hospitalization

2. If outcome/goal is not reached in specified time, the resident is reassessed to discover the reason

3. Reordering of priorities and new goal setting may be necessary

4. When diagnosis/problem is resolved, the date should be noted on care plan

F. Advantages of nursing process

1. Encourages thorough individual resident assessment by nurse

2. Determines priority of care

3. Provides comprehensive and systematic nursing care planning and delivery

4. Permits independent, creative, and flexible nursing intervention

5. Facilitates team cooperation by promoting

a. Contributions from all team members

b. Communication among team members

c. Coordination of care

d. Continuity of care

6. Provides for continuous involvement and input from resident or family members

7. Facilitates the "costing-out" of nursing services and care

8. Facilitates nursing research

9. Provides accurate legal document of resident care

10. Satisfies rules of regulatory agencies

Documentation In Long-Term Care

A. Universal principles of documentation
1. Professional responsibility
2. Accountability

B. Primary means of communication between members of the interdisciplinary team

C. Documentation must clearly communicate the following:

1. Nurse's decision-making process, assessments, diagnosis, planning, interventions, evaluations
2. Resident's response to nursing interventions
3. Resident/family education, discharge planning, and psychologic/psychosocial factors
D. Only approved abbreviations and medical terms should be used when charting in a resident's record. Knowledge of the common abbreviations and terms is required.
E. Purposes for written records include the following:
   1. Continuity of care
   2. Permanent record for accountability (i.e., for audits, accreditation, cost reimbursement)
   3. Legal record
   4. Teaching, research, and data collection
F. Two common formats for charting nurse's notes are narrative and focus. Focus charting has a data (D), action (A), and response (R) format.
G. Charting needs to be legible, clear, concise, accurate, and complete. These guidelines serve as a national standard for licensed nurses.
H. Each institution or unit may have specific forms and charting formats, but the general guidelines and rules for charting should be followed.
I. Medical records are legal documents. The physician or institution owns the original record.
J. Lawyers, courts, and residents can gain access to the record but must follow specified access procedures.
K. A health record is confidential information protected by the law and the Patient's Bill of Rights.
L. The nursing Kardex is a card-filing system used by nurses to condense all the orders and other care information needed quickly for each resident. It is kept at the nursing station for quick reference and is updated frequently.
M. The nursing care plan is a plan of care for a resident and a part of the health record. The nurse uses the assessment data to make nursing diagnoses of the resident's responses to illness and problems. This plan includes the nursing diagnosis, treatment goals, specific directions for care implementation, and evaluation guidelines. The care plan should serve as a guide for individualized nursing care delivery and recording.

N. Nursing access to computer terminals and care documentation systems has the potential to save time and energy needed for resident care services. These systems are expensive but are a great benefit to the nurses able to use them.
O. Fax machines are now used to send written documents over telephone lines to quickly transmit data between hospitals and other facilities.

LEGAL GUIDELINES

A. Do not erase, apply correction fluid, or scratch out errors made while recording.
B. Do not write retaliatory or critical comments about resident or care by other health care professionals.
C. Correct all errors promptly.
D. Record only facts.
E. Do not leave blank spaces in nurse's notes.
F. Record all entries legibly and in ink.
G. If order is questioned, record that clarification was sought.
H. Chart only for yourself.
I. Avoid using generalized, empty phrases such as "status unchanged" or "had good day."
J. Begin each entry with time, and end with your signature and title.

NANDA-approved Nursing Diagnoses

Activity intolerance
Activity intolerance, risk for
Adaptive capacity, decreased: intracranial
Adjustment, impaired
Airway clearance, ineffective
Anxiety
Aspiration, risk for
Body image disturbance
Body temperature, altered, risk for
Bowel incontinence
Breastfeeding, effective
Breastfeeding, ineffective
Breastfeeding, interrupted
Breathing pattern, ineffective
Cardiac output, decreased
Caregiver role strain
Caregiver role strain, risk for
Communication, impaired verbal
Community coping, potential for enhanced
Community coping, ineffective
Confusion, acute

Confusion, chronic
Constipation
Constipation, colonic
Constipation, perceived
Coping, defensive
Coping, family: potential for growth
Coping, ineffective family: compromised
Coping, ineffective family: disabling
Coping, ineffective individual
Decisional conflict (specify)
Denial, ineffective
Diarrhea
Disuse syndrome, risk for
Diversional activity deficit
Dysreflexia
Energy field disturbance
Environmental interpretation syndrome: impaired
Family processes, altered: Alcoholism
Family processes, altered
Fatigue
Fear
Fluid volume deficit
Fluid volume deficit, risk for
Fluid volume excess
Gas exchange, impaired
Grieving, anticipatory
Grieving, dysfunctional
Growth and development, altered
Health maintenance, altered
Health-seeking behaviors (specify)
Home maintenance management, impaired
Hopelessness
Hyperthermia
Hypothermia
Incontinence, functional
Incontinence, reflex
Incontinence, stress
Incontinence, total
Incontinence, urge
Infant behavior, disorganized
Infant behavior, disorganized: risk for
Infant behavior, organized: potential for enhanced
Infant feeding pattern, ineffective
Infection, risk for
Injury, perioperative positioning: risk for
Injury, risk for
Knowledge deficit (specify)
Loneliness, risk for
Management of therapeutic regimen, community:
  ineffective

Management of therapeutic regimen, families:
  ineffective
Management of therapeutic regimen, individuals:
  effective
Management of therapeutic regimen, individuals:
  ineffective
Memory, impaired
Mobility, impaired physical
Noncompliance (specify)
Nutrition, altered: less than body requirements
Nutrition, altered: more than body requirements
Nutrition, altered: risk for more than body require-
  ments
Oral mucous membrane, altered
Pain
Pain, chronic
Parent/Infant/Child attachment altered, risk for
Parental role conflict
Parenting, altered
Parenting, altered, risk for
Peripheral neurovascular dysfunction, risk for
Personal identity disturbance
Poisoning, risk for
Post-trauma response
Powerlessness
Protection, altered
Rape-trauma syndrome
Rape-trauma syndrome: compound reaction
Rape-trauma syndrome: silent reaction
Relocation stress syndrome
Role performance, altered
Self-care deficit, bathing/hygiene
Self-care deficit, dressing/grooming
Self-care deficit, feeding
Self-care deficit, toileting
Self-esteem disturbance
Self-esteem, chronic low
Self-esteem, situational low
Self-mutilation, risk for
Sensory/perceptual alterations (specify) (visual,
  auditory, kinesthetic, gustatory, tactile, olfactory)
Sexual dysfunction
Sexuality patterns, altered
Skin integrity, impaired
Skin integrity, impaired, risk for
Sleep pattern disturbance
Social interaction, impaired
Social isolation
Spiritual distress (distress of the human spirit)
Spiritual well-being, potential for enhanced

Suffocation, risk for
Swallowing, impaired
Thermoregulation, ineffective
Thought processes, altered
Tissue integrity, impaired
Tissue perfusion, altered (specify type) (renal, cerebral, cardiopulmonary, gastrointestinal, peripheral)
Trauma, risk for
Unilateral neglect
Urinary elimination, altered
Urinary retention
Ventilation, inability to sustain spontaneous
Ventilatory weaning process, dysfunctional (DVWP)
Violence, risk for: self-directed or directed at others

Physiologic Integrity

chapter three

General Nursing Management

In meeting the physiologic needs of residents, various measures are implemented that need not relate to a specific condition or problem. This chapter provides an overview of some of the common therapies and pertinent nursing considerations.

Nutrition and Diet Therapy

Nutrition is the combination of processes by which the body uses food for growth, energy, and maintenance. Nutrition is also the study of food and its relation to health and disease. The nurse plays an especially important role in the nutritional aspects of resident care. Because of close and continual contact with the resident, the nurse is able to evaluate and monitor the resident's nutritional status and inform the dietitian about the resident's nutritional needs and acceptance of the nutritional plan of care. Good nutrition is essential to good health throughout the life cycle, and the nurse is in an excellent position to encourage sound nutritional practices for each resident.

Principles of Nutrition

A. Functions of food
   1. Provides energy
   2. Builds and repairs body tissues
   3. Regulates and controls the body's chemical processes, which are essential for providing energy and building tissues
B. Evidence of good nutrition
C. Primary causes of nutritional deficiency
   1. Dietary lack of specific essential nutrients caused by
      a. Anorexia (resulting from a variety of causes)
      b. Alcoholism (and the resulting lack of proper nutrition)
      c. Poor food habits or eating nutritionally deficient foods
   2. Inability of the body to use a specific nutrient properly as a result of
      a. Diseases of the digestive tract such as ulcerative colitis
      b. Faulty absorption in digestive tract (such as the way in which the excessive use of mineral oil impedes the absorption of fat-soluble vitamins)
      c. Metabolic disorders such as diabetes
      d. Drug interactions and/or toxicity
D. Classification of nutrients
   1. Nutrients are chemical substances that are present in food and needed by the body to function
   2. Six prime nutrients
      a. Carbohydrates
      b. Fats
      c. Proteins
      d. Vitamins
      e. Minerals
      f. Water

FOUR BASIC FOOD GROUPS

A. Developed by the U.S. Department of Agriculture as a guide for planning a well-balanced diet
B. Milk group
   1. Milk, cheese, ice cream, and yogurt
   2. Daily recommended servings vary with age
      a. Adults, two servings
      b. Children under 9 years of age, two to three servings
      c. Children 9 to 12 years of age, three or more servings

3. Nutrients primarily supplied are calcium, protein, and riboflavin

C. Meat group
   1. Beef, veal, lamb, pork, organ meats, poultry, fish, eggs, dry peas and beans, nuts, and peanut butter
   2. Recommended servings, two or more per day
   3. Nutrients primarily supplied are protein, iron, and B vitamins

D. Vegetable and fruit group
   1. All fruits and vegetables except dry peas, beans, and lentils
   2. Recommended servings, four or more per day including
      a. One source rich in vitamin C (or two equal sources)
      b. One dark green or deep yellow vegetable or fruit rich in vitamin A
   3. Nutrients primarily supplied are vitamins A and C, carbohydrates (sugar), and most dietary fiber

E. Bread and cereal group
   1. All enriched and restored breads, cereals, pasta products, crackers, and other baked goods made with flour
   2. Recommended servings, four or more per day
   3. Nutrients primarily supplied are iron, B complex vitamins, and carbohydrates (starches); refined products contain fewer vitamins, whereas the enriched, fortified, or restored products contain many more vitamins

FOOD GUIDE PYRAMID

A. Emphasizes grains, fruits, and vegetables as the foundation of a balanced diet and downplays meats, dairy products, and fats; fats, oils, and sweets are recommended sparingly

B. Specific guidelines
   1. Breads, cereals, rice, pasta: six to eleven servings daily (1 serving = 1 slice of bread, 1 oz of ready-to-eat cereal, or $1/2$ cup of cooked cereal, rice, or pasta)
   2. Fruits: two to four servings daily (1 serving = 1 medium apple, banana, or orange or $1/2$ cup of cooked, chopped, or canned fruit)
   3. Vegetables: three to five servings daily (1 serving = 1 cup of raw, leafy vegetables or $1/2$ cup of other vegetables cooked, chopped, or raw)
   4. Milk, yogurt, cheese: two to three servings daily (1 serving equals 1 cup of milk or yogurt or $1^1/2$ oz of natural cheese)
   5. Meat, poultry, fish, dry beans, eggs, and nuts: two to three servings daily (1 serving equals 2 to 3 oz. of cooked lean meat, poultry, or fish; $1/2$ cup of cooked dry beans or 1 egg; 2 tbsp of peanut butter = 1 oz. of lean meat)

ASSIMILATION OF NUTRIENTS
Digestion and Absorption

A. Digestion: the process of changing foods to be absorbed and used by cells; mechanical digestion and chemical digestion occur simultaneously
   1. Mechanical digestion (chewing, swallowing, peristalsis) breaks food into small pieces, mixes it with digestive juices, and moves it along the digestive tract
   2. Chemical digestion occurs through the action of enzymes, which break large food molecules into smaller molecules
      a. Carbohydrate digestion begins in the mouth and occurs primarily in the small intestine; carbohydrates are reduced to simple sugars (monosaccharides), such as glucose, for absorption
      b. Protein digestion begins in the stomach and is completed in the small intestine; proteins are broken down into amino acids for absorption
      c. Fat digestion begins in the stomach but occurs primarily in the small intestine; fats are reduced to fatty acids and glycerol for absorption

B. Absorption: the process by which end products of digestion (fatty acids, glycerol, amino acids, and glucose) are absorbed from the small intestine into circulation (blood and lymph) to be distributed to the cells

Metabolism

A. Use of food by the body cells for producing energy and for building complex chemical compounds

B. Consists of two processes
1. Catabolism: the breakdown of food molecules into carbon dioxide and water, which releases energy; carbohydrates are primarily catabolized for energy
2. Anabolism: the process by which food molecules are built up into more complex chemical compounds; proteins are primarily anabolized (used for building)

Energy

A. Energy is required for the metabolic processes of catabolism and anabolism; energy needs of the body are based on three factors
1. Physical activity: the type of activity and how long it is performed
2. Basal metabolism: the energy required for the body to sustain life while in a resting state (1 calorie per kilogram [2 lbs.] of body weight per hour)
3. Thermic effects of food: energy required for the digestion, absorption, and metabolism of foods
B. Measurement of energy
1. The calorie (or kilocalorie) is the unit used to measure the energy value of food
2. Fuel values of basic nutrients
    a. Carbohydrate: 4 calories per gram
    b. Fat: 9 calories per gram
    c. Protein: 4 calories per gram
3. Total number of calories needed per day
    a. Moderately active man: 20.5 calories per pound (0.45 kg) of ideal weight
    b. Moderately active woman: 18 calories per pound (0.45 kg) of ideal weight

Nutrition in Childhood and Adolescence
PRESCHOOL CHILDREN

A. Growth rate is slower and more erratic, and food intake will vary accordingly
B. A variety of foods should be offered
1. "Finger foods" such as carrot sticks are enjoyed
2. Serve small amounts because too large a serving can discourage a child from eating
3. Avoid refined sweets
4. Do not coax a child to eat; if a food is refused, offer it at a later time
5. Nutritious snacks are a viable alternative for a child who is a poor eater
C. Teach healthy eating habits; avoid rewarding good behavior with food

SCHOOL CHILDREN (5 TO 10 YEARS OF AGE)

A. Gradual increase in growth at this age (approximately equal for boys and girls)
B. Proper nutrition is important to proper mental and physical development (adequate breakfast is important for alertness)
C. Children are usually good eaters at this age and should be encouraged by setting good examples

ADOLESCENTS

A. Tremendous growth spurt occurs at puberty (age of sexual maturity)
1. For girls, usually between 10 and 13 years of age
2. For boys, between 13 and 16 years of age
B. Diets are influenced by peers, with much empty-calorie foods being consumed
C. Boys gain mostly lean muscle tissue; they consume large amounts of food to meet energy requirements
D. Girls gain more fat tissue; their diets may be more influenced by a desire to remain thin; frequently require iron supplements to meet their needs; adequate nutrition during adolescence helps avoid complications in later years; promote healthy eating along with exercise

Nutrition in Adults
ADULTS

A. Adequate nutrition throughout the life span is important in avoiding many serious illnesses
B. Proper nutrition is based on guidelines set by U.S. government agencies (such as the four basic food groups)
C. Individuals who consume a balanced diet usually do not need vitamin supplements

GERIATRICS

A. Physiologic changes affect nutrition of older adults
1. Aging slows the basal metabolic rate (BMR); combined with decreased activity the result is decreased energy requirements and decreased number of calories needed

2. Taste may be adversely affected by gradual diminishment of the senses of smell, sight, and taste
3. Loss of teeth may affect food intake or the enjoyment thereof
4. Decreased body secretions make swallowing more difficult and digestion less efficient
5. Decreased movement of wastes through large intestine contributes to constipation
B. Economic and social considerations
   1. Decrease in income among older adults combined with an increase in the amount spent for medical care, leaves less for adequate nutrition; tendency is to eat less protein (which is expensive) and more carbohydrates (which are cheaper and easier to prepare)
   2. Loss of spouse, friends, or mobility results in isolation, depression, and often decreased will to obtain adequate nutrition
C. Planning diets
   1. Diet should be well-balanced in protein, vitamins, and minerals (especially calcium and iron) to allow for diminished absorption
   2. Calories sufficient to maintain energy and activity (reduced from those previously required)
   3. Soft bulk in diet to prevent constipation (cooked fruits and vegetables)
   4. Increased fluid intake required to eliminate metabolic wastes
   5. Meals should be light and easily digested, that is, contain only a small amount of fats; frequent small meals may be easier to digest than three large meals
   6. Individual preferences should be respected and the diet built around them; make changes slowly
   7. Meals eaten with others are often more appetizing than those eaten alone

Diet Therapy
NURSING RESPONSIBILITIES
A. Prepare the resident for mealtime
B. See that each person receives the correct tray unless foods are being withheld
C. Serve and remove tray promptly
D. Teach residents the value of proper nutrition and urge compliance with the nutritional care plan

PURPOSES
A. To increase or decrease weight
B. To allow a particular organ or system to rest (e.g., a low-fat diet in gallbladder disease)
C. To regulate the diet to correspond with the body's ability to metabolize a specific nutrient (e.g., diabetes)
D. To correct conditions caused by deficiencies
E. To eliminate harmful substances from the diet (e.g., caffeine, cholesterol, and alcohol)

DIET MODIFICATIONS
A. Calories may be increased or decreased
B. Nutrients may be adjusted (high or low protein)
C. Certain foods may be omitted
D. Modifications in texture (consistency—soft diet)
E. Frequency of meals: more than the standard three

STANDARD HOSPITAL DIETS (MODIFICATIONS IN CONSISTENCY)
A. Clear-liquid (surgical liquid) diet
   1. Temporary diet of clear liquids, non-residue, nonirritating, non–gas-forming; inadequate in protein, vitamins, minerals, and calories
   2. Used postoperatively to replace fluids, before certain tests, and to lessen amount of fecal matter in colon
   3. Includes water, coffee, tea, fat-free broth, pulp-free fruit juices (apple), sherbet, gelatin, and ginger ale
B. Full-liquid diet
   1. Foods liquid at room or body temperatures; may be adequate if carefully planned, although often deficient in iron
   2. Used postoperatively as a transition between clear and soft diet, in infections and acute gastritis; in febrile conditions; and for residents unable to chew or swallow or with an intolerance to food for other reasons
   3. Includes all clear liquids, milk, creamed soups, ice creams, plain puddings, and thin, strained cereal
C. Soft diet

1. Normal diet modified in consistency to have limited fiber; easily digested; nutritionally adequate
2. Used between full liquid and regular, for chewing difficulties, and in gastrointestinal disorders
3. Includes tender meats and tender, well-cooked vegetables (those with a great deal of fiber should be pureed or omitted); fruits (no fiber) and plain cakes are allowed; no spicy or coarse foods are allowed
D. Regular (general or house) diet
   1. Adequate, well-balanced diet designed to appeal to most people
   2. Used for those not requiring a modified or therapeutic diet
   3. Includes all foods from the four basic food groups

ADDITIONAL MODIFIED (OR THERAPEUTIC) DIETS

Table 3-1 lists diets, foods allowed and omitted, and when the diets are used.

Measures to Meet Nutritional Needs

A. Assessment: weight/height ratio, weight changes, skin and mucous membranes, food preferences, meal patterns, ability to eat, and appetite
B. Preparing for meals
   1. Environment
      a. Control odors, noise, and unpleasant sights; remove soiled equipment and linens
      b. Avoid stressful situations before and during mealtime
   2. Resident
      a. Provide oral hygiene and opportunity for elimination and hand washing
      b. Position comfortably, preferably in sitting position
   3. Meal tray
      a. Ensure appropriate temperature and correct tray for correct resident
      b. Arrange tray to be accessible to resident
      c. Assist in opening containers, removing covers, and cutting and preparing food
      d. Serve trays first to residents able to feed themselves

C. Assisting the resident to eat
   1. Place napkin across chest
   2. Explain what foods and liquids are on the tray
   3. Prepare foods and feed in order of resident's preference
   4. Encourage the resident to assist as much as possible
   5. Do not rush: allow time to chew and swallow
   6. Talk with the resident during meal
   7. Provide opportunity for handwashing and oral care
D. Gastric gavage (tube feeding or enteral feeding)
   1. Used when resident is unable to eat, swallow, or take in adequate quantities of food or fluids
   2. Blended foods and fluids (commercially or agency prepared) are passed to the stomach through a nasogastric tube either intermittently or by slow continuous drip
   3. Check amount, frequency, and type ordered by physician
   4. Feeding must be at room temperature before administering
   5. Placement of tube must be checked before feeding begins
      a. By aspirating stomach contents with a syringe
      b. Inject 10 ml of air into tube while simultaneously listening with a stethoscope over the stomach to hear a whooshing sound
   6. Place resident in sitting position
   7. Administer feeding slowly: 200 ml during 30- to 45-minute period
   8. Feeding should be followed by ordered amount of water
   9. Clamp tube after completion of feeding to prevent air entering stomach
   10. If nausea, vomiting, diarrhea, or cramps occur, rate may be too fast or resident may be intolerant of feeding, amount, or temperature
   11. Tube may be left in place between feedings or removed after each feeding as ordered by physician
   12. Have resident remain in sitting position for 45 minutes to help prevent aspiration
E. Nutritional supplements
   1. Vitamin supplements
   2. Mineral supplements

Table 3-1 Modified or therapeutic diets

Diet/Condition	Foods allowed	Purpose of diet
High calorie Underweight (10% or more) Anorexia nervosa Hyperthyroidism	Emphasis on increase in calories Easily digested foods (carbohydrates) recommended Full meals with high-calorie snacks	To meet the increased metabolic needs of the body or provide increased calories for weight gain
Low calorie Overweight	Fruits and vegetables especially recommended	To reduce the caloric intake below what the body requires so weight loss will occur
High protein Children who need additional protein for growth Following surgery Pregnancy and lactation Conditions that cause protein loss Extensive burns	Added amounts of poultry, meat, fish, milk, cheese, and eggs Nonfat dry milk added to soups and baked goods	To increase the intake of high-protein foods for maintaining and rebuilding tissues and correcting protein loss
Low protein Liver diseases Kidney diseases leading to renal failure	Fruits and vegetables Severely limited in amounts of meats, fish, poultry, eggs, and dairy products	To limit the end products of protein metabolism to avoid disturbing the fluid, electrolyte, and acid-base balances
Bland Gastric and duodenal ulcer Postoperative stomach surgery	Milk and protein foods Refined cereals Simple desserts Avoid Highly seasoned foods Raw foods Fried foods Alcohol and carbonated beverages Extremes in temperatures	To promote healing of the gastric mucosa by refraining from foods that are chemically or mechanically irritating To reduce peristalsis and excessive flow of gastric juices
High residue Constipation (atonic) Diverticulitis (when inflammation has ceased)	Increased whole grain cereals Increased fruits and raw vegetables Fibrous meats	Mechanically stimulate the gastrointestinal tract
Low residue Before and after bowel surgery Ulcerative colitis	Soft cheeses Tender meats	To soothe and be nonirritating to gastrointestinal tract

Table 3-1 Modified or therapeutic diets—cont'd

Diet/Condition	Foods allowed	Purpose of diet
Low residue—cont'd Diverticulitis (during inflammatory stage) Diarrhea	Refined cereals and breads Pureed fruits and vegetables Plain puddings	To soothe and be nonirritating to gastrointestinal tract
Low fat Gallbladder disease Obesity Cardiovascular disease	Vegetables and fruits Skim milk Sherbet Increased carbohydrates and proteins	To lower fat content in diet (may be deficient in fat-soluble vitamins)
Low cholesterol Cardiovascular disease	Lean meats and fish Poultry without the skin Liquid vegetable oils Skim milk	To decrease the blood cholesterol levels or maintain them at acceptable levels
High iron Anemias	Regular diet with high-iron foods Liver and organ meats Red meats Dried fruits Egg yolks	To correct an iron deficiency
Sodium restricted Kidney disease Cardiovascular disease Hypertension	Natural foods without salt Fruits and vegetables without salt Milk and meat in limited quantities	To control or correct the retention of sodium and water in the body by controlling sodium intake
High carbohydrate Preparation for surgery Liver disease Kidney disease	Emphasis on carbohydrate foods Full meals with high carbohydrate snacks	To provide increased energy and spare protein for tissue building
Low carbohydrate Dumping syndrome Hyperinsulinism Diabetes mellitus (although severe restriction of carbohydrates is currently considered unwarranted)	Proteins Only enough carbohydrate to maintain health and perform activities	To decrease the amounts of glucose in the bloodstream (increased blood glucose causes increased amounts of insulin to be produced by the body)
Lactose restricted Lactose intolerance	Avoid Foods containing lactose such as milk, cheese, and ice cream	To eliminate or cut down on lactose—a substance certain individuals cannot metabolize

From Saxton DF, et al: Mosby's review questions for NCLEX-RN, ed 2, St. Louis, 1994, Mosby.

F. Enteral feedings are commonly administered through
   1. Gravity
   2. Feeding pump
G. Complications and observations
   1. Observe for regurgitation and aspiration
   2. Check for abdominal distention
   3. Check for respiratory distress

Major Nursing Measures and Responsibilities in Caring for Residents With Special Needs

THE RESIDENT WITH A TRACHEOSTOMY

A. Assessment
   1. Location and security of tracheostomy tube
   2. Signs and symptoms of respiratory obstruction
   3. Condition of stoma: swelling, redness
   4. Amount, consistency, and color of secretions
   5. Vital signs and level of conciousness of resident
   6. Level of apprehension
B. Special considerations during care
   1. Factors
      a. Adequate and efficient humidity to keep secretions thin
      b. Regular chest therapy as ordered to aid in loosening secretions and preventing pneumonia
      c. Suctioning—to keep airway clear
   2. Key points
      a. Tube is either metal or plastic, which is usually cuffed
      b. Tube is held securely in place with cotton ties around the neck
      c. Ties are changed with extreme caution to prevent resident from coughing out tube
      d. A gauze dressing is placed under the tube to absorb secretions and must be changed as indicated
      e. Inner cannula is removed, cleaned with peroxide and pipe cleaners, and rinsed with normal saline at least once a shift by sterile technique; commercially prepared kits are available
      f. Skin around stoma is cleansed with peroxide, rinsed with saline, and assessed at least once a shift

g. Resident is often apprehensive and needs frequent reassurance
h. Tube must be suctioned frequently
i. Provide adequate amount of liquid intake
j. Conserve energy of resident during suctioning; allow periods of rest
k. Turn and position frequently, and promote sitting in upright position

C. Preventing complications
   1. Meticulous assessment
   2. Apply principles of aseptic technique
   3. Use principles of Universal Precautions
   4. Precut absorbent dressing around tube to keep dry and keep neck plate from digging into neck tissue
   5. Insure properly fitting inner cannula
   6. Provide adequate humidity to prevent mucous plug formation which may cause airway obstruction

THE RESIDENT WITH SUCTIONING, OXYGEN, AND INHALATION THERAPY

A. Assessment
   1. Abnormal lung sounds
      a. Crackles
      b. Wheezes
      c. Gurgling on inspiration or expiration
      d. Diminished breath sounds
   2. Ineffective coughing
   3. Rapid or difficulty breathing
   4. Pallor or cyanosis
   5. Excessive secretions
   6. Amount, consistency, and color of sputum
   7. Level of energy and conciousness of resident
B. General measures
   1. Encourage exercise and activity to help expand lungs, providing better oxygenation
   2. Bedridden patients must be turned and positioned every 2 hours (q2h) to prevent pooling of secretions in the lungs
   3. Encourage coughing and deep breathing at least q2h for inactive or bedridden patients to help with oxygenation and increasing secretions
   4. Ensure adequate fluid intake to keep secretions thin, thus making it easier for resident to expectorate
C. Suctioning: oral, nasopharyngeal, or tracheal

1. Necessary to remove accumulated secretions blocking airway or to obtain sputum specimen
2. Usually a sterile procedure
3. Introduce catheter gently; do not apply suction while introducing catheter
4. Suction intermittently for no more than 10 seconds
5. Slowly withdraw catheter by rotating motion while suctioning continues
6. Unless there are copious amounts of secretions, wait 30 seconds between suctionings
7. Repeat procedure until all excess secretions are removed
8. Administer oxygen before and between suctionings if needed
9. Place comatose or semi-alert residents in Sim's position to promote drainage of oral or nasal secretions
10. Check for signs of infection and inadequate hydration in residents with thick, sticky secretions
11. Employ principles of Universal Precaution
12. Allow for rest periods between suctioning
13. Always observe for tolerance and response to procedure
14. Always explain to and teach resident about this process

D. Administration of oxygen
  1. Safety precautions
    a. Caution residents and visitors that smoking is prohibited
    b. Post warning sign on door or bed: NO SMOKING—OXYGEN IN USE
    c. Do not use heating pads, electric blankets, or electric razors—safety hazard
    d. Do not use woolen blankets
    e. Secure oxygen tanks so they do not tip over
  2. Physician's order is required for method of administration, rate of oxygen flow, or concentration
  3. Oxygen must always be humidified
  4. Nasal cannula; prongs fit into nares
    a. Turn oxygen on and check flow through prongs before positioning on resident
    b. Adjust strap after placing cannula on resident
    c. Periodically check that there is sufficient water in humidity source
    d. Periodically check resident's nares and behind ears for pressure
    e. Periodically assess resident for changes in condition
  5. Oxygen by mask: simple; Venturi (delivers oxygen in precise concentrations)
    a. Proceed as with nasal cannula
    b. Fit mask snugly to face and adjust strap
    c. Periodically assess resident and equipment as with nasal cannula
  6. Provide humidity to minimize dryness of mucous membranes
  7. Air in croupette or tent must be checked periodically to be sure it is at desired temperature
  8. Nurse must open tent to assess respiratory status and check degree of dampness of resident's clothing/bedding
  9. Explain to resident and family the need for oxygen therapy and all related safety aspects

E. Use of nebulizer (aerosol)
  1. Method of delivering medications directly to the respiratory tract
  2. Nebulizer breaks liquids into a mist of droplets, which are inhaled

F. Incentive spirometer: to improve inspiratory volume
  1. With lips sealed around a mouthpiece, the resident takes a deep breath, holds it for 3 seconds, and slowly exhales
  2. The spirometer indicates with light or small plastic balls reaching an indicated level whether the resident has inhaled the desired volume

G. Intermittent positive pressure breathing (IPPB) therapy
  1. Forces the resident to inhale more deeply, allowing better oxygenation and loosening of secretions
  2. May be attached to oxygen or compressed air
  3. Humidity is provided, usually by normal saline solution
  4. Medications may be added
  5. Resident should be sitting up during treatment and encouraged to cough up secretions after treatment

H. Chest physical therapy
   1. Postural drainage: use of various positions so that gravity can assist in removal of secretions
   2. Percussion is a manual technique of striking the chest wall over the affected area with cupped hands in a rhythmic motion
   3. Vibration is a manual compression and tremorlike motion with hands or mechanical device against chest wall of affected area done during exhalation
   4. Nurse positions resident so affected areas are vertical and gravity can assist in drainage
   5. Position also depends on diagnosis and condition
   6. Nurse provides emesis basin and tissues, and gives oral hygiene after treatment
   7. This therapy is contraindicated in residents with lung abscess or tumors, pneumothorax, and diseases of the chest wall

THE RESIDENT WITH ELIMINATION PROBLEMS
Urinary Incontinence

A. Assessment: intake/output ratio, color, amount, and consistency of urine, frequency of urination, and continence
B. Common problems of urination
   1. Incontinence: inability to control voiding
      a. Requires frequent skin care and linen change
      b. May be reduced with scheduled toileting
      c. Kegel exercises—to strengthen the pelvic floor muscles, help hold back the flow of urine
   2. Retention: inability to void
      a. If adequate amounts of fluid have been taken in, no more than 8 hours should pass between voidings, except during sleeping hours
      b. Palpation of bladder can determine distention of full bladder
   3. Anuria: no urine being produced by the kidneys
   4. Dysuria: difficult or painful urination ("burning")
C. Assisting with urination
   1. Offer bedpan or urinal at regularly scheduled times

2. Keep bedpan or urinal and toilet paper within easy reach for residents who can assist themselves
3. Keep call signal within easy reach
4. Provide privacy
5. Hearing the sound of running water or having warm water poured over the perineum may induce voiding
6. Provide opportunity for hand washing after urination

D. Care of resident with retention catheter
   1. Presence of indwelling catheter greatly predisposes resident to urinary tract infection
   2. Opening a closed urinary system is to be avoided
   3. Drainage container must be kept below level of the bladder but must not touch the floor
   4. Drainage tubing must be free of kinks and taped to resident's leg
   5. Drainage container is emptied at end of shift or if container becomes nearly full; urine is measured and amount recorded
   6. Catheter care is given at least once per shift
      a. Meatus is cleansed with soap and water
      b. Removal of crusts and secretions from meatus and catheter may require use of hydrogen peroxide
      c. A bacteriostatic ointment is often ordered to be applied to the meatus
   7. Unless contraindicated, fluid intake should reach 2000 to 3000 ml per 24 hours
E. Bladder retraining
   1. Purpose: To reestablish partial to complete control of urinary elimination without urinary retention, overflow, or infection
   2. Actions
      a. Encourage good fluid intake during the day (at least 1500 ml unless contraindicated); reduce but do not eliminate fluid intake after 8 PM
      b. If diuretics are prescribed, administer early in the day
      c. Periodically ask resident if feeling wet or dry; monitor interval between voiding

d. Record resident's voiding pattern: time, amount voided, fluid intake, and related factors

e. Determine average time resident can hold urine

f. Establish schedule of expected voiding times based on resident's pattern

g. Toilet resident approximately 30 minutes before expected voiding time

h. Encourage voiding by measures such as running water, instructing resident to tighten and relax pelvic muscles or rock back and forth, or pouring a small amount of warm water over the vulva or penis

i. Measure the initial amount voided; then press the lower abdomen over the bladder to assist in expressing remaining urine (Crede's method); measure this amount

j. Praise resident for appropriate toileting

k. If incontinent episode occurs, discuss with resident to determine possible cause

l. Record results

F. Catheterization

1. *Straight*: catheter is removed at end of procedure

2. Indwelling, retention, or Foley: catheter is left in place in bladder

3. Assemble equipment: sterile catheterization tray or disposable kit containing catheter, basin, jar with lid (for specimen, if ordered), cotton balls, antiseptic solution, lubricant, sterile gloves, and drape

4. For indwelling catheterization, add Foley catheter, syringe, solution for inflating balloon, drainage bag with tubing, and tape for securing catheter

5. After explaining procedure to resident and ensuring privacy, place female resident in lithotomy position and male resident in dorsal recumbent position

6. Place equipment between resident's legs; using sterile technique open package, don gloves, and place drapes

7. For female resident, while holding labia apart, cleanse vulva and meatus well going from front to back toward vagina; use cotton ball for one stroke only before discarding

8. For male resident, cleanse glans then meatus in a circular motion

9. Insert catheter into meatus (3 to 4 inches [7.5 to 10 cm] in female and 6 inches [15 cm] in male) until urine flows; drain urine (no more than 750 ml at one time to prevent bleeding or shock); remove catheter (*straight*) or inflate balloon and connect drainage tubing (indwelling)

G. Intermittent bladder irrigation (hand bladder irrigation)

1. To rid bladder and tubing of clots or mucus; to instill antibiotic or other solutions

2. Open technique

a. Assemble equipment: sterile solution (type and amount as ordered), sterile container for solution, bulb syringe, and basin for return flow

b. Disconnect catheter from drainage tube over empty basin; protect ends from contamination

c. Allow solution to flow in by gravity or gentle pressure; drain by gravity or gentle suction; repeat until returns are clear or ordered amount of solution has been used

d. Subtract amount of solution used from amount of returns to note output to be recorded

Measures to Meet Needs for Bowel Elimination

A. Assessment: the individual's pattern of elimination; amount, color, consistency, odor, and shape of stool; resident's activity level; amount and type of food and fluid intake; passage of flatus; abdominal distention

B. Common problems of elimination

1. Constipation: passage of dry, hard feces

2. Diarrhea: frequent passage of liquid or unformed stools

3. Impaction: formation of a hardened mass of stool in the lower bowel forming an obstruction to the passage of normal stool; often characterized by the frequent seepage of small amounts of liquid stool

4. Abdominal distention: swollen abdomen caused by retention of flatus in the intestines

C. General nursing measures
   1. Encourage intake of roughage in the diet: fresh fruits and vegetables, as well as whole grain breads and cereals
   2. Encourage intake of adequate amounts of fluids unless contraindicated: 2000 to 3000 ml/day
   3. Encourage maximum amount of physical activity
   4. Encourage resident to respond to the urge to defecate
   5. Position resident comfortably and provide adequate time and privacy for elimination
   6. Provide access to call signal and toilet paper
   7. Provide opportunity for handwashing after elimination

D. Rectal tube
   1. To assist in expelling flatus
   2. Assemble equipment: rectal tube with flatus bag or waterproof pad, lubricant, glove, and tape
   3. After explaining procedure and providing privacy, position resident in side-lying position
   4. Insert lubricated tube 2 to 4 inches (5 to 10 cm) into rectum
   5. Tape tube to individual's buttock and leave in place no longer than 20 to 30 minutes
   6. Note passage of flatus or stool; report and record findings

E. Rectal suppository
   1. Purposes
      a. To stimulate peristalsis and stool elimination
      b. To soothe painful rectum or anus
   2. Assemble equipment: suppository as ordered, glove or finger cot, bedpan, and toilet tissue
   3. Suppository begins to melt at room temperature, providing its own lubrication
   4. Separate buttocks and with gloved index finger insert pointed end of suppository into anus
   5. Gently insert 3 to 4 inches (7.5 to 10 cm) into rectum
   6. Hold buttocks together until initial urge to defecate has passed

7. Best results occur within 30 minutes

F. Commercially prepared prefilled enema
   1. To promote bowel or flatus movement
   2. Assemble equipment: enema (usually 120 ml), underpad, bedpan, and toilet paper
   3. After explaining procedure and providing privacy, place resident in side-lying position
   4. Insert prelubricated tip of enema to the hub and squeeze container until most of solution is instilled
   5. Encourage resident to retain solution until urge to defecate is felt
   6. Place call signal, bedpan, and toilet paper within easy reach
   7. If resident uses toilet, instruct not to flush so that results can be assessed

G. Oil-retention enema
   1. To soften and lubricate stool, promoting easier passage
   2. Often followed by Fleet's or cleansing enema
   3. Equipment and administration are the same as for commercially prepared enema above
   4. Encourage resident to retain oil 30 to 60 minutes

H. Cleansing enemas
   1. To relieve constipation or flatus or cleanse the bowel before diagnostic procedures or surgery
   2. Solutions used as ordered by physician
      a. Tap water: can cause fluid and electrolyte imbalance
      b. Soap solution: 5 ml of liquid soap to 1000 ml water; can irritate mucous membranes of bowel
      c. Saline solution: can cause fluid and electrolyte imbalance
   3. Assemble equipment: disposable enema kit containing enema bag, tubing with clamp, liquid soap, and lubricant; waterproof underpad; solution at a temperature no greater than 105° F bedpan and toilet paper; intravenous (IV) fluids pole
   4. After explaining procedure and providing privacy, place resident in side-lying position (usually left)
   5. Insert lubricated tubing about 3 to 5 inches (7.5 to 12.5 cm) into rectum

6. With bottom of enema bag hanging 12 inches (30 cm) above anus or 18 inches (45 cm) above mattress, slowly administer 500 to 1000 ml of solution
7. If patient complains of cramping or has difficulty retaining solution
   a. Temporarily stop flow
   b. Slow administration rate
   c. Encourage slow, deep breathing through the mouth
8. After fluid has been administered, assist resident to bathroom or onto bedpan or commode; instruct resident not to flush toilet so that results can be assessed
9. If enemas are ordered "until clear," repeat procedure until returns are clear of stool (or of barium after barium enema)
10. Observe resident during procedure for signs of weakness or fatigue, which would necessitate stopping the procedure to allow rest

I. Digital removal of fecal impaction
1. Breaking up the hard fecal mass and removing it
2. Assemble equipment: gloves, waterproof underpad, lubricant, and bedpan
3. Liberally lubricate gloved index finger
4. With resident in side-lying position gently insert finger into hardened mass of stool
5. Gently break off small pieces of the stool, bringing them out and placing them in the bedpan
6. Assess resident for signs of weakness and fatigue; this is an uncomfortable, tiring procedure and may need to be intermittently stopped
7. Assist resident to bedpan: disimpaction may induce defecation

J. Colostomy irrigation
1. To regulate the discharge and drainage of fecal contents and flatus
2. Time of irrigation depends on physician's order and resident's own established routine; when colostomy has become regulated, irrigation may be only done every other day; some residents never irrigate their colostomies
3. Assemble equipment
   a. Irrigating appliance (types vary)
   b. Irrigating container (enema bag)
   c. Tubing and catheter (may be part of enema kit)
   d. Irrigating solution: usually 500 to 1000 ml tap water or physiologic saline solution at 100 °F (43.3 °C)
   e. Lubricant
   f. Drainage bag (may be part of irrigating appliance) and bedpan if not being performed on toilet
   g. Waterproof underpad if being performed in bed
   h. Fresh colostomy appliance, dressing, or stoma pad
   i. IV pole
4. After explaining procedure and ensuring privacy, place resident on toilet (most convenient) or in bed in side-lying position
5. Raise irrigation container 18 inches (45 cm) above stoma, clear catheter of air, lubricate catheter, introduce catheter through irrigating appliance, and insert catheter into stoma 2 to 6 inches (5 to 15 cm); do not advance if resistance is met
6. Allow solution to flow slowly and remove catheter; return is usually completed within 45 to 60 minutes
7. When return is completed, remove irrigating appliance, wash and dry abdomen, and apply fresh colostomy appliance, dressing, or stoma pad as indicated

Bowel Retraining: Fecal Incontinence
A. Causes
1. Physiologic changes
   a. External anal sphincter relaxation
   b. Perineal relaxation
   c. Muscle atony
2. Behavioral alterations
   a. Regression
   b. Rebellion
   c. Dependency
   d. Sensory deprivation
3. Central nervous system (CNS) injury
4. Obstruction
5. Impaction
6. Consciousness alterations
7. Immobility
8. Trauma
B. Intervention
1. Keep resident clean and dry
2. Absorbent, waterproof underpants

3. Skin care
4. Retraining
    a. Bowel retraining is easier than bladder retraining; if resident is incontinent of urine and stool, start bowel retraining program first
    b. Use no laxatives
    c. Ensure adequate fluid intake (2 L per day)
    d. Fluids and solids that promote resident's bowel movements (e.g., bran and orange juice) and roughage should be included in the diet
    e. Encourage physical activity
    f. Obtain bowel history
    g. Procedure
        (1) Establish regular day(s) and time to assist resident to the toilet for evacuation; preferably after a meal
        (2) After 20 minutes, if resident has not had a bowel movement, insert a lubricated glycerine suppository
            (a) Do not use directly from refrigerator
            (b) Do not insert into a bolus of stool (ineffective)
            (c) After ascertaining that resident requires the suppository for training, it can be inserted 1 to 2 hours before the scheduled training time and after a meal
        (3) Digital stimulation is recommended after 48 hours if the above procedure is not successful
        (4) Take resident to the bathroom at the scheduled time daily, even if a bowel movement has occurred between scheduled times

Management of Residents With Addictive Problems

A. General nursing diagnosis
    1. Anxiety, related to
        a. Threat to self-concept
        b. Inability to deal with responsibility
        c. Feelings of inadequacy
        d. Concern regarding continued source of abused substance
    2. Communication, impaired verbal, related to
        a. Inability to verbalize feelings and thoughts
        b. Mental confusion or CNS depression because of substance use
    3. Coping, ineffective family: compromised, related to
        a. Individual's preoccupation with abused substance
        b. Anger, frustration, and exhaustion associated with resident's negative response to attempts at assistance or support
    4. Coping, ineffective individual, related to
        a. Inability to meet basic needs or role expectations
        b. Inability to tolerate frustration
        c. Inappropriate use of defense mechanisms
        d. Excessive use of an abusing substance
    5. Coping, defensive, related to
        a. Denial of obvious problem
        b. Projection of blame/responsibility
        c. Rationalization of failures
        d. Lack of participation in treatment or therapy
    6. Denial, ineffective, related to inability to admit impact of problem on pattern of life
    7. Self-esteem disturbance, related to
        a. Inability to meet role expectations
        b. Feelings of inadequacy and expectation of failure
        c. Inability to accept strengths
        d. Negative feelings about self
    8. Management of therapeutic regimen, individuals; ineffective, related to
        a. Unhealthy lifestyle because of substance abuse
        b. Inability to take responsibility for health needs
        c. Failure to recognize that a problem exists
    9. Nutrition, altered: less than body requirements, related to
        a. A lack of interest in food
        b. Satiety of hunger by use of "empty calories" in alcohol

c. Chemical dependence
10. Injury, risk for, related to
  a. Altered cerebral or perceptual function
  b. Altered judgment
  c. Altered mobility
11. Noncompliance with abstinence and supportive therapy, related to inability to stop using substance because of dependence and refusal to alter lifestyle
12. Sensory-perceptual alterations (visual, kinesthetic, tactile), related to intake of mind-altering substances
13. Violence, risk for: self-directed or directed at others, related to
  a. Intake of mind-altering substances
  b. Misinterpretation of stimuli
  c. Feelings of suspicion or distrust of others
14. Self-mutilation, risk for related to intake of mind-altering substances

B. Nursing care of residents with alcohol dependence
1. Assessment
  a. History of alcohol use/abuse from resident and family if available
  b. Resident's perception of the problem
  c. Sleep patterns
  d. Physical and emotional status in relation to needs associated with nutrition, fluid and electrolyte status, and safety
  e. Why resident is seeking treatment at this time
2. Analysis/nursing diagnoses
Refer to General Nursing Diagnoses for Residents with Psychoactive Substance-Use Disorders
3. Planning/implementation
  a. Provide a well-controlled, alcohol-free environment
  b. Plan a full program of activities but provide for adequate rest
  c. Support the resident without criticism or judgment
  d. Expect and accept lapses as resident is changing a long-term habit
  e. Avoid attempting to talk resident out of problem or making resident feel guilty

  f. Accept the smooth facade that the resident may present while approaching the lonely and fearful individual behind it
  g. Accept failures without judgment or punishment
  h. Accept hostility without criticism or retaliation
  i. Recognize ambivalence and limit the need for decision making
  j. Maintain the resident's interest in a therapy program
4. Evaluation/outcomes
  a. Recognizes, accepts, and seeks treatment for problem
  b. Accepts responsibility for problem without blaming others
  c. Achieves optimal physiologic and nutritional status
  d. Learns new more self-preserving coping mechanisms
  e. Verbalizes feelings and emotions
  f. Enters into and continues with community-based self-help program

C. Nursing care of residents with drug dependence
1. Assessment
  a. History of drugs being used
  b. History of length and pattern of drug dependence
  c. Time since last dose was taken
  d. Physical status of the resident for signs and symptoms of drug dependence
  e. Symptoms of drug overdose or withdrawal
  f. Degree of difficulty sustained by resident in relation to family members, job, school, etc.
  g. Why resident is seeking treatment at this time
  h. Pending criminal charges
  i. Presence of hallucinations, paranoid ideation, and depression (often associated with cocaine use)
  j. Potential for violence toward others or self
2. Analysis/nursing diagnoses
Refer to General Nursing Diagnoses
3. Planning/implementation
  a. Set firm controls and keep area drug-free when the individual is hospitalized

b. Keep atmosphere pleasant and cheerful but not overly stimulating
c. Contribute to the resident's self-confidence, self-respect, and security in a realistic manner
d. Walk the fine line between a relatively permissive and a firm attitude
e. Expect and accept evasion, manipulative behavior, and negativism; but require the resident to shoulder certain standards of responsibility
f. Accept the resident without approving the behavior
g. Do not permit the resident to become isolated
h. Introduce the resident to group activities as soon as possible
i. Protect resident from themselves and others
4. Evaluation/outcomes
See Evaluation/outcomes under Nursing Care of Residents with Alcohol Dependence, p. 29

The Resident With a Pacemaker
PACEMAKERS

A mechanical pacemaker delivers an electrical impulse to the heart to stimulate contraction when the heart's natural pacemakers fail to maintain normal rhythm.

A. Indications for artificial pacemakers
1. Adams-Stokes attack (syncope)
2. Third-degree AV block with slow ventricular rate
3. Acute myocardial infarction
4. Right bundle branch block
5. Sinus bradycardia unresponsive to medical therapy
6. Carotid sinus sycope
7. Sick sinus rhythm
8. Prophylaxis before anesthesia and surgery in residents with history of cardiac arrest or AV block
B. Post-pacemaker insertion
1. Teach resident signs and symptoms that necessitate medical attention such as:
a. Decreasing pulse rate
b. Irregular pulse
c. Dizziness
d. Shortness of breath
e. Ankle swelling
f. Signs of infection

C. Resident education
1. Stress follow-up with pacemaker clinic
2. Confirm date of appointment
3. Teach resident expected life of pacemaker battery (approximately 5 to 10 yrs)
4. Know the manufacture of specific pacemaker
5. Medications dosage and precautions

THE RESIDENT EXPERIENCING PAIN

Types: *acute*—short lasting does not always require treatment; *chronic*—constant, lasts a long time and requires treatment

Measures to Meet Pain Relief Needs

Individuals (including nurses) vary in their perception of and response to pain. Pain is often intensified in the presence of anxiety and fatigue.

A. Assessment: intensity, onset, duration, quality, and location of pain, resident's nonverbal responses to pain, behavior, change in vital signs, and nausea; factors associated with the pain: activity and visitors; pain relief measures
B. Therapeutic relationship may help reduce anxiety, thus reducing pain level
C. Altering contributing factors: relieving constipation and nausea; eliminating environmental disturbances such as bright lights, odors, and noise
D. Providing diversional activities: television, radio, and visitors
E. Repositioning, back rub, and tightening linens
F. Application of heat or cold if ordered
G. Relaxation
1. To reduce muscle tension
2. First need
a. A comfortable position
b. A quiet environment
c. Focus on something outside the body, such as a word to repeat, an object to look at, or something to imagine
3. Techniques
a. Exercises in which various muscle groups are alternately tensed and relaxed
b. Exercises in which various muscle groups are alternately stretched and relaxed
c. Breathing techniques similar to those used in the Lamaze method of childbirth

d. Biofeedback: learning to control normally autonomic body functions
   (1) Muscle tension is monitored
   (2) Subject receives feedback as to the success of attempts to control functions

H. Medication classifications
   1. Placebo: inactive substance administered to satisfy the resident's need for a drug
      a. Pain relief after administration is probably a result of anxiety reduction
      b. Because relief is felt after placebo, it does not mean there was no pain
   2. Analgesics
      a. Narcotics
      b. Nonnarcotics

I. Assessment of responses to pain management
   1. Subjective—Ask resident if pain has been lessened or totally relieved
   2. Objective—Observe resident for facial expression, evidence of muscular relaxation or tension, ease or difficulty of motion

Review Questions

1. Which would be the most beneficial intervention in dealing with your resident's mobility impairment while unconscious?
   ① Get the resident out of bed to a chair for 2 hours
   ② Turn and reposition patient q2h
   ③ Give passive range-of-motion exercises twice each shift
   ④ Place the resident in Fowler's position once each shift

2. When first feeding residents in hyperextension who are lying on their backs, you should:
   ① Use suction on the residents first
   ② Offer sips of liquid to prepare them for solid food
   ③ Raise the head of the bed to facilitate swallowing
   ④ Offer soft food

3. With a tentative diagnosis of opiate addiction, the nurse should assess a recently hospitalized resident for signs of opiate withdrawal. These signs would include:
   ① Lacrimation, vomiting, drowsiness
   ② Nausea, dilated pupils, constipation
   ③ Muscle aches, pupillary constriction, yawning
   ④ Rhinorrhea, convulsions, subnormal temperature

4. The most important aspect of the nursing care for a resident with chest pain should be to:
   ① Elevate legs and note degree of pitting edema
   ② Note color, character, and amount of sputum
   ③ Monitor intake and output, and weigh daily
   ④ Evaluate/record onset, duration, and intensity of chest pain

5. A resident is placed on the "Prudent Diet" proposed by the American Heart Association. The nurse should be aware that the caloric distribution of this diet includes:
   ① 50% fat (20% saturated), 20% carbohydrate, 30% protein
   ② 10% fat (5% saturated), 80% carbohydrate (50% complex), 10% protein
   ③ 45% fat (15% saturated), 40% carbohydrate (20% complex), 15% protein
   ④ 30% fat (<10% saturated), 50% carbohydrate (35% complex), 20% protein

6. During a dressing change, the nurse observes the resident and the incision site for any signs of infection. Which of the following signs should the nurse report to the surgeon?
   ① An oral temperature of 99.2° F on the first postoperative day
   ② A small amount of clear, yellow exudate at the edges of the incision
   ③ Redness and swelling around the incision
   ④ A sudden drop in blood pressure on the day of surgery

7. A resident does not like to drink milk. To supply food of equal nutrient value, the nurse would encourage the resident to eat:
   ① Fresh pineapple
   ② Fish
   ③ Potatoes
   ④ Puddings

8. Which of the following juices should the nurse recommend to the resident to help keep the urine acid?
   ① Apple juice
   ② Tomato juice
   ③ Pineapple juice
   ④ Cranberry juice

9. A resident is placed on a clear-liquid diet. Which of these foods may be included in the resident's diet plan?
   1. Lime sherbet
   2. Cream of celery soup
   3. Oatmeal
   4. Weak tea with skim milk

10. The resident needs to be catheterized for residual urine. During the procedure, the nurse notes resistence to the catheter at the external urinary meatus. Which of the following actions is the most appropriate for the nurse to implement?
    1. Ask the resident to cough several times
    2. Remove the catheter, then try again
    3. Have the resident take several deep breaths
    4. Pull back the catheter, then push forward again

11. When caring for a resident in a full-leg cast, the nurse's main goal is:
    1. Application of support to prevent further injury
    2. Immobilization of the leg to promote healing
    3. Ensuring comfort and pain relief
    4. Prevention of hemorrhage and shock

12. When collecting a routine urine sample, the nurse should instruct the resident to:
    1. Completely fill the container
    2. Void 50 to 100 ml of urine
    3. Add a few drops of water to the empty container
    4. Use a sterile container

13. When assessing a resident's medication history, the nurse should:
    1. Only be interested in prescribed medication taken
    2. Know the names of all medications kept in the resident's home
    3. Record all nonprescription and prescription medication being taken
    4. Only be interested in nonprescription medication being taken

14. The nurse is aware that total parenteral nutrition is a more desirable therapy than just IV fluids for residents with gastrointestinal problems. The nurse understands that residents receiving only IV fluids lose weight because of:
    1. Lack of bulk in the diet
    2. Deficient carbohydrate intake
    3. Insufficient intake of water-soluble vitamins
    4. Increased concentrations of electrolytes in cells

15. The physician orders oxygen given in low concentration and intermittently, rather than in high concentration and continuously, for a resident with chronic obstructive pulmonary disease (COPD) to prevent:
    1. A decrease in red cell formation
    2. Rupture of emphysematous bullae
    3. Depression of the respiratory center
    4. An excessive drying of the respiratory mucosa

16. Besides an adequate diet with sufficient fluid intake, which of the following nursing interventions should be ordered to relieve a resident's constipation?
    1. Oil retention enema every other day
    2. Strong laxative every third day
    3. Stool softeners once a day
    4. Saline enema as needed

17. The nurse knows that the immediate rescuer response to a resident experiencing chest pain should be which of the following?
    1. Walk with the resident to help him remain conscious
    2. Start CPR before the resident's heart stops beating completely
    3. Put the resident in the car and drive to the hospital immediately
    4. Keep the resident at rest and call for emergency service.

18. For which of the following stool tests must the specimen still be warm when it reaches the laboratory?
    1. Culture and sensitivity
    2. Guaiac
    3. Hematest
    4. Ova and parasites

19. Suction apparatus is placed at the resident's bedside in case it is needed. You remember that in nasopharyngeal suctioning you:
    ① Suction only when introducing the catheter
    ② Suction continuously for 15 to 30 seconds followed by a 10-second rest period
    ③ Slowly withdraw suction catheter using rotating motion while suction continues
    ④ Use only medical asepsis

20. The nurse understands that the first activity of daily living that should be taught to a developmentally disabled resident is:
    ① Toileting
    ② Dressing
    ③ Self feeding
    ④ Combing hair

21. An important nursing action to institute when administering a sedative to a geriatric resident is to:
    ① Apply a posey jacket restraint
    ② Leave on the overhead light in the room
    ③ Raise the side rails on the bed and tell resident not to get out of bed unassisted
    ④ Check the resident every half hour to determine effectiveness of the medication

22. To help a resident retain tube feedings and avoid aspiration, the nurse should place the child in the:
    ① Prone position
    ② Left side-lying position
    ③ Semi-Fowler's position
    ④ Supine position with head turned

23. The nurse is aware that in administering routine oxygen therapy to a resident the oxygen:
    ① Should be labeled as flammable
    ② Is warmed before administration
    ③ Must be humidified before administration
    ④ May be administered without a prescription

24. In children with renal disease the best indicator of fluid balance is the daily measurement of:
    ① Body weight
    ② Urinary output
    ③ Abdominal girth
    ④ Urine osmolality

25. The nurse is asked to assist in the selection of a between-meal snack for a resident with second- and third-degree burns. The resident is ordered a diet high in protein. Of the following combinations of foods, which have the highest protein content?
    ① Cheese cubes and peanuts
    ② Cheese spread and potato chips
    ③ Jello with cream and glass of milk
    ④ Popcorn with butter and pretzels

ANSWERS AND RATIONALES FOR REVIEW QUESTIONS

1. **3** Primary intervention to maintain muscle tone.
   1 Inappropriate to transfer to chair in unconscious state; does not relate to increasing mobility.
   2 Necessary, but not the best.
   4 Inappropriate position and will promote skin breakdown.

2. **4** Soft foods are tolerated better by the resident and are easier to swallow.
   1 Use of suction is not necessary prior to feeding a resident in this position.
   2 Fluids tend to flow into the nasopharynx easily, with the danger of aspiration.
   3 Raising the head of the bed would not facilitate swallowing for a resident in this position.

3. **3** These symptoms are all associated with opiate withdrawal, which occurs after cessation or reduction of prolonged moderate or heavy use of opiates.
   1 Lacrimation and vomiting are present, but insomnia, not drowsiness, occurs with opiate withdrawal.
   2 Nausea is present, but diarrhea, not constipation and constricted pupils, rather than dilated pupils occur with opiate withdrawal.
   4 Rhinorrhea is present, but fever, rather than a subnormal temperature and muscle aches, rather than convulsions occur with opiate withdrawal.

4. **4** The description of the type of chest pain is significant to assist in diagnosing a myocardial infarction, angina pectoris, or congestive heart failure.
   1 These relate to symptoms of congestive heart failure.
   2 These relate to symptoms of congestive heart failure.
   3 These relate to symptoms of congestive heart failure.

5. **3** The Prudent Diet contains reduced fat with less saturated animal fat, increased carbohydrate with more of it in complex forms, and moderate protein with emphasis on lean forms.
   1 This caloric distribution does not represent the Prudent Diet proposed by the American Heart Association.
   2 This caloric distribution does not represent the Prudent Diet proposed by the American Heart Association.
   4 This caloric distribution does not represent the Prudent Diet proposed by the American Heart Association.

6. **3** Redness and swelling are common signs of a wound infection after surgery.
   1 An oral temperature of 101° F (38.3 °C) is more indicative of an infection.
   2 A small amount of clear, yellow drainage may be a normal part of the healing process. Cloudy, yellow or green drainage is not normal.
   4 A sudden drop in blood pressure on the day of surgery is more indicative of hemorrhage.

7. **4** Puddings are usually made with whole or skim milk.
   1 Fresh pineapple's main nutrient value is a high vitamin C content.
   2 Fish is high in protein and low in fat.
   3 Potatoes are high in vitamin B and carbohydrates.

8. **4** Cranberry juice acidifies the urine.
   1 This does not cause the urine to become acidic.
   2 This does not cause the urine to become acidic.
   3 This does not cause the urine to become acidic.

9. **1** Sherbet is made without milk and can be included on a clear-liquid diet.
   2 This contains milk. It may be included on a full-liquid diet.
   3 Oatmeal is considered a soft food, not a clear liquid.
   4 Skim milk makes this a full liquid.

10. **3** Having the resident take deep breaths will relax the external sphincter, allowing for easier passage of the catheter.
    1 Coughing would constrict the urinary meatus and sphincter.
    2 This technique would contaminate the catheter and increase the risk of introducing microorganisms into the bladder.
    4 This approach also increases the risk of contamination of the urinary tract.

11. **2** This provides good alignment and support for calcification and healing to the fracture.
    1 Proper support of the casted leg is essential for resident comfort; however, immobilization to aid the healing process is the main goal.
    3 Ensuring resident comfort and pain relief is a facet of all nursing care and is not specific to only this situation.
    4 Given a different situation, this response may be essential; however, this is not usually applicable to providing simple nursing care to a resident in a full-leg cast.

12. **2** It is suggested that 50 to 100 ml of urine be sent to the laboratory if possible, so that a thorough assessment can be performed.
    1 The size of the container has nothing to do with the suggested amount of urine to be collected.
    3 Water is contraindicated because it may dilute and/or contaminate the specimen.
    4 A routine urinalysis does not require the use of a sterile container; however, urine for culture and sensitivity does.

13. **3** Proper data collection
    1 Limiting
    2 Not necessary
    4 Limiting

14. **2** IV fluids supply minimal calories; a resident on only IV therapy will lose weight and become malnourished.
    1 This is not related to weight; lack of bulk in the diet results in constipation.
    3 Vitamins are not related to weight loss.
    4 Intracellular electrolytes are not related to weight loss.

15. **3** Residents with COPD must be given only low concentrations of oxygen; a decreased oxygen blood level is the only stimulus for breathing for these residents.
    1 Prolonged hypoxia will stimulate erythrocyte production; the goal of therapy is to relieve hypoxia.
    2 The pressure, rather than the concentration, at which oxygen is administered increases this risk.
    4 To prevent its drying effects on secretions and the mucosa, oxygen should be humidified.

16. **3** Stool softeners are more gentle to the gastrointestinal tract and promote regularity.
    1 Oil retention enemas are usually used for a fecal impaction.
    2 Strong laxatives are not routinely administered to relieve constipation, and they are not given on a regular basis.
    4 Saline enemas are only occasionally used to relieve constipation because there is the risk of inducing an electrolyte imbalance.

17. **4** The first rescuer should ascertain the presence of breathing and pulse. If it is not necessary to start cardiopulmonary resuscitation (CPR) immediately, the rescuer should call for help.
    1 The resident should not walk; he should lie down wherever he is.
    2 CPR is never initiated when the resident is still breathing and has a pulse.

    3 In the event of a heart attack, the rescuer should call for help rather than driving the victim to the hospital because there is no other assistance in the vehicle if it is needed for CPR.

18. **4** Cooling of environment may destroy ova and parasites.
    1 Although changes may take place in bacteria if specimens are held at room temperature, they may be stored in the refrigerator before being sent to the laboratory.
    2 Presence of blood in a stool specimen is not altered by cooling.
    3 Presence of blood in a stool specimen is not altered by cooling.

19. **3** Slowly rotating the catheter ensures that all areas are reached by the suction.
    1 Suction is not applied while the catheter is inserted to prevent unnecessary trauma to the mucous membranes.
    2 Each suction attempt should last no more than 15 seconds. While suctioning, you are preventing the resident from inhaling any oxygen.
    4 Most suctioning requires surgical asepsis.

20. **3** This follows the normal course of growth and development skills and is no different with a child who is mentally retarded.
    1 This would not be taught before self-feeding.
    2 This would not be taught before self-feeding.
    4 This would not be taught before self-feeding.

21. **3** Raising side rails on the bed, leaving the call bell within easy reach of the resident, and telling the resident to ring for assistance are general safety precautions for elderly receiving sedatives
    1 There is no need to restrain when administering a sedative
    2 While the light may prove helpful, the resident may still be unsafe getting out of bed alone because of the effects of the sedative
    4 This is also important, but safety precautions are priority.

22. **3** This position limits the potential for aspiration; the resident will be partially upright, and fluid is held in the stomach by gravity.
    1 This position allows gastric reflux and may lead to aspiration.
    2 This position allows gastric reflux and may lead to aspiration.
    4 This position allows gastric reflux and may lead to aspiration.

23. **3** Because of the drying nature of oxygen, most oxygen is humidified before it is administered.

    1 Oxygen is combustible and supports fire; it does not ignite; it is not flammable.

    2 Oxygen is not warmed before administration; it is cool on administration.

    4 Oxygen is considered a drug and therefore must be prescribed.

24. **1** With renal disease a large proportion of the child's body weight is composed of retained fluid; the loss of fluid would be readily reflected by a loss of weight.

    2 It is very difficult to get an accurate recording of output in a young child, especially if vomiting and diarrhea also occur.

    3 With renal disease, it would be difficult to evaluate return to fluid balance in this way because the edema is generalized, not concentrated, in the abdomen.

    4 Osmolality reflects kidney activity, not the reduction in edema.

25. **1** Cheese and nuts are high in protein content. A diet rich in protein helps to rebuild tissue destroyed by burns.

    2 Cheese spread contains protein but the potato chips contain little or no protein.

    3 Jello with cream contains little or no protein. Milk is a complete protein.

    4 Popcorn and pretzels contain little or no protein.

chapter *four*

Musculoskeletal System Overview

Musculoskeletal disorders may be acute or chronic. Acute problems are usually related to simple injuries. Chronic disorders may be more distressing to the resident because of loss of mobility and changes in self-image. The nurse needs to possess good skills in observation, positioning the resident safely as well as use and care of equipment. The nurse is probably the most important health care provider in preventive care associated with complications of immobility.

Nursing Assessment

A. Nursing observations
   1. General appearance
   2. Age
   3. Vital signs
   4. Loss of height
   5. Abnormal gait
   6. Impaired neurovascular status
   7. Comparisons between affected and nonaffected sides
   8. Absence of extremity
   9. Deformity
   10. Limb nonalignment
   11. Loss or inability to move body part
   12. Diminished handgrip
   13. Limited range of motion (ROM)
   14. Abnormal spinal curvature
   15. Bony joint enlargement
   16. Joint pain
   17. Presence of warmth, redness, or edema over skin
   18. Ability to perform activities of daily living (ADLs)
   19. Capillary refill
   20. Assistive devices; casts

B. Resident description (subjective data)
   1. Pain with or without movement
   2. Weakness
   3. Fatigue
   4. Feeling of joint stiffness
   5. Anorexia
   6. Weight loss or weight gain
   7. Limited movement/gait difficulty
   8. Recent injury

Diagnostic Tests/Methods

A. Serum laboratory studies
   1. Complete blood count (CBC): an aid in determining anemia or the presence of infection
   2. Erythrocyte sedimentation rate (ESR): elevation is evident during inflammatory processes
   3. Rheumatoid factor: a protein found in the blood of most individuals with rheumatoid arthritis
   4. Uric acid: high concentration is found in individuals with gout
   5. Systemic lupus erythematosus (LE) cell
      a. A cell identified in individuals with SLE
      b. Normally there are no LE cells in the blood

B. Procedures
   1. Radiograph (x-ray): a film to determine the presence of a deformity, fracture, or tumor of the skeletal system
   2. Aspiration: withdrawal of fluid from a joint to obtain a specimen for diagnostic purposes
   3. Bone biopsy: removal and examination of bone tissue

4. Myelogram: x-ray examination of the spinal cord after injection with radiopaque dye
5. Bone scan: isotope imaging of the skeleton
6. Computerized tomography (CT): use of x-ray to provide accurate images of thin cross sections of the body
7. Magnetic resonance imaging (MRI): aid for the diagnosis of musculoskeletal conditions through the clear differentiation of various types of tissue such as bone, fat, and muscle tissue
8. Arthroscopy: endoscopic examination that allows for direct visualization of a joint

C. Nursing intervention for myelogram
1. After procedure, have resident remain flat in bed 12 to 24 hours before allowing to resume usual activities
2. Encourage fluids of 2000 to 3000 ml every 24 hours
3. Observe for alterations in normal motor and sensory states
4. Observe for nausea and vomiting

Common Resident Problems and Nursing Care

A. Self-esteem disturbance; body image related to immobility
1. Provide atmosphere of acceptance
2. Express empathy, warmth, and friendliness
3. Encourage acceptance of self-limitations
4. Encourage self-performance

B. Skin integrity, impaired; potential breakdown related to immobility/assistive devices
1. Change the resident's position often
2. Keep the skin clean, dry, and lubricated
3. Massage bony prominences
4. Provide sheepskin or polyurethane foam pad

C. Joint contracture, potential for, related to incorrect body alignment
1. Place hands, feet, and knees in the natural position of function
2. Provide sandbags to protect against poor alignment of body part
3. Assist in performance of active and passive ROM exercises
4. Provide trapeze over the resident's bed
5. Avoid knee Gatch position/pillow under knee

D. Airway clearance, ineffective, related to potential respiratory secretion congestion

1. Change the resident's position often
2. Encourage coughing and deep breathing
3. Observe for coughing, fever, and green-yellow sputum

E. Mobility, impaired physical, related to edema and potential thrombus and emboli
1. Encourage resident to move lower extremities
2. Encourage adequate hydration
3. Avoid use of knee Gatch/pillow under knee
4. To avoid release of emboli, never rub legs

F. Pain: bone, related to bone fracture or disease
1. Inspect and palpate the painful site looking for inflammation, edema, bruising, tenderness, and skin warmth
2. Support the affected body part
3. Apply warm, moist compress to affected body part where prescribed
4. Give prescribed analgesic
5. Evaluate effectiveness of pain relief measures

G. Limited ROM, potential for, related to cast confinement, joint pain, stiffness, or inflammation
1. Explain the reason for and intended effect of ROM exercises
2. Maintain body alignment
3. Provide total exercising of muscles and joints except if severe pain or inflammation is present; contraindicated if recent surgery was performed on or near the joint

H. Pain, related to cast and alteration in comfort
1. Massage the area around the cast
2. Pad rough edges
3. Provide a scratching device
4. Inspect the skin for irritation
5. Observe for cyanosis of the extremity in a cast
6. Observe for complaints of numbness and tingling of extremity

I. Self-care deficits (feeding, bathing, and hygiene) related to impaired physical mobility
1. Assist with ADLs
2. Provide self-care aids/devices
3. Teach self-care activities

FRACTURES

A. Definition: a break in the continuity of bone that may be accompanied by injury of surrounding soft tissue, producing swelling and discoloration
B. Pathology

1. Most fractures are a result of trauma; pathologic fractures result from disorders such as osteoporosis, malnutrition, bone tumors, and Cushing's syndrome
2. Types of fractures
   a. Closed (simple): skin is intact over the site
   b. Open (compound): break in skin is present over the fracture site; the ends of the bone may or may not be visible
   c. Complete: fracture line extends completely through the bone
   d. Incomplete (partial): fracture line extends partially through the bone; one side breaks while the opposite side bends
   e. Comminuted: more than one fracture with bone fragments either crushed or splintered into several pieces
   f. Green-stick: splintering of one side of a bone (most often seen in children because of soft bone structure)
   g. Impacted: one bone fragment is driven into another bone fragment

C. Signs and symptoms
   1. Subjective
      a. Pain on movement of body part
      b. Tenderness
      c. Loss of function
      d. Muscle spasms
   2. Objective
      a. Deformity
      b. Edema
      c. Bruising
      d. Crepitus
D. Diagnostic test: x-ray examination to confirm location and direction of fracture line
E. Treatment
   1. Reduction of the fracture consists of pulling the broken bone ends to correct alignment and regain continuity; usually a cast is applied or the part may be placed in a traction device
      a. Closed reduction: manual manipulation to bring ends into contact
      b. Open reduction: surgical intervention to cleanse the area and attach devices to hold the bones in position
   2. Cast application to immobilize, support, and protect the part during the healing process

3. Traction to apply a pulling force in two directions to realign the bones
F. Nursing intervention
   1. Provide emergency nursing care of fractures
   2. Provide nursing care for the resident with a cast
      a. Observe for circulatory impairment of limb: color, temperature, pulse, and motor function
      b. Elevate extremity in cast on pillow
      c. Promote drying of cast by exposing it to air
      d. Inspect for skin irritation under edges of cast: apply lotion, pad edges, and apply tape to edge of cast
      e. If drainage is present on the cast, measure and note
      f. Observe for possible infection: increased temperature, foul odor from cast, edema, and "hot spots" over the cast
      g. Observe for complications of pulmonary embolisms, fat embolism, and compartment syndrome

FRACTURED HIP

A. Definition: fracture of the hip joint
B. Pathology
   1. Site of fracture
      a. Inside the joint (intracapsular or neck of the femur)
      b. Outside the joint (extracapsular or base of the neck of the femur)
   2. Older adult women experience high incidence because of osteoporosis
C. Signs and symptoms
   1. Subjective: pain
   2. Objective
      a. Leg appears shorter than nonaffected extremity
      b. Foot points upward and outward on affected side
      c. Edema
      d. Discoloration
D. Diagnostic test: x-ray study confirms discontinuity of the bone
E. Treatment
   1. Russell traction or Buck's extension: before open reduction to prevent muscle spasms if surgery is not contraindicated

2. Closed reduction with application of hip spica cast if the fracture occurred in the intertrochanteric site
3. Open reduction and implantation of a prosthesis to replace head and neck of femur or fixation device to secure fragments of the fracture
   a. Austin Moore prosthesis
   b. Neufeld nail and screws
   c. Smith-Petersen nail
F. Nursing intervention
   1. Considerations for the geriatric resident
      a. Complications of immobility
      b. Reduced tolerance to drugs
      c. Delayed healing because of nutritional problems related to the older adults
   2. Keep side rail up and provide trapeze to facilitate movement
   3. Encourage resident to participate in activities of daily living: eating, bathing, and combing hair

ARTHROPLASTY

A. Definition: replacement of a joint, which may be necessary to restore function, relieve pain, and correct deformity
B. Pathology: arthritic changes damage the joint, resulting in impaired mobility, pain, and deformity; hip, knee, elbow, and shoulder are commonly affected
C. Signs and symptoms
   1. Subjective
      a. Pain
      b. Limited ROM
      c. Limited weight-bearing ability
   2. Objective
      a. Limited ROM
      b. Edema and skin character changes around affected joint
D. Diagnostic tests/methods
   1. X-ray studies confirm joint changes and damage
   2. Arthroscopy provides direct visualization and inspection of joint changes
E. Treatment: a prosthetic device used to replace the articulating joint surfaces (hip, knee, shoulder, elbow, and fingers)
F. Nursing intervention
   1. Proper positioning: (maintain affected leg in abduction)

2. Assist with prescribed activity and encourage prescribed exercise
3. Monitor pain; provide pain control
4. Assess neuromuscular function
5. Monitor skin integrity

AMPUTATION

A. Definition: surgical removal of part or all of an extremity
B. Pathology
   1. Majority of amputations result from blood vessel disorders causing inadequate oxygen supply to the tissue
   2. Other indications for amputation are gas gangrene, malignant tumors, septic wounds, severe trauma, and burns
   3. Usually a skin flap is constructed for prosthetic equipment
C. Signs and symptoms
   1. Subjective
      a. Gas gangrene and septic wounds: pain
      b. Peripheral vascular diseases
         (1) Pain
         (2) Tingling
   2. Objective
      a. Gas gangrene and septic wounds
         (1) Fever
         (2) Edema
         (3) Foul odor
         (4) Bronze or blackened wound
         (5) Necrosis
      b. Peripheral vascular diseases
         (1) Edema
         (2) Pallor
         (3) Cyanosis
         (4) Diminished pulses
         (5) Hyperpigmentation
         (6) Ulcer formation
D. Diagnostic tests/methods
   1. Oscillometry
   2. Arteriography
   3. Skin temperature studies
   4. X-ray examination
E. Treatment
   1. Psychologic preparation
   2. Rehabilitation preparation
   3. Nutritional status buildup
   4. Prosthetic device
F. Nursing intervention
   1. Prepare resident

a. Encourage expression of feelings by providing honesty concerning loss of limb

b. Explain to the resident the possibility of experiencing pain in the amputated limb (called phantom limb pain)

c. Explain to the resident that he or she will undergo a program of exercises that includes strengthening of upper extremities, transferring from bed to chair, and ambulating with a walker

SYSTEMIC LUPUS ERYTHEMATOSUS (SLE)

A. Definition: a chronic inflammatory disorder involving the connective tissues, such as the muscles, kidneys, heart, and serous membranes

B. Pathology
1. Cause is unknown; is believed to be an autoimmune disorder
2. Inflammation produces fibroid deposits and structural changes in connective tissue of organs and blood vessels
3. Results in problems with mobility, oxygenation, and elimination

C. Signs and symptoms
1. Subjective
   a. Abdominal, joint, and muscle pain
   b. Weakness
   c. Depression
2. Objective
   a. Low-grade fever
   b. Weight loss
   c. Butterfly skin rash over bridge of nose and cheeks
   d. Anemia

D. Diagnostic test: positive LE cell test

E. Treatment
1. Corticosteroids, analgesics, and medications for anemia
2. Avoidance of exposure to sunlight

F. Nursing intervention
1. Provide emotional support to resident and family in coping with poor prognosis
2. Encourage alternative activity and planned rest periods

3. Instruct on avoidance of residents with infections, undue exposure to sunlight, and emotional stress, which can cause exacerbations
4. Encourage intake of foods high in iron content: liver, shellfish, leafy vegetables, and enriched breads and cereals

SCLERODERMA

A. Definition: fiberlike changes in the connective tissue throughout the body

B. Pathology
1. An insidious, chronic, progressive disorder usually beginning in the skin
2. Skin becomes thick and hard; fingers and toes becomes fixed in a position
3. Other disorders that occur are difficulty in swallowing, gastrointestinal (GI) impaired mobility, cardiac and renal problems, and osteoporosis

C. Signs and symptoms
1. Subjective
   a. Sweating of hands and feet
   b. Stiffness of hands
   c. Muscle weakness
   d. Joint pain
   e. Dysphagia
2. Objective
   a. Increased pigmentation or dyspigmentation
   b. Dilated capillaries of lips, fingers, face, and tongue

D. Diagnostic tests/methods
1. Positive LE cell test
2. False-positive syphilis test

E. Treatment
1. Skin care to prevent formation of decubiti
2. Physical therapy
3. Analgesics for joint pain

F. Nursing intervention
1. Provide emotional support to resident and family to promote physical and psychologic needs
2. Encourage moderate exercise to promote muscular and joint function

Review Questions

1. A resident recently admitted to your unit had two diagnostic tests performed: white blood cell (WBC) count and erythrocyte sedimentation rate (ESR). In an individual with rheumatoid arthritis you would expect the results to be:
   1. Within normal range
   2. Below normal
   3. Elevated
   4. Absent

2. Important in preventing complications of immobility would be a diet high in:
   1. Fluids
   2. Calcium
   3. Fats
   4. Sodium

3. The dietitian and resident have already discussed the dietary restrictions related to gout. Later the resident tells the nurse that he forgot which foods to avoid. The nurse should instruct the resident to avoid:
   1. Cheese, milk, and dairy products
   2. Marbled hamburger, lean steaks, and pork
   3. Potatoes, breads, and sugar
   4. Liver, kidney, and sardines

4. Following a below-the-knee amputation, the resident received instructions about care of the residual limb. Which of these comments by the resident indicates the need for further teaching?
   1. "I'll rub my residual limb with alcohol twice a day."
   2. "I'll press my residual limb against a pillow when the wound is healed."
   3. "I'll bathe my residual limb with soap and water every day."
   4. "I'll be sure to exercise the joints above and below my residual limb every day."

5. Four weeks following a total hip replacement, a resident asks when daily walks can be resumed. The nurse bases the answer on the knowledge that after surgery:
   1. Full-weight bearing is usually permitted after 6 weeks
   2. Full-weight bearing is usually restored after 4 months
   3. Partial weight-bearing restrictions will be enforced for at least 12 weeks
   4. Partial weight-bearing and positional restrictions will be in effect for 2 months

6. Body functions decline with age, thus making an individual prone to which of the following reactions to medication?
   1. Developing a tolerance to medications
   2. Metabolizing medications more rapidly
   3. Developing more frequent adverse effects
   4. Experiencing more cumulative effects

7. When assessing a resident using a prosthesis following an above-the-knee amputation, the finding that indicates that the prosthesis fits correctly is:
   1. Shrinking of the stump
   2. Absence of phantom pain
   3. Darkened skin areas on the stump
   4. Uneven wearing down of the heels

8. The nurse must stress which of the following when caring for a resident with rheumatoid arthritis?
   1. Continuous activity during the day
   2. Self-performance activities
   3. Use of the semifirm mattress for greater comfort
   4. ROM exercises beyond limits of pain tolerance

9. To avoid urinary complications associated with decreased mobility the nurse should encourage residents to:
   1. Increase intake of citrus fruits
   2. Decrease intake of fluids
   3. Decrease intake of dairy products
   4. Increase urine acidity

10. To best assist a resident who has been on bed rest to prepare for ambulation the nurse should:
    1. Dangle the resident's legs, and swing them back and forth daily
    2. Have the resident push the popliteal space against the bed to the count of five, several times daily
    3. Perform passive ROM exercises three times daily
    4. Have the resident perform push-ups and use the bed trapeze bar as much as possible

11. The nurse should teach a resident with an above-the-knee amputation a variety of postoperative activities. The activity designed to aid in the use of crutches is:
    1. Stump care
    2. Weight lifting
    3. Changing bed position
    4. Phantom-limb exercise

ANSWERS AND RATIONALES FOR REVIEW QUESTIONS

1. **3** The WBC count would be slightly elevated, and the ESR would be elevated because of the inflammatory process present in rheumatoid arthritis.

   1, 2 WBC and ESR within and below normal limits would not indicate inflammatory process as seen in rheumatoid arthritis.

   4 Absence of either, especially a WBC count, indicates a disease process in which the body was unable to defend itself (e.g., an autoimmune process).

2. **1** Fluids, if not contraindicated, help to prevent several complications of immobility, including constipation, urinary infection, and urinary calculi.

   2 Too high a calcium diet may predispose a resident to urinary calculi.

   3 Adequate but high fats are not recommended.

   4 Adequate amounts but high sodium is not recommended for the diet.

3. **4** Organ meats are high in purines, which break down into uric acid.

   1,2,3 These foods would not be restricted.

4. **1** Alcohol is drying and will promote skin breakdown on the residual limb.

   2 This is a good exercise to toughen the residual limb.

   3 Good hygiene with mild soap and water is appropriate skin care.

   4 ROM exercises for the joints above and below the residual limb is important to prevent contractures.

5. **4** Avoidance of strain is essential to provide time for the prosthesis to sit adequately in the socket and not become dislodged; this usually takes 2 months.

   1 This is an inadequate time for healing to take place.

   2 This is too long; it is usually up to 2 months for partial weight-bearing, although positional restrictions may go beyond 2 months.

   3 Same as answer 1.

6. **4** Older adults metabolize drugs slower because of declining body functions.

   1 Anyone can develop a tolerance to medications; age is not specific to developing tolerance to medications.

   2 Older adults metabolize drugs slower not faster

   3 Older adults can be prone to more adverse drug reactions because of the number of medications they consume, not because of declining body functions.

7. **3** The even distribution of hemosiderin (iron-rich pigment) in the tissue in response to pressure of the prosthesis indicates proper fit.

   1 This would result in an improper fit.

   2 This has nothing to do with a proper fit.

   4 This indicates that the prosthesis is too long or too short.

8. **2** Correct; such activities would include combing hair, feeding self, and brushing teeth.

   1 Periods of undisturbed rest should be provided.

   3 A firm mattress is recommended for proper body alignment.

   4 ROM exercises should not exceed limit of pain tolerance.

9. **3** Ingestion of dairy products increase calcium intake. Excessive calcium in the body during periods of decreased mobility increases the chance of kidney stone formation.

   1 Vitamin and mineral requirements are important, as is fiber, which promotes proper elimination.

   2 Unless fluid restrictions are necessary, at least 2000 ml of fluid should be consumed on a daily basis.

   4 Increase in urine acidity will decrease incidence of urinary tract infections; however this is not applicable to urinary complications resulting from decreased mobility.

10. **2** Quadriceps setting exercises improve the strength of muscles needed for walking.

    1,3,4 These actions will not strengthen the muscles needed for walking.

11. **2** Preparation for crutch walking includes exercises to strengthen the arm and shoulder muscles.

    1 This is important in healing and preparation for the prosthesis, not for crutch walking.

    3 Position changes are to prevent hip flexion contractures, not to prepare for crutch walking.

    4 Phantom-limb phenomenon is a sensation that the absent limb is present; there are no such exercises.

chapter *five*

Respiratory System Overview

All cells of the body are dependent on adequate oxygenation and removal of carbon dioxide for health. The respiratory system is dependent on central nervous system (CNS) regulation and on the cardiovascular system for blood supply. Respiratory distress or dysfunction may be secondary to disease in another system. Many pulmonary diseases are chronic. Therefore it is essential that the nurse make a complete respiratory assessment of all residents and include this in nursing care planning, even when the primary diagnosis is unrelated to the respiratory system.

Physiology of Respiration

A. Mechanism of inspiration
1. Respiratory muscles contract
2. Thorax increases in size
3. Lungs increase in size
4. Air rushes in from the atmosphere due to positive pressure and enters the alveoli
5. Inspiration is completed
6. Oxygen enters the blood stream
B. Mechanism of expiration
1. Respiratory muscles relax
2. Thorax decreases in size
3. Lungs decrease in size
4. Carbon dioxide is released from the blood stream into the lungs
5. Air is expelled out of the lungs into the atmosphere
6. Expiration is complete

The following are terms used to describe respirations:

- **bradypnea** slow respirations
- **Cheyne-Stokes** periods of apnea alternating with rapid respirations
- **DOE** dyspnea on exertion
- **dyspnea difficulty** breathing; may be subjective or objective

- **Kussmaul breathing** fast, deep, and labored respirations
- **orthopnea** difficulty breathing in a supine position; relieved by sitting up
- **paroxysmal nocturnal dyspnea** transient episodes of acute dyspnea that occur a few hours after falling asleep
- **SOB** short of breath
- **tachypnea** rapid respirations
- **wheeze** sound as air moves out through bronchi and bronchioles that have been narrowed by spasm, swelling, and secretions

Nursing Assessment

A. Nursing observations (objective data)
1. Respirations
   a. Rate
   b. Depth
   c. Characteristics, and any difficulty
2. Oxygen deprivation (note any)
   a. Restlessness
   b. Yawning
   c. Anxiety
   d. Drowsiness
   e. Confusion
   f. Disorientation
3. Cough
   a. Frequency
   b. Relationship to activity and precipitating factors
   c. Production of sputum
   d. Describe completely (e.g., dry, productive, nonproductive, hoarse, barking, moist, or hacking)
4. Lung sounds (adventitious)
   a. Crackles
   b. Wheezes
   c. Friction rub
5. Sputum (note the following)

a. Consistency (e.g., thick, tenacious, watery, or frothy)
b. Amount (e.g., scant, moderate, or copious)
c. Color (e.g., white, yellow, pink, rust, blood-tinged, or green)
d. Odor
6. Skin color
a. Pallor, ashen, or ruddy
b. Cyanosis (bluish discoloration): observe lips, nail beds, and mucous membranes
7. Skin
a. Temperature
b. Diaphoresis
8. Vital signs
a. Pulse: note rate, quality, and characteristics
b. Blood pressure
c. Temperature (rectal)
9. Nasal discharge
10. Voice: huskiness
B. Resident description (subjective data)
1. Cough
2. Pain
3. Difficulty breathing
4. Fatigue or weakness
5. Sputum
C. Patient history
1. Use of extra pillows needed to sleep
2. Respiratory illness or difficulty
3. Injuries
4. Use of medications or respiratory aids
5. Smoking

Diagnostic Tests/Methods

A. Chest x-ray examination: a picture of lung tissue from different angles; based on a knowledge of normal anatomy and usual changes in disease, diagnosis of many conditions can be made (e.g., tumors, pneumonia); there is no preparation and no special care or observations after x-ray examination
B. Bronchoscopy
1. Direct inspection of the trachea and bronchi through a scope passed through the nose or mouth; with this procedure specimens are obtained for biopsy and culture; foreign bodies can be removed (e.g., fish bones)
2. Nursing responsibilities: provide general preparation as that for a surgical procedure; after procedure, monitor vital signs, provide oral hygiene, and observe for cough and blood-streaked sputum; do not allow patient to eat or drink until gag reflex returns
C. Bronchogram
1. Visualization of bronchial tree through x-ray examination after introducing radiopaque dye; patient is given sedative and antispasmodic
2. Nursing responsibilities: provide postural drainage to aid in removal of dye; encourage deep breathing and coughing; do not allow patient to eat or drink until gag reflex returns
D. Computed tomography (CT) scan: produces clear, anatomic images of the chest cavity
E. Ultrasound: image of area is created by high-frequency sound; used for specific data relative to lung capacities
F. MRI: image created by magnetic resonance, a noninvasive procedure
G. Thoracentesis
1. Needle aspiration of fluid from pleural cavity (space); local anesthesia is used
2. Nursing responsibilities: maintain proper positioning; support and reassure resident during the procedure; monitor vital signs during and after the procedure
H. CBC: WBC count changes from normal values indicate type of infection
I. Arterial blood gases
1. Measurement of the partial pressure of oxygen and carbon dioxide in the blood; arterial puncture is performed
2. Nursing care: once the blood sample is obtained, apply constant pressure to the site for 5 minutes; apply pressure dressing; inspect site frequently for hematoma and pain
J. Culture and sensitivity
1. Throat or nasopharynx
2. Sputum
a. Identifies organisms and specific medication to which resident will respond
b. Nursing responsibilities: obtain before starting antibiotics; first sputum in the morning usually has the most organisms

K. Sputum analysis
   1. Acid-fast bacillus (AFB): determines presence of mycobacterium tuberculosis
   2. Cytology: assist in the diagnosis of lung carcinoma
L. Pulmonary function tests: determine extent of respiratory difficulty and evaluate function of respiratory system; measure vital capacity, tidal volume, and total lung capacity; no special preparation or nursing care after testing
M. Lung scan: positron emission tomography (PET): radioisotopes are inhaled or administered intravenously; a scanning device records the pattern of radioactivity; used in diagnosing vascular diseases (e.g., pulmonary embolism); no special preparation or nursing care
N. Biopsy examination
   1. Removal of a small amount of tissue to identify disease; biopsy may be of a lymph node to determine if the disease has spread into the lymphatic system
   2. Nursing care: provide general preoperative and postoperative care

NURSING OBSERVATIONS OF SIGNIFICANT CHANGES IN THE RESIDENT'S RESPIRATORY STATUS

The resident's expression, chest movements and respirations all provide valuable visual clues. There may be times when residents cannot verbalize distress, however, the keen observations of the nurse will provide vital information indicating significant respiratory changes. The following are the signs and symptoms to observe:
- Wheezing
- SOB, orthopnea, dyspnea
- Apprehension, anxiety, restlessness
- Decreased ability to concentrate
- Decreased level of consciousness
- Increased fatigue
- Vertigo
- Behavioral changes
- Increased pulse rate
- Increased rate and depth of respiration
- Elevated blood pressure; if O_2 deficiency is not correct, blood pressure will decrease
- Cardiac dysrhythmias
- Pallor
- Cyanosis
- Clubbing

- Flared nostrils

Nursing measures the nurse must implement to improve respiratory status:
- Assure a clear airway
- Put resident in upright position to support expansion of the thorax and gaseous exchange
- Provide oxygen to support and replenish tissue oxygenation and prevent cyanosis
- Administer antianxiety medication to allay apprehension

Special nursing considerations:
- Monitor resident's color, alertness
- Observe for signs of fatigue and low activity tolerance
- Be alert for signs of symptoms of respiratory infections

Common Resident Problems And Nursing Care

A. Activity intolerance related to fatigue and weakness: body cells' demand for oxygen is not met; the resident tires easily and becomes short of breath
   1. Protect from exertion; provide care
   2. Plan care to include rest periods
   3. Leave bed in low position
   4. Leave call bell and all personal belongings within easy reach
   5. Provide oxygen with humidity as ordered
   6. Limit conversation
B. Risk for injury related to dizziness: caused by diminished oxygen to the brain cells
   1. Provide all care as in preceding list
   2. Maintain safety; use side rails
   3. Make neurologic assessment every 4 hours (q4h)
C. Altered oral mucous membrane related to mouth breathing
   1. Force fluids if allowed
   2. Provide oral hygiene q2h
   3. Lubricate lips
D. Altered breathing pattern related to orthopnea
   1. Place a pillow longitudinally under back
   2. Provide table with pillow for headrest in extreme difficulty
   3. Use footboard to prevent slipping down in bed
   4. Semi- to high-Fowler's position
E. Ineffective airway clearance; impaired gas exchange related to dyspnea and coughing

1. Oxygen therapy: maintain safety of equipment and proper care and observations
2. Organize care and work efficiently to conserve resident's energy
3. Plan rest periods
4. Position in semi- to high-Fowler's position; use two pillows
5. Provide soft diet and small, frequent feedings
6. Avoid gas-forming foods
7. Prevent constipation and straining
8. Use rectal thermometer
9. Make accurate observations about cough and sputum
10. Obtain specimens as needed
11. Provide tissues and bag for disposal in easy reach
12. Provide sputum cup if needed
13. Change position q2h
14. Encourage deep breathing
15. Force fluids q2h
16. Provide oral hygiene q2h
17. Provide postural drainage if ordered
18. Give expectorants as ordered

F. Anxiety related to dyspnea, fatigue, and weakness
   1. Maintain quiet environment
   2. Remain calm
   3. Explain everything slowly and carefully
   4. Provide physical and mental rest
   5. Answer call lights promptly
   6. Provide frequent contacts
   7. Offer realistic encouragements
   8. Provide restful diversion (e.g., music)
   9. Encourage residents to express feelings and concerns

G. Nutrition, altered: less than body requirements, related to dry mouth from mouth breathing, foul taste and odor from sputum, and fatigue; may affect desire for food
   1. Make mealtime pleasant
   2. Provide oral hygiene before each meal
   3. Remove used tissues and sputum cups
   4. Request food preferences
   5. Give small, frequent, attractively served meals

Major Medical Diagnoses
PNEUMONIA

A. Description: an inflammation of the lungs or part of the lung (e.g., left lower lobe [LLL] pneumonia) secretions fill the alveolar sacs, which is a good medium for bacterial growth; the inflammation spreads to adjacent sacs; spaces of the lung consolidate with thick exudate; irritation may cause bleeding, and sputum has the characteristic rusty color; exchange of air is difficult and, in advanced conditions, not possible

B. Causes: (1) Bacterial infections and viruses are spread by respiratory secretions (droplets); chemical irritation; fungi and other organisms; residents with poor health and low natural resistance to infection are more susceptible (e.g., older adults, those with chronic illness, and immunocompromised individuals) (2) Aspiration—an accidental inhalation of food or fluids into the lungs during breathing. This is a common problem in the older adult or unconcious individual with absent gag reflex or decreased cough mechanism

C. Signs and symptoms
   1. Dyspnea, short of breath, pain on inspiration, shallow breathing, signs of air hunger, orthopnea, and oxygen deprivation
   2. Marked elevation in temperature
   3. Cough: painful and dry at first, then productive with copious amounts of thick sputum (color according to organism)

D. Diagnostic tests/methods
   1. Resident history
   2. Physical assessment with auscultation of chest
   3. Chest x-ray examination
   4. Sputum culture and sensitivity
   5. CBC

E. Treatment
   1. Specific and broad-spectrum antibiotics
   2. Antipyretics, analgesics (codeine), expectorants, and bronchodilators
   3. Intravenous (IV) fluids; force oral fluids
   4. Oxygen with humidity; incentive spirometer

F. Nursing intervention
   1. Provide optimum rest: provide care; help resident conserve energy; schedule rest periods; limit conversation; keep personal items and call bell within easy reach; alleviate anxiety
   2. Maintain oxygen with humidity
   3. Isolate as indicated, especially residents with oral and nasal secretions; provide for proper disposal

4. Liquefy secretions: force fluids (3000 ml daily or more); observe and document production of sputum; suction as necessary
5. Provide oral hygiene q2h
6. Monitor vital signs q4h; use rectal thermometer; monitor lung sounds
7. Assist with loosening of secretions: have resident turn, cough, and deep breathe q2h (splint chest if painful); observe and document cough
8. Maintain adequate nutrition: provide liquid-to-soft diet high in protein and calories
9. Maintain IV fluids and medication schedule to ensure continued blood levels
10. Position for comfort (high-Fowler's or lying on affected side)

INFLUENZA

A. Description: acute disease that may occur as an epidemic; recovery is usually complete; no permanent immunity results; complications and death may occur in residents with chronic or debilitating conditions, especially cardiac or pulmonary
B. Cause: virus
C. Signs and symptoms
   1. Headache, chest pain, nuchal rigidity, and muscle ache
   2. Elevated temperature
   3. Coughing, sneezing, dry throat, nasal discharge, and herpetic lesions
   4. Gastrointestinal symptoms: nausea, vomiting, and anorexia
   5. Weakness
D. Diagnostic tests/methods: resident history and physical assessment
E. Treatment
   1. Prevention with vaccines
   2. Symptomatic
F. Nursing intervention
   1. Provide rest; assist with care; provide quiet environment and dim lighting
   2. Force fluids
   3. Relieve symptoms: provide antipyretics, analgesics

PULMONARY TUBERCULOSIS

A. Description: a chronic, progressive infection; alveoli are inflamed, and small nodules are produced called primary tubercles; the tubercle bacillus is at the center of the nodule (these become fibrosed); the area becomes calcified and can be identified on x-ray film; the person who has been infected harbors the bacillus for life; it is dormant unless it becomes active during physical or emotional stress
B. Cause: *Mycobacterium tuberculosis*, Koch's bacillus, an acid-fast bacillus (AFB) spread by droplets from an infected person
C. Signs and symptoms
   1. Malaise; resident is easily fatigued
   2. Chest pain, cough, and hemoptysis (coughing up blood from the respiratory tract)
   3. Elevation of temperature and night sweats
   4. Anorexia and weight loss
   5. Anxiety, fear of chronic disease, and fear of public rejection
D. Diagnostic tests/methods
   1. Resident history and physical assessment
   2. Chest x-ray examination
   3. Sputum specimen for AFB; aspiration of gastric fluid for AFB if unable to obtain specimen
   4. Tuberculin skin testing (e.g., tine or Mantoux test)
E. Treatment
   1. Antituberculin drugs for 18 to 24 months
   2. Rest (physical and emotional)
   3. Diet high in carbohydrates, proteins, and vitamins (especially B_6)
   4. Surgical resection of affected lung tissue or involved lobe (only when necessary)
F. Nursing intervention
   1. Provide rest; assist with or provide care; plan rest periods; limit conversation; leave personal items in easy reach
   2. Prevent transmission: ensure respiratory isolation; provide tissues and bag for disposal; encourage proper use of tissues; insist on resident covering mouth and nose when coughing or sneezing
   3. Provide frequent, small meals and nutritious snacks
   4. Avoid chills; keep skin dry and clean; protect from drafts, especially at night
   5. Allay fears of resident and family about transmission: encourage proper adherence to drug maintenance; explain how organism is carried, transmitted, and destroyed (nurse must be aware that a tuberculin test

is recommended for all contacts with a person with tuberculosis (TB); a positive test result does not mean the disease has manifested but indicates that the organism has entered the body and that the body has produced antibodies at some point

CHRONIC OBSTRUCTIVE PULMONARY DISEASE

Chronic obstructive pulmonary disease (COPD) includes chronic and frequently progressive pulmonary disorders that affect expiratory air flow; asthma, chronic bronchitis, and pulmonary emphysema may occur independently or together.

ASTHMA

A. Description: spasms of the bronchial muscle occur; edema and swelling of the mucosa produce thick secretions; air flow is obstructed; air enters and is trapped; a characteristic wheeze accompanies attempts to exhale through narrowed bronchi; breathing is labored; coughing is attempted, but resident fails to expectorate satisfactory amounts; resident experiences great anxiety; the attacks last 30 to 60 minutes, often with normal breathing between attacks; if attack is difficult to control, and is resistant to all forms of treatment, it is called status asthmaticus
B. Causes
   1. Recurrent respiratory infection
   2. Allergic reaction
   3. Physical or emotional stress may provoke attack in a person with asthma
C. Signs and symptoms
   1. Shortness of breath, expiratory wheeze, labored respirations, and diaphoresis
   2. Thick, tenacious sputum (after acute attack)
   3. Anxiety or feeling of suffocation
D. Diagnostic tests/methods: patient history and physical examination
E. Treatment
   1. Removal of cause (source of allergy) or desensitization
   2. Low-flow, humidified oxygen
   3. Bronchodilators, mast cell inhibitors, corticosteroids, or sedatives
F. Nursing intervention
   1. Reduce anxiety: provide time to listen; do not leave patient alone during attack

2. Remove cause: keep environment free from dust and other allergens
3. Provide continuous humidity as ordered
4. Force fluids; maintain IV as ordered
5. Position for maximum comfort and breathing: have resident sit in high-Fowler's position with arms supported by over-bed table
6. Prevent secondary infections: avoid staff and visitors with upper respiratory infections
7. Teach abdominal breathing
8. Do not allow smoking; refer resident for help in quitting

CHRONIC BRONCHITIS

A. Description: chronic, progressive infection accompanied by hypersecretion of mucus by the bronchioles; without treatment and prevention of acute attacks, the alveolar sacs and capillaries will extend and destruct
B. Causes
   1. Asthma
   2. Acute respiratory tract infections (e.g., pneumonia, influenza, smoking, and air pollution contribute to incidence)
   3. Familial tendency
C. Signs and symptoms
   1. Problems related to acute infection
   2. Cough, productive with thick, white sputum; sputum is blood-tinged as disease progresses (cough is greatest on arising)
D. Diagnostic tests/methods
   1. Resident history
   2. Pulmonary testing to rule out other disease (e.g., tuberculosis or malignancy)
E. Treatment
   1. Prevent irritation of bronchial mucosa: encourage resident to discontinue smoking and change aggravating conditions in occupation or home environment
   2. Prevent upper respiratory tract infection: maintain optimum health, adequate rest, and high-protein, high-vitamin diet
   3. Provide bronchodilators, antibiotics, corticosteroids, and influenza vaccine during epidemics
F. Nursing intervention
   1. Provide care to relieve resident problems (see discussion on common resident problems and nursing care outlined on pp. 46-47)

2. Loosen, liquefy, and remove secretions: provide postural drainage and chest percussion as ordered; force fluids
3. Involve resident and family in care and care planning
4. Do not allow smoking; refer resident for help in quitting

EMPHYSEMA

A. Description: a chronic, progressive condition in which the alveolar sacs distend, rupture, and destroy the capillary beds; the alveoli lose elasticity, inspired air is trapped; inspiration is difficult and expiration is prolonged; the lung tissue becomes fibrotic; exchange of gases is not possible; anxiety increases; signs of oxygen deprivation are evident
B. Cause (see discussion on bronchitis)
C. Signs and symptoms
   1. Dyspnea on exertion (later, dyspnea on slightest exertion and orthopnea); inspiration is difficult; expiration is prolonged, accompanied by wheeze
   2. Chronic cough; productive, purulent sputum in copious amounts
   3. Difficulty talking: speaks in short, jerky sentences
   4. Cerebral anoxia: is drowsy and confused; may become unconscious and go into coma
   5. Barrel chest
   6. Anorexia, weight loss, and weakness
D. Diagnostic tests/methods
   1. Resident history and physical examination
   2. Chest x-ray examination
   3. Pulmonary function tests
   4. Arterial blood gases; CBC
   5. Sputum analysis
E. Treatment (see discussion on bronchitis)
F. Nursing intervention
   1. Loosen, liquefy, and remove secretions: provide postural drainage and chest percussion as ordered; force fluids; administer expectorants as needed
   2. Promote respiratory function: breathing exercises and coughing
   3. Administer oxygen; oxygen is administered in low concentrations only (1 to 2 L); oxygen can be dangerous when the carbon dioxide level of the blood is high; the respiratory center of the brain becomes accustomed to the low blood oxygen level; if oxygen increases, respiratory rate will slow significantly
   4. Prevent and control infections: administer antibiotics; avoid contact with people with upper respiratory tract infections; avoid smoking
   5. Provide rest: limit exertion of any type; provide care; minimize conversation; assist with all movements (e.g., turning and getting into chair)
   6. Include family in care and care plan; be understanding that this condition is chronic
   7. Teach pursed-lip breathing; abdominal breathing

CANCER OF THE LUNG

A. Description: primary or secondary (from metastasis [e.g., from prostate]) malignant tumor; bronchogenic carcinoma is the most common primary tumor; is usually without symptoms until late stages when metastasis has occurred to brain, spinal cord, or esophagus; treatment is difficult in late stages and usually is symptomatic; prognosis is poor unless detected and treated early
B. Cause: exact cause is unknown, but strongly related to smoking, air pollution, and chemical irritants
C. Signs and symptoms (occur in late stages)
   1. Productive cough with blood-streaked sputum
   2. Dyspnea and chest pain
   3. Fatigue, anorexia, and weight loss
D. Diagnostic tests/methods
   1. CT scan; MRI
   2. Examination of sputum for cells
   3. Bronchial biopsy examination
E. Treatment
   1. Surgery: procedure depends on size and location of tumor (lobectomy or pneumonectomy)
   2. Radiation
   3. Chemotherapy

Review Questions

1. A resident's serum cholesterol level is 260 mg/100 L. Which of the following recommendations by the nurse is the best nutritional counseling for this resident?
   ① Eat only foods low in cholesterol
   ② Eat a soft, high-protein diet
   ③ Maintain a low-fat diet
   ④ Eat only easily digestible foods

2. The nurse notes that a resident, who has a diagnosis of COPD, is more comfortable after:
   ① Being placed in low-Fowler's position
   ② Having postural drainage
   ③ Fluids are restricted
   ④ The resident has provided all personal care

3. Your resident's care plan indicates he has orthopnea; nursing intervention will include:
   ① Keeping the bed in high-Fowler's position
   ② Maintaining oxygen at 40% by Venturi mask
   ③ Taking vital signs q2h
   ④ Using the log-rolling technique to turn resident on side

4. A resident is to be taught to monitor blood glucose level using the capillary glucose test (Dextrostix). Because of his insulin prescription, it would be most important to teach this resident to check blood glucose level:
   ① After strenuous activity
   ② Two hours after meals
   ③ Before lunch
   ④ Before strenuous activity

5. A resident has emphysema. Which of the following characteristics would the nurse expect the resident to exhibit?
   ① Thin body build and a pigeon chest
   ② Cyanotic skin color and dry, sparse hair
   ③ Peripheral edema and moist, shiny skin
   ④ Barreled chest and clubbing of the fingers

6. A resident has a diagnosis of asthma. When planning care for this resident, the nurse should know that asthma is defined as:
   ① A chronic, progressive condition that involves destruction of the elastic tissues of the alveolar walls
   ② A chronic dilation of a bronchus or bronchi, with secretions of large amounts of purulent sputum
   ③ A respiratory disorder characterized by recurring episodes of labored breathing with wheezing on expiration
   ④ An infectious disease caused by a tubercle bacillus

7. When suctioning secretions of a resident with a tracheostomy, suction is turned off as the catheter is inserted to prevent:
   ① Irritation of the lining of the trachea and loss of additional oxygen
   ② Blocking of the catheter with mucus
   ③ Infection of the oral cavity
   ④ "Kinking" of the catheter

8. A resident who has had emphysema (COPD) for many years develops an enlarged liver. The nurse understands that this results from:
   ① Liver hypoxia
   ② Hepatic acidosis
   ③ Esophageal varices
   ④ Portal hypertension

9. In assessing a resident with pneumonia, which of the following observations takes immediate priority?
   ① Rectal temperature 100° F
   ② Skin pale, moist
   ③ Urinal is full
   ④ Weight gain of 1 lb since yesterday

10. Based on the problems associated with bronchiolitis, the treatment of choice for a resident with this illness should consist of:
    ① Croupette and adequate hydration
    ② Postural drainage and corticosteroids
    ③ Adequate hydration and bronchodilators
    ④ Croupette and broad-spectrum antibiotics

ANSWERS AND RATIONALES FOR REVIEW QUESTIONS

1. **3** The resident should be on a low-fat diet to help lower cholesterol level.
   1 Some foods may not contain cholesterol (found in animal foods) but may have a high level of fat content such as vegetable oil. A low-fat diet best reduces cholesterol levels.
   2 A soft, high-protein diet is not needed.
   4 This diet is not necessary.

2. **2** Postural drainage helps drain sections of the lung, aids in coughing and removing secretions, and improves breathing.
   1 High-Fowler's position (45- to 90-degree elevation) is most effective in relieving dyspnea.
   3 Fluids should be forced to liquefy secretions.
   4 Resident should have rest and conserve energy.

3. **1** High-Fowler's position allows better lung expansion, thus promoting better oxygenation.
   2 Oxygen therapy would require a physician's order.
   3 Vital sign frequency is determined by a complete assessment of the resident.
   4 Log-rolling technique is used to turn the resident whose back cannot be flexed.

4. **4** Capillary blood glucose should always be tested before strenuous activity. Because exercise burns glucose and lowers blood glucose levels, it is important to assess the blood glucose level before exercising so that food and insulin could be adjusted to prevent hypoglycemia.
   1 Although testing the blood glucose level after exercise could be done, it is not the most important time to do this.
   2 Two hours after meals, blood glucose levels would be at their highest; this is not the best time.
   3 Although the level could be taken before lunch, this is not the best time.

5. **4** Because of chronic hypoxia and labored breathing, the chest develops a barrel-like configuration and the fingertips become blunted and clubbed.
   1 Pigeon chest is a congenital deformity; it is not usually the result of a chronic respiratory disease.
   2 The hair would become dry and sparse as a result of conditions other than emphysema.
   3 Moist shiny skin is not a manifestation of emphysema.

6. **3** Asthma involves recurring episodes of increased tracheal/bronchial responsiveness to various stimuli.
   1 This is the definition of emphysema.
   2 This is the definition of bronchiectasis.
   4 This is the definition of pulmonary tuberculosis.

7. **1** The suction is turned off as the catheter is inserted to avoid irritation of the trachea and additional loss of oxygen.
   2 Suctioning does not relate to blocking of the catheter.
   3 Having the suction on or off does not relate to an infectious process.
   4 Having the suction on or off does not relate to "kinking" of the catheter.

8. **4** The enlarged liver is caused by long-term respiratory acidosis with increased pulmonary pressures that eventually cause right heart enlargement and failure (corpulmonale); the elevated pressures cause backup pressure in the hepatic circulation.
   1 Liver hypoxia would cause atrophy and necrosis of cells, not enlargement.
   2 Right ventricular heart failure with increased pressure in the ascending vena cava causes increased pressure in the hepatoportal system, resulting in an enlarged liver, not hepatic acidosis.
   3 These are the result of hepatic portal hypertension, not the cause of an enlarged liver.

9. **2** May indicate change in condition, requiring further assessment.

    1 Normal range.

    3 Not a priority.

    4 With no indication of heart failure; would not be a priority.

10. **1** Adequate hydration and high humidity are essential to loosen tenacious secretions and minimize fluid loss.

    2 Corticosteroids are not used because they have not been proven effective.

    3 Bronchodilators are not used because the bronchial tree is not in spasm.

    4 Antibiotics are ineffectual because the etiologic agent is viral.

Chapter Five Answers

chapter six

Circulatory System Overview

A. Functions
  1. Major function: transports oxygen, carbon dioxide, cell wastes, nutrients, enzymes, and antibodies throughout the body
  2. Secondary function: contributes to the body's metabolic functions and maintenance of homeostasis
B. Heart: hollow, cone-shaped muscular organ the size of a man's fist; functions as pump
C. Conduction system: initiates heartbeat; conducts electrical impulses around heart; coordinates heartbeat
D. Blood vessels
  1. Arteries: elastic, muscular-conducting tubes; carry blood away from the heart and to the capillaries; all arteries (except pulmonary) carry oxygenated blood
    a. Aorta: the largest artery, from which all other arteries branch out and become smaller and smaller
    b. Arterioles: extremely small arteries; branch into the capillaries
  2. Veins: thin-walled tubes that have one-way valves to prevent backflow of blood; transport blood back to the heart; all veins (except pulmonary) carry deoxygenated blood
    a. Venae cavae: largest veins; enter the right atrium
      (1) Superior vena cava: returns blood from the head, arms, and thoracic region
      (2) Inferior vena cava: returns blood from body regions below the diaphragm
    b. Venules: extremely small veins; collect blood from the capillaries
  3. Capillaries: microscopic vessels; carry blood from arterioles to venules; exchange of nutrients and waste products occurs in capillaries

Problems
ANGINA PECTORIS

A. Definition: episodes of acute chest pain resulting from insufficient oxygenation of myocardial tissue, caused by decreased blood flow to the area
  1. Episodes occur most often during periods of physical or emotional exertion
    a. Exercise
    b. Eating a heavy meal
    c. Environmental temperature extremes
  2. Episodes seldom last more than 15 minutes
B. Causes
  1. The major cause is atherosclerosis
  2. Narrowed coronary arteries obstruct blood flow; thus oxygen carried by the blood cannot sufficiently meet tissue demands, particularly during periods of exertion
C. Signs and symptoms
  1. Substernal chest pain, usually brought on by exertion
  2. Radiation of pain to the jaw or an extremity
  3. Dyspnea
  4. Anxiety or feeling of impending doom
  5. Tachycardia
  6. Diaphoresis
  7. Sensation of heaviness, choking, or suffocation
  8. Indigestion
D. Diagnostic tests/methods
  1. Resident history and physical examination
  2. Electrocardiogram (ECG)
  3. Holter monitoring

4. Coronary angiography
5. Stress testing
6. Chest x-ray examination
7. Serum lipid and enzyme values

E. Treatment
 1. Relief of chest pain through the use of vasodilating drugs (e.g., nitrates, beta blockers, calcium channel blockers), sedatives, and analgesics
 2. Dietary restriction of fat and cholesterol
 3. Planned exercise
 4. Weight management
 5. Stress management
 6. If conservative measures are unsuccessful, coronary bypass surgery or an angioplasty may be considered

F. Nursing intervention
 1. Assess and document signs and symptoms and reactions to treatment
 2. Administer vasodilating medication and monitor for side effects
 3. Instruct resident to inform the nursing staff at the onset of an anginal attack
 4. Provide emotional support and assurance
 5. Provide prompt relief of pain
 6. Monitor vital signs, particularly during an attack
 7. Educate resident and family regarding diet, activity, drug therapy, and avoidance of risk factors

HYPERTENSION (HIGH BLOOD PRESSURE)

A. Definition: characterized by persistent elevation of blood pressure in which the systolic pressure is above 140 mm Hg and the diastolic pressure is above 90 mm Hg
 1. Primary hypertension (essential): a persistent elevation of blood pressure without an apparent cause
  a. Actual cause is unknown
  b. Primarily, small blood vessels are affected; peripheral resistance increases; and blood pressure rises
  c. Constricted blood vessels eventually cause damage to organs that rely on a blood supply from these vessels
 2. Secondary hypertension: a persistent elevation of blood pressure associated with another disease state
  a. Renal disease
  b. Adrenal dysfunction
  c. Atherosclerosis
  d. Coarctation of the aorta

B. Predisposing factors
 1. Smoking
 2. Obesity
 3. Heavy salt and cholesterol intake
 4. Heredity
 5. Aggressive, hyperactive personality
 6. Age: develops between 30 and 50 years of age
 7. Sex: primarily men over 35 years of age and women over 45 years of age
 8. Race: blacks have twice the incidence of whites

C. The heart, brain, kidney, and eyes can be damaged if the hypertensive state continues without correction

D. Signs and symptoms may be insidious and vague; a person can have the disorder and not know it
 1. Tinnitus
 2. Light-headedness
 3. Blurred vision
 4. Irritability
 5. Fatigue
 6. Tachycardia and palpitations
 7. Occipital, morning headaches
 8. Nosebleeds (epistaxis)
 9. Dyspnea on exertion

E. Diagnostic tests/methods
 1. Resident history and physical examination
 2. Series of resting blood pressure readings
 3. Routine urinalysis, blood urea nitrogen (BUN), and serum creatinine to screen for renal involvement
 4. Serum electrolytes to screen for adrenal involvement
 5. Blood sugar levels to screen for endocrine involvement
 6. Lipid profile
 7. Chest x-ray examination
 8. ECG
 9. Holter monitoring
 10. Funduscopic eye examination

F. Treatment
 1. Lowering blood pressure through the use of anti-hypertensive drugs
 2. Sodium-restricted diet
 3. Cholesterol-controlled diet
 4. Weight management

5. Stress management
6. Reduction or elimination of smoking
7. Planned exercise

G. Nursing intervention
1. Assess and document signs and symptoms and reactions to treatments
2. Administer prescribed medication
3. Observe for and report drug-related side effects
4. Monitor weight every day (qd) to evaluate initial diuretic therapy
5. Monitor intake and output to evaluate initial diuretic therapy
6. Monitor vital signs, particularly blood pressure, under the same conditions qd
7. Provide planned activity and rest periods
8. Provide prescribed diet; calorie controlled

MYOCARDIAL INFARCTION (HEART ATTACK)

A. Definition: the obstruction of a coronary artery or one of its branches
1. The obstruction results in the death of the myocardial tissue supplied by that vessel
2. The myocardial tissue dies because of oxygen deprivation
3. The heart's ability to regain or maintain its function depends on the location and size of the area of infarction

B. A myocardial infarction can occur whenever a coronary artery or branch of the artery becomes occluded by a thrombus, emboli, or the atherosclerotic process.

C. Signs and symptoms
1. "Crushing" chest pain lasting longer than 15 minutes and unrelieved by rest or drugs
2. Shortness of breath
3. Nausea and vomiting
4. Tachycardia
5. Diaphoresis and pallor
6. Temperature rise after 48 hours
7. Elevation of the cardiac enzymes
8. Dysrhythmias
9. Anxiety

D. Diagnostic tests/methods
1. Resident history and physical examination
2. ECG
3. Cardiac enzyme studies (SGOT, LDH, CPK-MB)
4. Chest x-ray examination

E. Treatment
1. Analgesic drugs to relieve pain
2. Oxygen to relieve respiratory distress
3. Vasopressor drugs to prevent circulatory collapse (cardiogenic shock)
4. Cardiac monitoring to detect dysrhythmias
5. Hemodynamic monitoring: internal monitoring of the blood pressure and pulmonary artery pressure
6. Bed rest with progressive activity to allow the damaged myocardium to heal
7. Intravenous (IV) fluids to provide for IV drug administration
8. Cardiopulmonary resuscitation in the event of cardiac standstill (arrest)
9. Pacemaker insertion
10. Anticoagulant therapy
11. Thrombolytic therapy to dissolve blood clot and restore blood flow

F. Nursing intervention
1. Provide pain relief
2. Provide ongoing assessment and documentation of symptoms and reactions to treatment
3. Administer and monitor oxygen
4. Record vital signs qh during the acute period
5. Record intake and output qh during the acute period
6. Provide best rest during the acute period and progressive activity as prescribed
   a. Apply antiembolism stockings
   b. Allow resident out of bed to use bedside commode (less taxing to the cardiovascular system)
   c. Monitor pulse during periods of activity
7. Avoid activities that produce straining (Valsalva maneuver) to avoid taxing the cardiovascular system
   a. Administer stool softeners as prescribed
   b. Caution resident against straining when attempting a bowel movement
8. Provide diet as prescribed
   a. May start out on liquids and then progress

b. Sodium and cholesterol may be restricted
c. Caffeine may be restricted
9. Give prescribed antidysrhythmics and monitor for side effects
10. Give prescribed cardiotonics and diuretics and monitor for side effects
11. Monitor for complications
   a. Cardiogenic shock: circulatory collapse caused by decreased cardiac output (the amount of blood pumped out by the heart to the body per minute) the vital organs are not being perfused
      (1) Monitor vital signs every 15 minutes
      (2) Record intake and output qh
      (3) Report changes in rate, rhythm, and conductivity
      (4) Observe and report signs and symptoms of restlessness, diaphoresis, pallor, low blood pressure, and tachycardia
      (5) Administer and monitor prescribed vasopressors and antidysrhythmics
      (6) Administer oxygen as prescribed
      (7) Provide cardiac and hemodynamic monitoring (hemodynamic monitoring refers to the internal monitoring of blood pressure and pulmonary artery pressure) hospital setting
   b. Pulmonary edema: left ventricle failure (pumping mechanism) caused by strain on a diseased heart; cardiac output is reduced, resulting in lung congestion
      (1) Observe and report symptoms of anxiety, dyspnea, orthopnea, frothy, pink-tinged sputum, rales, decreased urine output, and dependent edema
      (2) Record vital signs every 15 minutes
      (3) Record intake and output qh
      (4) Place bed in high-Fowler's position
      (5) Administer cardiotonics and diuretics as prescribed and monitor for side effects
      (6) Administer and monitor oxygen therapy
      (7) Use rotating tourniquets: to reduce the circulatory volume to the right side of the heart (seldom used)
      (8) Be prepared to administer analgesics to allay anxiety and reduce respiratory rate
      (9) Provide emotional support to resident and family

CONGESTIVE HEART FAILURE

A. Definition: failure of the pumping mechanism of the heart resulting in an insufficient blood supply to meet the body's needs
B. Causes
   1. The underlying mechanism in congestive heart failure (CHF) involves the failure of the pumping mechanism of the heart to respond to the metabolic changes of the body
   2. The end result is a heart that cannot supply a sufficient amount of blood in relation to the body's needs and to the amount of blood returning to the heart (venous return); pressure builds up in the vascular beds on the affected side of the heart
C. CHF is described in terms of left-sided or right-sided failure, depending on which side is affected
D. Signs and symptoms are divided into left-sided failure and right-sided failure, although both sides may be affected
   1. Left-sided failure leads to pulmonary congestion
      a. Dyspnea
      b. Orthopnea
      c. Nonproductive cough that worsens at night
      d. As severity of failure increases, frothy, blood-tinged sputum is noted
      e. Anxiety and restlessness
      f. Fatigue
   2. Right-sided failure may follow left-sided failure and results in systemic venous congestion
      a. Weight gain caused by fluid accumulation in the tissues
      b. Dependent edema in the form of ankle edema or sacral edema

c. Ascites caused by the collection of fluid in the abdominal cavity; ascites may also hinder respiration
d. Fatigue
e. Gastrointestinal symptoms such as nausea, vomiting, and anorexia
f. Decreased urine output

E. Diagnostic tests/methods
1. Resident history and physical examination including the findings of edema, abnormal heart sounds, and the presence of rales with dyspnea (orthopnea)
2. Chest x-ray examination
3. ECG
4. Arterial blood gas studies
5. Liver function studies
6. Renal function studies

F. Treatment
1. Drug therapy: digitalization, diuretics, and sedatives
2. Recording of weight qd
3. Monitoring intake and output
4. Oxygen therapy
5. Rotating tourniquets (seldom used)
6. Restricting fluids
7. Restricting dietary sodium
8. Bed rest with progressive activity
9. Elevate the head of the bed
10. Monitor vital signs

G. Nursing intervention
1. Provide ongoing assessment and documentation of signs, symptoms, and reactions to treatment
2. Monitor oxygen therapy
3. Record vital signs every 15 minutes to 2 hours during the acute phase
4. Record intake and output qh during the acute phase
5. Weigh resident qd
6. Administer and monitor prescribed cardiotonics, diuretics, and sedatives; observe for side effects
7. Determine the amount of activity that produces the least discomfort to the resident
8. Monitor for dependent edema
a. Ankle edema when sitting upright
b. Sacral edema when in supine position
9. Raise the head of the bed as prescribed
10. Observe for complications of bed rest
a. Have resident turn, cough, and take deep breaths

b. Apply antiembolism stockings
11. Provide emotional support to the resident and family
12. Provide a diet low in sodium if prescribed
13. Educate the resident and family concerning dietary management, drug therapy, and activity
14. Restrict fluids as ordered

EMBOLISM

A. Definition: a blood clot circulating in the blood
B. Causes
1. The clot may be a fragment of an arteriosclerotic plaque, or it may have originated in the heart
2. If large, an embolism may lodge in a vessel bifurcation and obstruct the flow of blood to vital organs or tissues
3. Most emboli arise from deep vein thrombi; the embolis travels in the bloodstream until it lodges in a narrowed area, usually the lungs

C. Signs and symptoms: depend on the area involved
1. Pain at the site
2. Shock
3. Areas supplied by the involved vessel evidence pallor, coldness, numbness, tingling, and cyanosis
4. Sudden onset of dyspnea
5. Cough and hemoptysis
6. Chest pain
7. Tachycardia
8. Tachypnea

D. Diagnostic tests/methods
1. Resident history and physical examination
2. Lung scan
3. Chest x-ray examination
4. Arterial blood gases

E. Treatment
1. Oxygen therapy
2. IV fluids
3. IV anticoagulants
4. Analgesics
5. Thrombolytic agents

F. Nursing intervention
1. Assess and document signs and symptoms and reactions to treatments
2. Monitor vital signs
3. Monitor arterial blood gas reports and notify the physician

4. Administer prescribed analgesic and monitor for side effects
5. Administer anticoagulants as prescribed and monitor for bleeding tendencies
6. Monitor oxygen therapy
7. Give range-of-motion (ROM) exercises
8. Provide antiembolism stockings
9. Educate resident and family concerning drug therapy, monitoring for bleeding tendencies, and restriction of activities

ARTERIOSCLEROSIS/ATHEROSCLEROSIS

A. Definition
   1. Arteriosclerosis: a process in which the arterial walls harden, thicken, and lose their elasticity, resulting in restricted blood flow
   2. Atherosclerosis: one form of arteriosclerosis; fatty plaques form on the intima (inner layer) of the arteries
B. Pathology
   1. The underlying mechanism is the formation of fatty plaque deposits in the arteries
   2. The plaque increases in size and ultimately obstructs blood flow to vital areas
C. Arteriosclerosis is associated with the following health problems
   1. Coronary artery disease
   2. Angina pectoris
   3. Myocardial infarction
   4. Hypertension
   5. Peripheral vascular disease
   6. Cerebrovascular accidents (strokes)
D. Signs and symptoms vary, depending on the arteries affected by the sclerosing process
   1. Extremity involvement
      a. Cramping pain (intermittent claudication)
      b. Numbness and tingling
      c. Reduced circulation causing ulceration or pain
      d. Outward changes: skin pallor, cool skin, reduced or absent pulses, loss of leg hair, and skin ulceration
   2. Coronary involvement
      a. Chest pain
      b. Dyspnea
      c. Palpitations
      d. Fainting (syncope)
      e. Fatigue

INTERNAL BLEEDING

A. Description
   1. Potentially life-threatening situation
   2. Difficult to diagnose
   3. Progresses rapidly
B. Signs and symptoms
   1. Symptoms of shock
   2. Vertigo
   3. Hemoptysis (vomiting or expectorating blood)
   4. Hematuria
   5. Pain
   6. Tenderness
   7. Obvious bleeding from mouth, rectum, or any other body part.
C. Nursing intervention
   1. Priority medical emergency
   2. Place resident with legs slightly elevated if this is not contraindicated
   3. Monitor vital signs
   4. Maintain body temperature with blankets
   5. Keep NPO
   6. Oxygen as ordered by physician

SHOCK

A. Description: depressed state of vital body functions that, if untreated, could result in death
B. Types
   1. Hypovolemic: decrease in circulating blood volume (e.g., hemorrhage)
   2. Vasogenic: disturbance in tissue perfusion caused by circulating blood volume alterations
   3. Cardiogenic: faulty pumping resulting in reduced cardiac output
   4. Neurogenic: disruption of vasomotor tone resulting in decrease of circulating blood volume (e.g., spinal cord injury)
   5. Septic: massive bacterial infection, for example, gram-negative organisms
C. Assessment
   1. Shallow, rapid respirations
   2. Cool, pale, clammy skin
   3. Thirst
   4. Tachycardia
   5. Decreased blood pressure
   6. Weak, thready pulse
   7. Restlessness
   8. Decreased urine output
   9. May become confused or disoriented

D. Intervention
   1. Priority medical emergency
   2. Ensure adequate airway and ventilation
   3. Control bleeding if present
   4. Place in supine position with legs elevated unless contraindicated (e.g., head injuries)
   5. Insert urinary catheter
   6. Monitor vital signs
   7. Cover victim to conserve body heat
   8. Administer oxygen

Review Questions

1. An important nursing assessment for an ambulatory resident receiving care for CHF would include monitoring for:
   ① Ankle edema when sitting upright
   ② Sacral edema when sitting upright
   ③ Swelling of the hands and face
   ④ Abdominal distention and diarrhea

2. Mild exercises of the legs and wearing antiembolitic stockings are prescribed for a resident with CHF. When applying the stockings, the nurse explains that the purpose for these is to:
   ① Reduce circulation to the legs and ease the workload of the heart
   ② Prevent abdominal edema
   ③ Prevent clot formation in the lower extremities
   ④ Reduce edema of the extremities

3. A resident has developed thrombophlebitis after being confined to bed for several weeks. To explain the diagnosis to the resident the nurse's best statement would be that thrombophlebitis is:
   ① An ulcer that becomes infected
   ② A traumatic inflammation of blood vessels
   ③ An inflammation of the vein with clot formation
   ④ An inflammation of an artery with clot formation

4. Residents with pulmonary edema associated with CHF may benefit from the use of the alpha-adrenergic blocking agents because these drugs:
   ① Have a direct diuretic action on lung tissue
   ② Enhance the absorption of carbon monoxide
   ③ Lower elevated pulmonary arterial pressure

   ④ Achieve an indirect cardiotonic effect and thereby improve general circulation

5. A resident with a diagnosis of CHF is on a 500-g sodium-restricted diet. Which tray would be most appropriate for this resident?
   ① Fresh beef, salt-free cottage cheese, one small sweet potato, and one large tangerine
   ② Smoked fish, prepared muffins, frozen lima beans, and an apple
   ③ Corned beef on rye sandwich, dill pickle, and pear
   ④ Ham and cheese on regular bread, unsalted hard-boiled egg, and an orange

6. A resident with CHF is placed in a high-Fowler's position. What is the rationale for placing the resident in this position?
   ① To reduce the volume of blood returning to the heart
   ② To increase the volume of blood returning to the heart
   ③ To increase cardiac output and stroke volume
   ④ To reduce ankle edema and prevent dysrhythmias

7. Pulmonary edema is a complication of CHF. Which of the following findings suggests pulmonary edema?
   ① Angina, nausea, vomiting, and dyspnea on exertion
   ② Confusion, diaphoresis, bradycardia, and hypotension
   ③ Angina, cough, bradycardia, and cyanosis
   ④ Restlessness; frothy, pink-tinged sputum; and dyspnea

8. Physical examination reveals that a resident is suffering from systemic hypertension. Possible causes of hypertension include:
   ① Loss of fluid and electrolytes
   ② Overstimulation of the sympathetic nervous system
   ③ Decreased elasticity of the arterioles
   ④ Decreased blood volume

9. Initial treatments that the nurse may anticipate for a resident with thrombophlebitis include:
   ① Warm, moist heat applications to the affected extremity
   ② Exercise to the affected leg four times daily
   ③ Keeping the affected leg lower than the rest of the body
   ④ Administering Coumadin (warfarin sodium) to help dissolve the clot

10. The nurse should observe the resident with deep vein thrombosis for the possibility of an embolism, as indicated by:
    ① Pain at the site
    ② Warm affected areas
    ③ Bradycardia
    ④ Decreased respirations

11. In assessing a resident with hypertension, the nurse is aware that a sign of primary hypertension, as opposed to other types of hypertension, is an elevation of:
    ① Atrioventricular pressure
    ② Diastolic pressure
    ③ Systolic pressure
    ④ Pulse pressure

12. If a resident's diagnosis is thrombophlebitis, what other signs or symptoms might the nurse expect to find?
    ① Decreased pedal pulses on the affected leg
    ② Ecchymosis on the area that has pain
    ③ Dry, flaky skin particularly on the foot
    ④ Redness, edema of the affected leg

13. The nurse must recognize that the primary symptoms of superficial thrombophlebitis include:
    ① Fever, nausea, and vomiting
    ② Pain, heat, and redness
    ③ Diarrhea or constipation, and abdominal discomfort
    ④ Anorexia, and pain when walking

14. When performing a physical assessment, the nurse identifies bilateral varicose veins. The symptom the nurse should expect the resident to report is:
    ① Increased sensitivity to cold
    ② Pallor of the lower extremities
    ③ Calf pain when foot is dorsiflexed
    ④ Increasing ankle edema over the day

15. For a resident with cardiac disease, a low-salt diet is prescribed. Which of the following foods contain the least amount of sodium?
    ① Baking soda
    ② Citrus fruits
    ③ Milk and cheese
    ④ Canned meats

16. In planning care for a resident with CHF, the nurse should know that the condition is:
    ① An occlusion of a major coronary artery or one of its branches
    ② An infection or inflammation of the inner membranous lining of the heart, particularly the valves
    ③ A decrease of blood flow through the heart and great vessels
    ④ An enlargement or ballooning of an artery

17. A resident has a diagnosis of angina pectoris. This condition is best described by which of the following?
    ① An area of necrosis of the myocardium
    ② Rubbing of an enlarged epicardium against the pericardial sac
    ③ Inability of the coronary arteries to meet the oxygen needs of the myocardium
    ④ Generalized vasospasm throughout the endocardium and surrounding structures

18. A resident has been experiencing intermittent chest pain for the last 6 months. The resident seems to be more aware of the pain during exertion, takes nitroglycerin sublingual, and rests. The pain seems to subside. The outstanding symptom of angina pectoris is:
    ① Acute pain that is often mistaken for indigestion
    ② Severe cyanosis
    ③ Elevation of blood pressure
    ④ Chest pain that radiates down the left arm

19. When a resident complains of anginal pain, the nurse would expect the resident to describe it in which of the following ways?
    ① Mild midepigastric pain
    ② Sharp, burning, substernal pain
    ③ Severe, crushing chest pain
    ④ Dull, ache-like pain in the arm

20. The pain associated with a myocardial infarction differs from that of angina in that the pain is:
    ① Relieved with rest
    ② Not relieved by rest
    ③ Considerably less severe
    ④ Quickly relieved with nitroglycerin

21. A resident with peripheral vascular disease suddenly develops pain in the left foot. Which of these assessments of the resident's foot would the nurse report immediately to the team leader?
    ① Numbness and tingling
    ② Warm to the touch
    ③ Brisk capillary refill
    ④ Absent pedal pulse

22. In planning care for residents with hypertension, the nurse knows that the treatment is usually directed toward:
    1. Preventing further damage to the blood vessels
    2. Increasing the urine output
    3. Lowering the blood pressure below normal level
    4. Repairing the damaged blood vessels

23. If a resident has an angina attack, the nurse should record:
    1. Onset, duration, and intensity of the pain
    2. Activity, vital signs, and intensity of the pain
    3. Onset, duration of pain, vital signs, and activity
    4. Duration, intensity of the pain, and activity

24. Nursing interventions on the care plan of a resident with thrombophlebitis would most likely include:
    1. Increasing foods containing vitamin C
    2. ROM exercises to all extremities
    3. Bed cradle and cold compresses to the extremities
    4. Continual use of elastic stockings

25. When auscultating respirations of a resident with CHF, the types of sounds the nurse would expect to hear are:
    1. Diminished or absent breath sounds
    2. Crackling
    3. Expiratory wheezing
    4. Inspiratory sounds louder than expiratory sounds

26. In planning the nursing care of a resident with acute CHF, the nurse should consider which of the following?
    1. Provide a high-calorie diet; prevent deformities; provide exercise
    2. Prevent infection; force fluids; encourage exercise and activity
    3. Provide gradual return to activity; maintain skin integrity; provide a sodium-restricted diet
    4. Provide bed rest during hospitalization; force fluids; provide a high-calorie, nutritious diet

ANSWERS AND RATIONALES FOR REVIEW QUESTIONS

1. **1** Swelling appears in the dependent parts of the body.
    2 Swelling appears in the dependent parts of the body; the sacral area is not a dependent body part.
    3 Not classic presentations for CHF.
    4 Not classic presentations for CHF.

2. **3** Exercise and support hose help reduce the complication and possibility of clots in the lower extremities.
    1 Exercise usually increases rather than decreases circulation.
    2 Exercise does not prevent abdominal edema.
    4 Exercise does not necessarily reduce edema of the extremities.

3. **3** The inflammation and clot formation are associated with venous stasis.
    1 There is no ulcer present.
    2 There is inflammation, but the condition involves a clot.
    4 Phlebitis is an inflammation of the vein.

4. **3** One of the actions of this classification of drugs.
    1,2,4 Drugs such as prazosin (minipress) block synaptic receptors that regulate vasomotor tone and reduce peripheral resistance by dilating arterioles and venules

5. **1** Fresh or frozen beef is permitted. Also fresh fruits and vegetables have little sodium.
    2 All smoked, processed, and canned meats are high in sodium. Most frozen foods have sodium added.
    3 Corned beef and dill pickles are high in sodium.
    4 Ham, cheeses, and regular bread are high in sodium.

6. **1** Blood return to the right atrium is delayed.
    2 Blood return is delayed.
    3 Will not directly affect either.
    4 Positioning has no effect on dysrhythmias.

7. **4** Symptoms of pulmonary edema are the result of pulmonary congestion and fluid in the interstitial spaces and alveoli.
    1 May have chest pain, not necessarily angina; nausea and vomiting are not usually associated symptoms; there is dyspnea not necessarily associated with exertion.
    2 Individual is restless but not necessarily confused; tachycardia and hypertension are usually present.
    3 Angina and bradycardia are not associated symptoms.

8. **2** Although there is no generally accepted cause, high blood pressure is usually considered a hereditary disease in which increased stimulation of sympathetic nerve fibers leads to greater vasoconstrictor activity.
    1 Loss of fluid and electrolytes can cause hypokalemia, hyperkalemia, and hypocalcemia
    3 Arteriolar changes can occur as a direct result of the hypertension, but are not usually the initial cause of the condition.
    4 Blood volume is not in question; increase in blood pressure is a result of vasoconstrictor activity.

9. **1** Causes vasodilation and reduces edema.
    2 Inappropriate treatment for this resident because this would aggravate the condition.
    3 Inappropriate treatment for this resident because this would aggravate the condition.
    4 Coumadin does not dissolve clots, but prevents their formation; may not be an initial treatment.

10. **1** Chest pain is exhibited if the embolism is lodged in the lungs. Severe pain can lead to shock and depletion of proper circulation.
    2 Areas involved would be cyanotic and cold; resident would complain of a tingling sensation or numbness.
    3 The resident's pulse would be elevated.
    4 The resident would show apprehension and sudden onset of dyspnea.

11. **2** A typical sign of primary hypertension is a chronically elevated diastolic pressure. Usually a diastolic pressure of 90 mm Hg is the cutoff.
    1 Measurement of atrioventricular pressure can be used to assist in diagnosing valve defects; this pressure is not related to a symptom of hypertension.
    3 Diastolic pressure is primarily involved.
    4 Pulse pressure is the difference between the systolic and diastolic pressures, normally 30 to 40 mm Hg.

12. **4** Thrombophlebitis, as do other venous disorders, causes edema and redness of the lower extremity because of venous pooling.
    1 A sign of arterial, not venous, disease.
    2 Redness, not ecchymosis, would be present.
    3 A sign of arterial, not venous, disease.

13. **2** The cardinal symptoms of a blood clot in a vein are pain, heat, redness, and swelling.
    1 Fever, nausea, and vomiting may be associated with an infectious process, but they are not specific for thrombophlebitis.
    3 These gastrointestinal symptoms are not related to venous obstruction.
    4 Anorexia may occur as a result of the pain involved in vascular obstruction. This answer, however, is not inclusive of the primary symptoms of thrombophlebitis.

14. **4** When the legs are dependent, gravity and incompetent valves promote increased hydro-

static pressure in leg veins and, as a result, fluid moves into the interstitial spaces.

1 This reflects inadequate arterial blood supply; arterial circulation is not affected by varicose veins.

2 This reflects inadequate arterial blood supply; arterial circulation is not affected by varicose veins.

3 This pain is referred to as Homans' sign and is most often associated with thrombophlebitis.

15. **2** Citrus fruits in their natural state are least likely to contain large amounts of sodium.

1 Baking soda has a high sodium content.

3 These choices contain sodium.

4 Canned meats are high in sodium.

16. **3** This comes from the inability of the heart to function as a pump resulting in an insufficient amount of blood to meet the body's demand.

1 This is a symptom of myocardial infarction.

2 This is a symptom of endocarditis.

4 This is a symptom of an aneurysm; an aneurysm can result from trauma, congenital weakness, arteriosclerosis, or infection.

17. **3** Angina pectoris is characterized by the inability of the coronary arteries to meet the oxygen demand of the myocardial muscle, a condition leading to pain (angina).

1 Necrosis would be indicative of myocardial infarction, not angina.

2 Although the friction of an enlarged epicardium rubbing against the pericardial sac may cause pain, it is not typical of anginal discomfort.

4 Vasospasm of a coronary artery is transient and reversible; it is not generally relieved by decreasing activity, as it is in the case of angina.

18. **4** Angina means pain, and pectoris refers to the chest.

1 This symptom most likely occurs in a heart attack.

2 Cyanosis is not necessarily a symptom of angina.

3 Exercise usually precedes an angina attack.

19. **2** Sharp, burning substernal pain radiating to the jaw, shoulder, or left arm are most common descriptions of anginal pain.

1 This is not descriptive of anginal pain; wrong location.

3 This is more descriptive of a myocardial infarction.

4 This is not descriptive of anginal pain; wrong location.

20. **2** The pain associated with an acute myocardial infarction is usually not relieved with rest, nitroglycerin, or changes in position.

1 The pain of a myocardial infarction is typically not relieved with rest.

3 Pain is often described as severe, squeezing, or crushing.

4 The pain of a myocardial infarction is usually not relieved with the administration of nitroglycerin.

21. **4** Lack of pedal pulse means that there is a gross lack of blood supply to the extremity. This must be reported immediately.

1 This is an indicator of arterial insufficiency, but it is not as severe as No. 4.

2 This is normal.

3 This is normal.

22. **1** The purpose in treating hypertension is to minimize the damage that has occurred to the blood vessels.

2 This will be the outcome of diuretic therapy and is part of the overall treatment plan.

3 It is not advisable to lower blood pressure below normal level because of adverse effects of hypotension.

4 Because there are no early symptoms, some damage has already occurred and cannot be repaired.

23. **3** This would most accurately and completely document an anginal episode. It is especially important to document activity in relation to the anginal episode.

1 These do not completely document all areas.

2 These do not completely document all areas.

4 These do not completely document all areas.

24. **4** Elastic stockings support the leg and encourage venous blood return. They should be worn at all times.

1 This is not necessary, because no wound is present.

2 The affected extremity should not have change of motion. Inflamed parts must be at rest.

3 Warm compresses are preferred to encourage venous circulation.

25. **2** This is most characteristic when lungs are congested.

1 These sounds are associated with pneumothorax.

3 These are sounds of chronic obstructive pulmonary disease.

4 This is not expected when auscultating.

26. **3** Resident may fatigue easily; skin is fragile; sodium and fluid may be restricted to reduce blood volume.

1 Sodium is restricted; there is gradual return to activity, and rest periods are a consideration.

2 Fluid may be limited; there is a gradual return to activity along with rest periods.

4 Rest and activity are balanced; fluids and dietary sodium may be restricted.

chapter seven

Hematologic System Overview

Disorders of hemopoiesis refer to problems of the blood-forming tissues. These include the blood cells, bone marrow, spleen, and lymph system. This discussion includes descriptions of the anemias, leukemia, and acquired immunodeficiency syndrome (AIDS).

Nursing Assessment

A. Nursing observations
1. Mouth ulcerations
2. Incoordination
3. Tachycardia
4. Tachypnea
5. Hypotension
6. Pallor and jaundice
7. Pruritus
8. Smooth tongue
B. Resident description (subjective data)
1. Weakness and fatigue
2. Irritability
3. Anorexia
4. Nausea and vomiting
5. Dyspnea
6. Bleeding from the mouth and nose
7. Numbness, tingling, and burning of the feet
8. Headache
9. Incoordination
10. Easy bruising
11. Nonhealing cuts
12. Swollen, tender lymph nodes

Diagnostic Tests/Methods

A. Red blood cell (RBC) count
1. RBCs are formed in the bone marrow
2. RBCs transport oxygen to cells and take carbon dioxide to the lungs
3. Circulating RBC counts elevate in conditions such as anemia and hypoxia
4. The blood study is used in routine screenings
B. Erythrocyte indexes (mean cell volume, mean cell hemoglobin concentration, and mean cell hemoglobin)
1. Aid in describing the anemias
2. Provide a relationship between the number, size, and hemoglobin content of the RBCs
C. Hemoglobin and hematocrit levels
1. Provide an index to the severity of the anemia
2. Hematocrit refers to the number of packed RBCs found in 100 ml of blood
3. Hemoglobin is the oxygen-carrying component of the RBC and is more reliable in determining the severity of the anemia
D. Reticulocyte count
1. Provides information concerning the cause of the anemia
2. Indicates whether the anemia is a result of diminished production or excessive loss or destruction of RBCs
E. Sedimentation rate
1. Not specific to anemias
2. Elevated erythrocyte sedimentation rate (ESR) suggests the presence of an underlying disease process; therefore further workup may be indicated
F. Serum iron
1. Helpful in classifying the anemia
2. Useful in differentiating an acute from a chronic disorder
G. Total iron-binding capacity (TIBC): helpful in classifying the anemia and differentiating between an acute and a chronic disorder
H. Serum bilirubin
1. Useful in evaluating the degree of RBC hemolysis

2. Bilirubin is formed from the hemoglobin of destroyed RBCs
3. Elevations may indicate the increased destruction of RBCs caused by a particular disease process

I. Schilling test
1. Used in classifying anemias, particularly a vitamin B_{12} disorder
2. Helps differentiate between an intrinsic factor deficiency and an intestinal absorption disorder
3. Resident preparation
   a. The resident may be instructed to take nothing by mouth (NPO) before the test
   b. Oral radioactive vitamin B_{12} is administered
   c. Nonradioactive parenteral dose is given 2 hours later
   d. Urine collection follows
   e. A third of the vitamin appears in the urine; little or no radioactivity in the urine suggests a gastrointestinal malabsorption problem
   f. Procedure may be repeated with the addition of intrinsic factor to the oral vitamin B_{12}
   g. Nonabsorption of vitamin B_{12} without intrinsic factor but absorption with the intrinsic factor is suggestive of pernicious anemia
4. Nursing intervention
   a. Explain the basic procedure to the resident
   b. Maintain NPO
   c. Collect the urine at the specified time

J. Vitamin B_{12} level
1. Used to help classify the anemias
2. Provides an index for determining the adequacy of vitamin B_{12} levels and the need for further evaluation
3. Vitamin B_{12} is important for normal hematopoiesis

K. Serum folate level
1. Folic acid is another important factor in hematopoiesis
2. Useful in classifying the anemias

L. Gastric analysis
1. Nasogastric tube is inserted and then histamine is injected to stimulate gastric secretions

2. Gastric contents are aspirated and analyzed
3. Achlorhydria (absence of hydrochloric acid) is a feature of pernicious anemia

M. Sickle cell preparation
1. The reaction of the blood specimen in hypoxia is observed
2. Sickling of cells in hypoxia suggests sickle cell trait or sickle cell anemia

N. Hemoglobin electrophoresis
1. An electric field separates the specimen into the various types of hemoglobin present
2. Hemoglobins S and A suggest sickle cell anemia or trait
3. Hemoglobin F suggests thalassemia

O. Bone marrow biopsy
1. Bone marrow aspiration provides information about blood cell production
2. Test may be used in residents suspected of having leukemia, aplastic anemia, and other hematologic disorders
3. Sample of marrow may be obtained from the sternum, iliac crest, vertebrae, or vertebral body

P. White blood cell (WBC) count and differential
1. Determines the total number of leukocytes
2. The differential helps analyze each type of WBC and determine if the amount present is in proper proportion
3. Aids in the diagnosing of infection and blood disorders such as leukemia

Q. Platelet count
1. Evaluates adequacy of platelet levels
2. If platelet levels drop below a certain level, spontaneous hemorrhage is possible

R. Serum for human immunodeficiency virus (HIV): determines the presence of the AIDS virus

S. Lymphangiography: radiologic examination used to detect lymph node involvement

Common Resident Problems and Nursing Care

A. Activity intolerance related to weakness and fatigue
1. Provide planned activity and rest periods
2. Monitor for signs of fatigue
3. Reinforce resident teaching of planned activity and exercise
4. Assist resident with activities of daily living
5. Assess vital signs as ordered

B. Risk for alteration in tissue perfusion related to hypotension
 1. Observe for evidence of postural hypotension
 2. Assist resident to dangle legs over the side of the bed before standing
 3. Instruct resident to get up slowly
 4. Assess resident's pulse when standing
C. Ineffective breathing pattern related to dyspnea on exertion
 1. Note the degree or kind of activity that causes dyspnea
 2. Note character and rate of respirations during the episodes
 3. Instruct the resident to stop the activity and relax when dyspnea is experienced
 4. Assist the resident in planning activities so that dyspnea will not occur
 5. Reinforce resident teaching regarding planned exercise and rest periods
D. Impaired swallowing caused by ulcerations of the mouth and tongue
 1. Assess the ulcerated areas qd
 2. Provide mouth care with a soft-bristle brush or cotton swab
 3. Offer soothing mouthwashes q2-4h
 4. Instruct the resident to avoid ingesting food or drink that may aggravate the ulcers
E. Fluid volume deficit related to hemorrhage
 1. Assess for signs of bleeding
 a. Tarry stools
 b. Hematuria
 c. Bleeding gums
 d. Bleeding tendency
 e. Petechiae
 f. Epistaxis
 2. Protect from trauma and injury
 3. Avoid parenteral injections
 4. Have resident use soft-bristle brush for mouth care
 5. Monitor vital signs at least q4h
 6. Monitor hemoglobin and hematocrit values
 7. Encourage intake of fluids and the prescribed diet
F. Risk for infection related to interference with the immune system
 1. Prevent exposure to others with infection
 2. Monitor for signs and symptoms of infection

3. Give prescribed drugs and monitor for side effects
4. Place in protective isolation if ordered

Major Medical Diagnoses
ANEMIA CAUSED BY DECREASED RBC PRODUCTION

A. Normally there is a balance between RBC production and RBC destruction; however, alterations do occur that significantly affect RBC production
 1. Iron deficiency anemia
 a. Results from insufficient dietary intake of iron, which is needed for the formation of hemoglobin and RBCs
 b. Other causes: malabsorption, blood loss, and hemolysis
 2. Pernicious anemia
 a. Caused by a lack of intrinsic factor in the gastrointestinal (GI) tract
 b. Intrinsic factor is needed for the absorption of vitamin B_{12}
 c. Anemia usually results from a loss of the mucosal surface of the GI tract, which secretes intrinsic factor
 d. Residents undergoing total gastrectomies and small bowel resections are at risk
 3. Folic acid deficiency anemia
 a. Folic acid is required in the synthesis of DNA, which in turn is necessary for the production of RBCs
 b. Common causes: poor diet (lacking in green, leafy vegetables; citrus fruits; liver; grains; and dried beans), malabsorption, and drugs that interfere with the absorption of folic acid
 4. Thalassemia
 a. Unlike the other three anemias, thalassemia is a genetic disorder resulting in abnormal hemoglobin synthesis
 b. The main problem is an inadequate production of normal hemoglobin; hemolysis is a secondary problem
 c. People of Mediterranean ancestry are at risk
 d. Mild forms of this anemia (thalassemia minor) may be asymptomatic
 e. Residents with a more severe hemolytic form (thalassemia major)

may experience hepatomegaly, splenomegaly, jaundice, and bone marrow hypertrophy
B. Signs and symptoms
1. Skin changes
   a. Pallor
   b. Jaundice
   c. Pruritus
   d. Dermatitis
2. Eye and visual disturbances
   a. Blurred vision
   b. Scleral icterus
3. Mouth
   a. Glossitis
   b. Smooth tongue
   c. Ulcerations of the mucosa
4. Cardiovascular
   a. Tachycardia
   b. Murmurs
   c. Angina
   d. Congestive heart failure (CHF)
   e. Hypotension
5. Respiratory
   a. Tachypnea
   b. Dyspnea on exertion
   c. Orthopnea
6. Neurologic
   a. Dizziness
   b. Headaches
   c. Irritability
   d. Depression
   e. Incoordination
   f. Impaired thought processes
7. Gastrointestinal (GI)
   a. Nausea and vomiting
   b. Anorexia
   c. Hepatomegaly
   d. Splenomegaly
8. General
   a. Weight loss
   b. Weakness and fatigue
   c. Bone pain
   d. Numbness, tingling, and burning of the feet
C. Diagnostic tests/methods
1. Resident history and physical examination
2. Routine chest x-ray examination
3. Routine electrocardiogram (ECG)
4. Schilling test
5. Gastric analysis
6. Complete blood count (CBC)
7. Bone marrow aspiration or biopsy
8. Serum iron level
D. Treatment
1. Iron therapy
2. Increase dietary iron intake
3. Vitamin B_{12} replacement (pernicious anemia)
4. Folic acid replacement
5. Use of hematinics
6. Blood transfusions (thalassemia)
E. Nursing intervention
1. Assess and document signs and symptoms and reactions to treatment
2. Provide planned activity alternated with rest periods
3. Assist resident with activities of daily living to avoid fatigue
4. Monitor supplemental oxygen therapy in use
5. Administer prescribed drugs and monitor for side effects
6. Monitor blood transfusions
7. Provide oral hygiene, particularly if mouth ulcers are present
8. Provide the prescribed diet
9. Instruct resident to get up from bed or chair slowly to avoid dizziness
10. Instruct resident on avoiding and preventing exposure to infection
11. Support resident and allay anxiety
12. Educate resident and family concerning drugs, diet therapy, and planned activity

ANEMIA CAUSED BY RBC DESTRUCTION

A. Definition: a process in which RBCs are being destroyed faster than they are produced
B. Known causes of RBC destruction
1. Snake venom
2. Infections
3. Drugs or chemicals
4. Heavy metals or organic compounds
5. Antigen-antibody reaction
6. Splenic dysfunction
7. Congenital causes
   a. Thalassemia: a group of hereditary hemolytic anemias characterized by a defect or defects in one or more of the hemoglobin polypeptide chains
   b. Sickle cell anemia: a severe chronic, incurable anemia that occurs in people homozygous for hemoglobin S

c. Spherocytosis: a hemolytic anemia characterized by spherocytes (small, globular erythrocytes without the characteristic central pallor) in the blood; the abnormal cells are destroyed by the spleen

d. Glucose-6-phosphate dehydrogenase (G6PD) deficiency: a hemolytic disorder brought on by stressors such as infection, certain drugs, acidosis, and toxic substances; individuals with this genetic disorder are relatively symptom free until they experience the stressor that initiates the hemolytic process

C. Signs and symptoms
1. Anemia
2. Jaundice
3. Splenomegaly
4. Hepatomegaly
5. Weakness and fatigue
6. Skin pallor
7. Anorexia
8. Weight loss
9. Dyspnea
10. Tachycardia
11. Tachypnea
12. Hypotension
13. Cholelithiasis (gallstones): caused by excessive bilirubin

D. Diagnostic tests/methods
1. Resident history and physical examination
2. Laboratory studies
3. Routine chest x-ray examination
4. Routine ECG
5. Bone marrow biopsy
6. Renal studies to monitor kidney status

E. Treatment
1. Identify the causative agent
2. Blood or blood product replacement
3. Supportive care
4. Genetic counseling
5. Splenectomy to halt the destruction of abnormal RBCs by the spleen
6. Maintain renal function
7. Maintain fluid and electrolyte balance

F. Nursing intervention
1. Assess and document signs and symptoms and reactions to treatment
2. Monitor vital signs as ordered and report abnormalities

3. Allay fears and anxieties
4. Provide planned exercise and rest periods
5. Caution resident to get up slowly from the bed or chair to avoid postural hypotension
6. Assist resident with activities of daily living
7. Monitor intake and output
8. Monitor laboratory studies
9. Encourage intake of fluids
10. Provide prescribed diet
11. Administer prescribed drugs and monitor for side effects
12. Educate resident and family concerning drugs, diet, activity, and compliance to the prescribed regimen

APLASTIC ANEMIA (HYPOPLASTIC)

A. Definition: a failure of the bone marrow to produce adequate amounts of erythrocytes, leukocytes, and platelets

B. Exact cause is unclear (idiopathic)
1. May be congenital
2. Related to radiation exposure
3. Results from a disorder that suppresses bone marrow (cancer)
4. Exposure to toxic substances may be a contributing factor

C. Signs and symptoms
1. General symptoms of anemia; refer to the preceding outlines in this section
2. Susceptibility to infection
3. Fever
4. Bleeding tendencies

D. Diagnostic tests/methods
1. Resident history and physical examination
2. Laboratory studies, particularly WBC count and platelet count; a reduced WBC count predisposes resident to infection; a low platelet count predisposes resident to a bleeding disorder
3. Bone marrow biopsy examination to evaluate blood cell production
4. Routine chest x-ray examination
5. Routine ECG

E. Treatment
1. Identify the causative agent
2. Supportive care
3. Administration of blood or blood products
4. Hydration with intravenous (IV) fluids
5. Protect from injury and infections
6. Prevent hemorrhage
7. Splenectomy

8. Bone marrow transplant

F. Nursing intervention
1. Assess and document signs and symptoms and reactions to treatment
2. Monitor vital signs at least q4h
3. Monitor for and report signs of bleeding
4. Give prescribed medication and monitor for side effects
5. Avoiding fatiguing the resident; provide planned exercise and rest periods
6. Prevent injury and exposure to infection
7. Neutropenic precautions may be necessary
8. Monitor supplemental oxygen if ordered
9. Provide and encourage the prescribed diet
10. Allay fears and anxiety
11. Provide oral hygiene, avoiding aggravation of bleeding gums
12. Provide skin care using protective devices and frequent repositioning
13. Educate resident and family concerning drug therapy, diet, planned activity, avoidance of injury and infection, monitoring for bleeding tendencies, and compliance with the regimen

LEUKEMIA

A. Definition: a disorder of the hematopoietic system characterized by an overproduction of immature WBCs
1. As the disease progresses, fewer normal WBCs are produced
2. The abnormal cells continue to multiply and eventually infiltrate and damage the bone marrow, spleen, lymph nodes, and other organs

B. Classification of leukemias
1. Two major categories are acute and chronic
   a. Acute leukemia has a rapid onset; cells in this phase are young, undifferentiated, and immature
   b. Chronic leukemia has a gradual onset; cells are mature and differentiated
2. Further classification: identifying the type of WBC involved
   a. Acute granulocytic leukemia: the myeloblasts proliferate; myeloblasts are the precursors of granulocytes
   b. Acute lymphoblastic leukemia: immature lymphocytes proliferate in the bone marrow

   c. Chronic granulocytic leukemia: excessive neoplastic granulocytes are found in the bone marrow
   d. Chronic lymphocytic leukemia: characterized by inactive, mature-appearing lymphocytes

C. Leukemia is considered a neoplastic process; cause is unknown

D. Predisposing factors
1. Familial tendency
2. Viral origin
3. Exposure to chemicals
4. Exposure to radiation

E. Once leukemia is diagnosed, the aim of therapy is to prolong survival by attaining a state of remission
1. Management of acute leukemia is aggressive
2. Management of chronic leukemia aims to control the disorder and maintain remission
3. All forms of leukemia are fatal if untreated

F. Signs and symptoms
1. General symptoms of anemia
2. Decreased resistance to infection
3. Fever
4. Bleeding tendencies
5. Enlarged lymph nodes
6. Splenomegaly
7. Hepatomegaly
8. Elevated WBC count
9. Low platelet count and low hemoglobin and hematocrit levels
10. Poor appetite
11. Mouth ulcers
12. Diarrhea

G. Diagnostic tests/methods
1. Resident history and physical examination
2. Laboratory studies to evaluate peripheral blood
3. Bone marrow biopsy
4. Routine chest x-ray examination
5. Routine ECG
6. Lymph node biopsy examination

H. Treatment
1. Drug therapy: chemotherapeutic agents, analgesics, sedatives, and antibiotics
2. Radiation therapy
3. Bone marrow transplants are still under investigation
4. Hydration with IV fluids

5. Replacement of blood and blood products
6. Monitoring renal status
7. Protection against infection (neutropenic precautions if needed)
8. Prevention of hemorrhage

I. Nursing intervention
1. Assess and document signs and symptoms and reactions to treatment
2. Prevent resident from being exposed to infection
   a. Screen visitors
   b. Monitor WBC counts
3. Avoid fatigue
   a. Provide planned exercise and rest periods
   b. Assist resident with activities of daily living
4. Monitor for bleeding tendencies
5. Encourage intake of fluids
   a. Keep fluids at the bedside
   b. Provide resident with favorite fluids
6. Administer prescribed medication as ordered and monitor for side effects
   a. Analgesics and sedatives
   b. Antiemetics
7. Monitor IV fluids
   a. Monitor the IV site for infiltration
   b. Monitor rate
8. Allay anxieties and fears
9. Monitor vital signs at least q4h and report abnormalities
10. Monitor supplemental oxygen if ordered
11. Provide and encourage the prescribed diet
12. Provide oral hygiene, which avoids aggravation of bleeding and drying of the mouth
13. Provide skin care to include the use of protective devices and frequent repositioning
14. Educate resident and family concerning drug therapy, diet, activity, monitoring for bleeding tendencies, avoidance of injury and infection, and compliance with the regimen

ACQUIRED IMMUNODEFICIENCY SYNDROME (AIDS)

A. Definition: a viral disorder that disrupts the balance of T lymphocytes and ultimately destroys them, rendering the body incapable of defending itself against infection; course is progressive and fatal

B. Causes
1. The virus is spread by sexual contact, sharing of infected needles by drug abusers, and blood and blood products
2. Infected mothers can pass on the virus to the unborn baby
3. The virus may also enter the body when contaminated blood or body fluids come in contact with broken skin surfaces
4. Symptoms may occur 2 to 6 weeks after exposure; seroconversion may not occur until 8 to 12 weeks or longer

C. Signs and symptoms (vary with each resident; may harbor the virus but be asymptomatic for months)
1. Swollen lymph glands
2. Recurrent fever; night sweats
3. Weight loss; diminished appetite
4. Chronic diarrhea
5. Fatigue
6. White patches or lesions in the mouth
7. Presence of opportunistic infections such as *Pneumocystis carinii* (pneumonia) and Kaposi's sarcoma (purplish skin lesions)
8. Dry cough; shortness of breath

D. Diagnostic tests/methods
1. Resident history and physical examination
2. Serum for HIV
3. Presence of opportunistic infections
   a. *Pneumocystis carinii* pneumonia
   b. Kaposi's sarcoma
4. Bronchial biopsy
5. Lumbar puncture
6. CT scan
7. Enzyme-linked immunosorbent assay (ELISA); detects antibodies for HIV; false positives may occur
8. Western blot test: used to confirm the results of a positive ELISA test; detects HIV antibodies

E. Treatment
1. Treatment is instituted according to the symptoms
2. Protect the resident from opportunistic infections
3. Vaccines are still in experimental stages (e.g., azidothymidine [AZT] interferes with replication of HIV virus/may slow disease process)
4. Nutritional support

F. Nursing care
1. Assess and document signs and symptoms and reactions to treatment
2. Monitor vital signs
3. Monitor arterial blood gas, CBC, and platelet count
4. Administer prescribed medication and monitor for side effects
5. Employ blood and body fluid precautions
    a. Wear protective clothing (e.g., gloves, masks, goggles, gowns) as needed for the procedure
    b. Wash hands thoroughly
    c. Label specimens accordingly
    d. Dispose of contaminated articles properly
6. Plan activity followed by rest periods
7. Encourage physical independence
8. Monitor oxygen therapy
9. Monitor pain status and provide analgesia and comfort measures
10. Support resident and allay anxiety
11. Educate the resident and family concerning mode of spread, protective measures, and home care

Review Questions

1. Which nursing assessment is most appropriate for the resident with iron deficiency anemia?
    ① Pain
    ② Anxiety
    ③ Fluid volume deficit
    ④ Activity intolerance
2. A resident's diagnosis is anemia. Which statement indicates that the resident understands the dietary plan related to the treatment of anemia?
    ① "I won't drink tea or coffee with my meals."
    ② "I will include eggs in my diet daily."
    ③ "I'll drink a quart of milk every day."
    ④ "I'll include green, leafy vegetables every day."
3. The most serious adverse reaction to anticoagulant therapy is:
    ① A rapid fall in blood pressure
    ② Formation of thrombi in major blood vessels
    ③ Hemorrhage
    ④ Infection
4. A resident has a daily prothrombin time level ordered. The nurse gives the anticoagulant warfarin sodium (Coumadin). The main action of this drug is to:
    ① Prevent hemorrhage
    ② Prevent infection in the blood
    ③ Interfere with clotting mechanisms
    ④ Stimulate the heart action
5. In addition to *Pneumocystis carinii,* a resident with AIDS also has an ulcer 4 cm in diameter on a leg. Considering the resident's total health status, the most critical nursing diagnosis would be:
    ① Social isolation
    ② Impaired skin integrity
    ③ Impaired gas exchange
    ④ Altered nutrition: less than body requirements
6. A resident with AIDS and cryptococcal pneumonia is incontinent of feces and urine and is producing copious sputum. When providing care for this resident the nurse's priority should be to:
    ① Wear goggles when suctioning the resident
    ② Wear gown, mask, and gloves when bathing the resident
    ③ Wear gloves to administer oral medications to the resident
    ④ Wear a gown when assisting the resident with the bedpan
7. Blood screening tests of the immune system of a resident with AIDS would indicate:
    ① A decrease in CD4 and T cells
    ② An increase in thymic hormones
    ③ An increase in immunoglobulin E
    ④ A decrease in the serum level of glucose-6-phosphate dehydrogenase
8. The nurse knows that a positive diagnosis for HIV infection is made based on:
    ① A history of high-risk sexual behaviors
    ② A positive ELISA and Western blot test
    ③ Evidence of extreme weight loss and high fever
    ④ Identification of an associated opportunistic infection

9. When giving nursing care to a child with leukemia, the nurse notes blood on the pillow case and several bloody tissues. The nurse should check the child's laboratory report for the:
   1. Platelet count
   2. Uric acid level
   3. Prothrombin time
   4. Red blood cell count

10. The drug of choice in the treatment of AIDS is:
    1. Acetylsalicylic acid (ASA) (aspirin)
    2. Azidothymidine (AZT)
    3. Pralidoxime chloride (PAM)
    4. Phencyclidine hydrochloride (PCP)

ANSWERS AND RATIONALES FOR REVIEW QUESTIONS

1. **4** Fatigue is a common symptom associated with iron deficiency anemia. Because of chronic tissue hypoxia, the resident has an activity intolerance.
   1 Pain is not associated with iron deficiency anemia.
   2 This is not specific for iron deficiency anemia.
   3 This is not specific for iron deficiency anemia.

2. **4** Green, leafy vegetables are a good source of iron.
   1 These are not a problem for iron deficiency anemia.
   2 Although eggs do contain some iron, green vegetables are a higher source.
   3 Milk does not contain iron. A quart of milk is unnecessary for adults.

3. **3** Major adverse reaction.
   1 A rapid fall in BP would be the result of hemorrhage; hemorrhage would occur first, followed by a rapid fall in BP.
   2 The therapy in question is anticoagulant therapy, which is the opposite of the formation of thrombi; therapy is aimed at preventing thrombi from forming.
   4 Infection is unlikely with anticoagulant therapy and if it did occur would not be the direct result of the therapy.

4. **3** Warfarin sodium (Coumadin) is an anticoagulant. *Anti* means against; coagulation refers to blood clotting.
   1 An anticoagulant used in excess would cause bleeding.
   2 Warfarin sodium is used for blood infection.
   4 This is not an action of warfarin sodium (Coumadin). This drug is an anticoagulant, not a cardiac stimulant.

5. **3** *Pneumocystis carinii* is a protozoan that causes pneumonia in immunosuppressed hosts, which can cause death in 60% of the residents; the resident's respiratory status is the priority.
   1 Although this is a concern, the resident's respiratory status is the priority.
   2 Although this is a concern, the resident's respiratory status is the priority.
   4 There are no data to support this diagnosis.

6. **2** These items prevent contact with feces, sputum, or other body fluids during intimate body care.

   1 Goggles and a mask would be required because the resident is producing copious sputum.
   3 Gloves are not necessary, because touching body fluids when giving oral medication is not likely.
   4 Only gloves are necessary when assisting the resident with a bedpan.

7. **1** The HIV selectively infects helper T cell lymphocytes; therefore, 300 or fewer CD4/T4 cells per cubic millimeter of blood or T4/CD4 cells accounting for less than 20% of lymphocytes is suggestive of AIDS.
   2 The thymic hormones necessary for T-cell growth are decreased.
   3 This finding is associated with allergies and parasitic infections.
   4 This finding is associated with drug-induced hemolytic anemia and hemolytic disease of the newborn.

8. **2** These tests confirm the presence of HIV antibodies that occur in response to the presence of the human immunodeficiency virus.
   1 This places someone at risk but does not constitute a positive diagnosis.
   3 These do not confirm the presence of HIV; these adaptations are related to many disorders.
   4 HIV infection is confirmed with the ELISA and Western blot tests; an opportunistic infection (included in the CDC surveillance case definition for AIDS) in the presence of HIV antibodies and T4/CD4 lymphocyte counts below 300 cells/µl indicates that the individual has AIDS.

9. **1** The platelet count is reduced as a result of the bone marrow depression associated with leukemia.
   2 The uric acid level affects urinary output, not blood clotting.
   3 Prothrombin time is influenced by vitamin K factors, not lack of platelets.
   4 The red blood cell count will indicate the hematocrit and hemoglobin levels, which would neither provide the reason for nor cause the bleeding.

10. **2** Most promising; other drugs are being tested.
    1 This is aspirin, which is an antiflammatory agent.
    3 This is used to restore depressed cholinesterase activity resulting from organophosphate poisoning.
    4 This is a substance of abuse used for its hallucinogenic properties; the hydrochloride has analegsic and anesthetic propereties.

chapter *eight*

Gastrointestinal System Overview

The gastrointestinal (GI) system provides a means by which food and fluids enter the body and are converted into elements that help maintain the human organism. It is important to note that other systems of the body influence this system. The endocrine system, central nervous system, and autonomic nervous system all serve as regulators to the GI system.

Digestion and Absorption

A. Digestion: the process of changing foods to be absorbed and used by cells; mechanical digestion and chemical digestion occur simultaneously
   1. Mechanical digestion (chewing, swallowing, peristalsis) breaks food into small pieces, mixes it with digestive juices, and moves it along the digestive tract, ending with elimination
   2. Chemical digestion occurs through the action of enzymes, which break large food molecules into smaller molecules
      a. Carbohydrate digestion begins in the mouth and occurs primarily in the small intestine; carbohydrates are reduced to simple sugars (monosaccharides), such as glucose, for absorption
      b. Protein digestion begins in the stomach and is completed in the small intestine; proteins are broken down into amino acids for absorption
      c. Fat digestion begins in the stomach but occurs primarily in the small intestine; fats are reduced to fatty acids and glycerol for absorption

B. Absorption: the process by which end products of digestion (fatty acids, glycerol, amino acids, and glucose) are absorbed from the small intestine into circulation (blood and lymph) to be distributed to the cells

Nursing Assessment

A. Nursing observations
   1. Gingivitis
   2. Stomatitis
   3. Hematemesis
   4. Stool changes: melena, clay-colored, or frothy stool
   5. Constipation or diarrhea
   6. Hemorrhoids
   7. Distention
   8. Jaundice
   9. Edema
   10. Dark urine
B. Resident description (subjective data)
   1. Nausea and vomiting
   2. Difficulty chewing
   3. Dysphagia
   4. Appetite change: increase or decrease
   5. Weight changes
   6. Indigestion and dyspepsia
   7. Intolerance to certain foods
   8. Pain
   9. Gas
   10. Changes in bowel habit
   11. Bruising easily
   12. Medical history of GI-related problems
   13. Family history of GI-related problems

Diagnostic Tests/Methods

A. Resident history and physical examination
B. Examination of stool
  1. Examination of stool for occult (hidden) blood
  2. Fecal analysis: analysis of stool for mucus, pus, blood, parasites, and fat content
  3. Nursing intervention
    a. Instruct the resident on the proper collection of the specimen
    b. Take the specimen to the laboratory promptly
C. Radiographic examination
  1. Upper GI series
    a. Resident ingests contrast medium (barium), and the movement of the medium through the esophagus and into the stomach is observed by fluoroscopy; x-ray films are also taken
      (1) Aids in identification of esophageal and stomach pathology
      (2) Nursing intervention
        (a) Explain procedures to the resident
        (b) Resident is usually NPO before the examination
        (c) Enemas or cathartics may be given before and after the examination
        (d) Allay resident's anxiety
  2. Lower GI series (barium enema)
    a. The filling of the colon with barium is observed by fluoroscopy; x-ray films of the colon are also taken
    b. Aids in the detection of abnormalities or defects in the colon such as lesions, polyps, tumors, and diverticula
    c. Nursing intervention
      (1) Explain procedures to the resident
      (2) Resident is usually NPO before the examination
      (3) Enemas or cathartics may be given before and after the examination
      (4) Allay resident's anxiety
  3. Gallbladder series (oral cholecystography)
    a. Resident is given an oral radiographic dye to ingest the evening before the examination
    b. The gallbladder is visualized to detect gallstones and obstruction of the biliary tract
    c. Nursing intervention
      (1) Explain procedures to the resident
      (2) Administer the radiographic dye as prescribed
      (3) Maintain NPO after the dye is given
      (4) Allay resident's anxiety
  4. Cholangiography
    a. Aids in the visualization of the biliary duct system
    b. Three methods
      (1) Intravenous cholangiography (IVC): a radiographic dye is administered intravenously, and x-ray films are taken
      (2) Percutaneous transhepatic cholangiography: under fluoroscopy a cannula is inserted into the liver and bile duct; a radiographic dye is injected into the duct, and filling is observed
      (3) Operative or T-tube cholangiography: contrast medium is instilled into the common bile duct, cystic duct, or gallbladder using a fine needle or catheter during surgery or via an existing T-tube postoperatively
    c. Nursing intervention
      (1) Explain procedures to the resident
      (2) Maintain NPO as ordered
      (3) Monitor the resident for bleeding or bile leakage if the percutaneous approach was used
  5. Barium swallow: barium contrast study used to detect esophageal abnormalities
D. Endoscopy
  1. Endoscopy of the upper GI tract (esophagoscopy, gastroscopy, gastroduodenoscopy, esophagogastroduodenoscopy)
    a. Visualization of the esophagus, stomach, or duodenum with a lighted scope
    b. Useful in detecting inflammation, ulceration, tumors, and other lesions
    c. Nursing intervention

(1) Explain procedures to the resident

(2) Obtain signed consent

(3) Maintain NPO as ordered

(4) Administer preoperative medication as ordered

(5) After the examination, maintain NPO until the gag reflex returns

2. Colonoscopy/sigmoidoscopy

   a. Visualization of the internal structures of the colon with a fiberoptic scope

   b. Lesions, tumors, and polyps may be visualized, and a biopsy may be performed

   c. Nursing intervention

     (1) Explain procedures to the resident

     (2) Prepare resident with enemas and cathartics as ordered

     (3) After the examination, observe for rectal bleeding and signs of perforation (malaise, distention, and tenesmus)

E. Ultrasonography

1. Noninvasive test that uses echoes from sound waves to visualize deep structures of the body

2. No special preparation is needed

3. Useful in detecting masses, fluid accumulation, cysts, tumors, etc.

F. Scans (liver and pancreas)

1. Assessment of size, shape, and position of the organ

2. Radionuclide is injected intravenously, and a scanning device picks up the radioactive emissions, which are recorded on paper

3. Nursing intervention

   a. No preparation is required for liver scanning

   b. Fasting and dietary preparation may be ordered for pancreatic scanning

   c. Explain procedures to the resident

   d. Allay resident's anxiety

G. Computerized tomography (CT scan)

1. Noninvasive, radiologic imaging technique that takes exposures of the body or body part at different depths

2. No special preparation is necessary

H. Liver biopsy

1. Invasive procedure in which a needle is inserted into the liver through a small incision in the skin and a sample of liver tissue is obtained

2. The incision is usually made on the right side, at the sixth, seventh, eighth, or ninth intercostal space

I. Laboratory studies

1. Serum amylase

   a. Measures the secretion of amylase by the pancreas

   b. Useful in diagnosing pancreatitis

2. Serum lipase

   a. Measures the secretion of lipase by the pancreas

   b. Useful in diagnosing pancreatitis

3. Serum bilirubin and spot urine amylase: indicates the liver's ability to conjugate and excrete bilirubin

4. Coagulation studies (prothrombin time [PT] and partial thromboplastin time [PTT]): useful in analyzing hemostatic functions

5. Liver enzyme studies (serum glutamic-oxaloacetic transaminase [SGOT], serum glutamate-pyruvate transaminase [SGPT], and lactate dehydrogenase [LDH]): elevations usually indicate liver damage

6. Hepatitis-associated antigen (HAA): presence suggests hepatitis

7. Ammonia levels: elevated in advanced liver disease

8. Urine amylase: elevated amylase levels indicate pancreatic dysfunction

J. Gastric analysis

1. Gastric contents are analyzed primarily for hydrochloric acid content

2. Acidity (pH), volume, and cytology may also be determined

K. D-xylose tolerance test

1. This study evaluates absorption

2. Xylose in water is given orally

3. A urine collection of several hours follows; the amount of D-xylose in the urine is measured

4. Abnormal amounts of D-xylose in the urine indicate a malabsorption problem

5. Nursing intervention

   a. Explain procedure to the resident

   b. Maintain NPO before the examination

   c. Give resident instructions on collecting the urine

Common Resident Problems And Nursing Care

A. Pain related to stomatitis
1. Give soft, bland foods
2. Encourage intake of fluids that do not aggravate the condition
3. Encourage the use of soothing mouth rinses
4. Administer topical medication as prescribed
B. Impaired swallowing related to gingivitis
1. Give mouth irrigations as prescribed
2. Offer soft, bland foods and liquids
3. Instruct the resident on the benefit of good oral hygiene and professional dental cleaning
C. Risk for fluid volume deficit related to nausea and vomiting
1. Observe character and quantity of emesis
2. Observe for associated symptoms
3. Observe for precipitating factors
4. Administer antiemetics as prescribed
5. Offer ice chips
6. Maintain cool environment
7. Apply a cool compress to the neck and forehead for comfort
8. Offer sips of clear liquids such as 7-Up
9. Reduce environmental stimuli such as noise, unpleasant odors, and unpleasant sights
10. Encourage rest and deep breathing
11. Serve resident's favorite foods
12. Limit food servings
13. Provide mouth care after episodes of emesis
D. Impaired swallowing related to dysphagia
1. Provide resident with favorite foods arranged attractively
2. Provide soft, bland foods that can easily be chewed
3. Provide small, frequent feedings
4. Avoid irritating food and fluids
5. Monitor intake
6. Administer topical medication as ordered
E. Altered in nutrition: less than body requirements, related to anorexia
1. Assess status of the anorexia
2. Monitor intake of food and fluid
3. Determine resident's food likes and dislikes
4. Prepare resident for meals

a. Relieve pain
b. Provide mouth care
c. Assist resident to a comfortable position
d. Use screen for privacy
e. Remove unpleasant stimuli from resident's view
5. Prepare food tray
a. Serve food at the proper temperature
b. Make the tray attractive
c. Serve appropriate quantities (large quantities may reduce the appetite)
F. Risk for fluid volume deficit related to diarrhea
1. Document character, consistency, and number and appearance of stools
2. Assess for associated symptoms
3 Monitor intake and output
4. Administer antidiarrheals as prescribed and monitor for side effects
5. Cleanse the anal area to avoid excoriation
6. Avoid milk and milk products
7. Increase fluid intake to at least 3000 ml daily
8. Monitor vital signs at least q4h
9. Identify symptoms of electrolyte imbalance
10. Monitor laboratory reports for electrolyte values
G. Constipation related to decreased peristalsis/activity
1. Administer enemas, stool softeners, and cathartics as ordered
2. Force fluids to at least 3000 ml daily
3. Provide hot drinks to stimulate peristalsis
4. Encourage a diet high in fiber
5. Check for an impaction
6. Encourage exercise
7. Instruct resident concerning proper diet, increased fluid intake, exercise, and avoidance of laxative abuse

Major Medical Diagnoses
GASTRITIS

A. Definition: an inflammation in the mucosal lining of the stomach; the condition may be acute or chronic
B. Gastritis may be caused by bacteria, drugs, or toxins that cause the lining of the stomach to become inflamed and edematous
C. Signs and symptoms
1. Nausea and vomiting

2. Anorexia
3. Epigastric tenderness
4. Feeling of fullness
5. Cramping
6. Diarrhea
7. Fever
D. Diagnostic tests/methods
   1. Resident history and physical examination
   2. Identification of a causative agent
   3. Laboratory studies
   4. Stool culture
   5. Endoscopy with biopsy
   6. Gastric analysis
E. Treatment
   1. Supportive care
   2. Bed rest
   3. NPO if nausea or vomiting is severe
   4. Hydration with IV fluids
   5. In severe cases a nasogastric tube is inserted
   6. Drug therapy: antiemetics, antacids, and H_2 receptor antagonists
   7. Progressive diet when acute symptoms subside
   8. Restriction of smoking
F. Nursing intervention
   1. Assess and document signs and symptoms and reactions to treatment
   2. Monitor vital signs at least q4h
   3. Monitor intake and output
   4. Provide the prescribed diet
   5. Administer medication as prescribed and monitor for side effects
   6. Note amount and character of emesis and diarrhea

CANCER OF THE STOMACH

A. Cancer can develop anywhere in the stomach
B. Causes
   1. Exact cause is unknown
   2. Familial tendency is suspected
   3. Predisposing conditions: chronic gastric ulcers and gastritis
C. Signs and symptoms
   1. Loss of appetite; early satiety
   2. Weight loss
   3. Weakness and fatigue
   4. Pain
   5. Melena
   6. Anemia
   7. Hematemesis

8. Dizziness
9. Indigestion or dysphagia
10. Constipation
D. Diagnostic tests/methods
   1. Resident history and physical examination
   2. Laboratory studies
   3. Stool analysis
   4. Gastric analysis
   5. Barium studies
   6. Gastroscopy
E. Treatment
   1. Preoperative therapy
      a. Correct nutritional deficiencies
      b. Treat anemias
      c. Blood replacement
      d. Gastric decompression with a nasogastric tube
   2. Surgery: removal of the cancerous lesion or tumor along with a margin of normal tissue
   3. Radiation therapy and chemotherapy may be used if the resident is not expected to undergo surgery
      a. Combination therapy has a better response rate
      b. Single-agent therapy has proved to be of little value
F. Nursing intervention
   1. Preoperative care
      a. Support the resident and family
      b. Assess and document signs and symptoms and reactions to treatment
      c. Provide and encourage the prescribed diet
      d. Monitor vital signs at least q8h
   2. Postoperatively educate resident and family regarding drug therapy, dietary restrictions, activity and compliance with the prescribed regimen

PEPTIC ULCERS

A. Definition: ulcerations in the mucosal lining of the distal esophagus, stomach, or small intestine (duodenum or jejunum); duodenal ulcers are more common than gastric ulcers, and men are more prone to ulcers than women
B. Cause: exact cause is unknown
C. Predisposing factors
   1. Stress
   2. Smoking
   3. Heavy caffeine ingestion
   4. Ingestion of certain drugs

D. Signs and symptoms
1. Loss of appetite
2. Weight loss or gain
3. Pain (gnawing, burning)
4. Melena
5. Anemia
6. Hematemesis; coffee-ground emesis
7. Occasional nausea or vomiting
8. Dark, tarry stools
E. Diagnostic tests/methods
1. Resident history and physical examination
2. Gastroscopy and duodenoscopy
3. Barium studies
4. Gastric analysis
5. Laboratory studies
F. Treatment
1. Conservative
a. Rest
b. Drug therapy: antacids, anticholinergics, histamine receptor antagonists, sedatives, and analgesics
c. Elimination of smoking and caffeine
d. Reduction of stress
e. Bland diet with small, frequent feedings
f. In acute situations the resident may be NPO and have nasogastric tube inserted
2. Surgical intervention
a. Closure if perforation has occurred
b. Pyloroplasty and vagotomy if the gastric outlet is obstructed
c. Total or partial resection of the stomach to remove the ulcerated area(s)
G. Nursing intervention
1. Conduct ongoing assessment of signs and symptoms and reactions to treatment
2. Monitor vital signs at least q4h
3. Administer the prescribed medication and monitor for side effects
4. Provide the prescribed diet
5. Provide physical and emotional rest
6. Monitor for signs and symptoms of complications (perforation, hemorrhage, and obstruction)
7. Instruct resident regarding elimination of smoking, avoidance of certain foods, and reduction of stress
8. Educate resident and family concerning drug therapy, diet and dietary restrictions, avoidance of stress, and the need for compliance with the prescribed regimen

OBSTRUCTION

A. Definition: a mechanical or neurologic abnormality inhibiting the normal flow of gastric or intestinal contents
B. Obstructions may result from scar tissue formation, cancer, or strangulated hernias; all are mechanical barriers to the normal flow of gastric or intestinal contents
C. A neurologic obstruction, in the form of a paralytic ileus, causes interference with innervation, thus hindering normal peristaltic activity
D. Signs and symptoms
1. Abnormal pain and distention
2. Projectile vomiting
3. Nausea
4. Possible absence of bowel sounds or increase in bowel sounds
5. Cramping
6. Abdomen may be tense (distended)
7. Obstipation (chronic constipation)
E. Diagnostic tests/methods
1. Resident history and physical examination
2 Flat plate of the abdomen
3. Laboratory studies
F. Treatment
1. Surgery is the treatment for mechanical obstructions
2. Gastric or intestinal decompression to decrease nausea and vomiting
3. Hydration with IV therapy
4. Prophylactic antibiotics
5. Monitor intake and output
6. Supportive care

ULCERATIVE COLITIS

A. Definition: an inflammatory disorder of the large bowel; the inflammatory process begins in the distal segments of the colon and ascends
1. The mucosa ulcerates, bleeds, and becomes edematous and thickens
2. Perforations and abscesses can occur
3. The colon eventually loses its elasticity, and its absorptive ability is reduced
B. Cause is unknown, although it has been associated with stress, autoimmune factors, and food allergies
C. Signs and symptoms
1. Abdominal cramping pain with diarrhea
2. Nausea
3. Dehydration
4. Cachexia
5. Weight loss

6. Anorexia
7. Bloody diarrhea
8. Anemia
D. Diagnostic tests/methods
   1. Resident history and physical examination
   2. Laboratory studies reveal anemia and electrolyte imbalance: CBC, electrolytes
   3. Stool examination
   4. Proctosigmoidoscopy
   5. Barium studies
E. Treatment
   1. Drug therapy: sedatives, antidiarrheals, antibiotics, steroids, hematinics, anticholinergics, and analgesics
   2. Correction of malnutrition
   3. Hydration with IV therapy
   4. Colectomy with ileostomy if other medical treatment fails
   5. Provide symptomatic relief
   6. Monitor weight
   7. Monitor intake and output
   8. Parenteral hyperalimentation may be necessary
   9. Psychotherapy
F. Nursing intervention
   1. Assess and document signs and symptoms and reactions to treatment
   2. Provide emotional as well as physical rest
   3. Monitor number, amount, and characteristics of stools
   4. Provide skin-care measures to avoid anal excoriation
   5. Monitor intake and output
   6. Monitor vital signs q4h
   7. Weigh patient qd
   8. Increase intake of fluids
   9. Provide the prescribed diet
   10. Administer prescribed medication and monitor for side effects
   11. Assess bowel sounds q4h
   12. Assist with activities of daily living
   13. Provide emotional support

DIVERTICULOSIS/DIVERTICULITIS

A. Definition: diverticulum—an outpouching of the mucosa of the colon
   1. Diverticulosis: the existence of diverticula in the large intestine
   2. Diverticulitis: an inflammation of the diverticulum

B. Cause of diverticulosis is unknown; theories include a congenital weakness of the colon, colon distention, constipation, and inadequate dietary fiber
C. Signs and symptoms
   1. Abdominal cramps
   2. Lower-quadrant tenderness
   3. Constipation or constipation alternating with diarrhea
   4. Fever
   5. Occult bleeding
   6. Elevated WBC count
D. Diagnostic tests/methods
   1. Resident history and physical examination
   2. Laboratory studies
   3. Stool examination for occult blood
   4. Sigmoidoscopy
   5. Colonoscopy
   6. Barium studies
E. Treatment
   1. High-residue diet
   2. Drug therapy: bulk laxatives, antibiotics, stool softeners, and anticholinergics
   3. In more severe cases the resident may be NPO and require IV therapy
   4. Surgery: colon resection for obstruction and hemorrhage
F. Nursing intervention
   1. Assess and document signs and symptoms and reactions to treatment
   2. Provide increased roughage in the diet
   3. Increase intake of fluids
   4. Administer prescribed medication and monitor for side effects
   5. Instruct resident to avoid activity that increases intraabdominal pressure (straining at stool, lifting, bending, and wearing restrictive clothing)

COLON/RECTAL CANCER AND POLYPS

A. Definition: the cancerous process can invade the large intestine; cancer of the colon and rectum may take the form of well-defined tumor or cancerous polyp: a polyp is pouchlike structure projecting from the wall of the bowel; polyps may be cancerous or benign
B. Cause of colon cancer is unknown; persons with colon polyps, lesions, diverticula, or ulcerative colitis are monitored closely for malignant changes in the bowel
C. Signs and symptoms

1. Changes in bowel pattern
2. Rectal bleeding
3. Changes in the shape of stool
4. Weakness and fatigue
5. Weight loss
6. Rectal pain
7. Abdominal pain
8. Anemia
D. Diagnostic tests/methods
   1. Resident history and physical examination
   2. Laboratory studies
   3. Barium studies
   4. Proctosigmoidoscopic examination
E. Treatment
   1. Surgical resection of the affected area/creation of a colostomy if necessary
   2. Chemotherapy
   3. Radiation therapy
   4. Supportive therapy
F. Nursing Intervention
   1. Assess and document reactions to treatment
   2. Monitor vital signs
   3. Monitor colostomy site
   4. Monitor hydration status
   5. Provide psychologic support
   6. Educate resident and family relative to diet, activity and colostomy care

HEPATITIS

A. Definition: inflammation of the liver
B. Causes
   1. Drugs or chemicals (toxic hepatitis)
   2. Viral origin (hepatitis A virus [HAV] and hepatitis B virus [HBV])
   3. Multiple blood transfusions (hepatitis non-A or non-B)
C. The most common forms of HAV and HBV
   1. HAV: infectious hepatitis
      a. Transmitted by the fecal-oral route
      b. Incubation period is approximately 2 to 7 weeks
      c. May be spread by contaminated food, water, milk, and shellfish
   2. HBV: serum hepatitis
      a. Associated with contaminated needles and syringes
      b. Transmitted through blood or blood products and pricking of the skin with contaminated equipment

c. May also be spread through feces, urine, saliva, and semen
d. Residents are prone to exacerbations and complications (cirrhosis) from the disease
e. Incubation period is approximately 6 to 26 weeks
   3. Non-HAV, non-HBV
      a. Name given to forms of hepatitis caused by a virus genetically different than hepatitis A or B
      b. Associated with blood transfusions, particularly from paid donors
      c. No specific antigen is associated with the form
      d. Similar to hepatitis B in characteristics
D. Signs and symptoms (early symptoms of HAV may be more severe)
   1. Fever and chills
   2. Headache
   3. Respiratory symptoms
   4. Anorexia
   5. Nausea and vomiting
   6. Liver tenderness
   7. Jaundice and itching
   8. Elevated liver enzymes
   9. Elevated PT values
   10. Elevated bilirubin levels
   11. Presence of HAV in feces and serum
   12. Presence of the hepatitis B surface antigen (HB$_s$Ag)
   13. Clay-colored stools and dark-colored urine
E. Diagnostic tests/methods
   1. Resident history and physical examination
   2. Laboratory studies: HAA; liver profile
   3. Stool examination
   4. Urinary bilirubin and urobilinogen
   5. Liver biopsy
F. Treatment
   1. Monitor liver function studies
   2. Bed rest with bathroom privileges
   3. High-calorie, high-carbohydrate, high-protein, moderate-fat diet
   4. Topical lotions to alleviate dry, itchy skin
   5. Hydration with IV therapy
   6. Administration of vitamin K preparations
   7. Monitor for bleeding tendencies and progression of the illness
   8. Blood and body fluid precautions
   9. Passive immunity

G. Nursing intervention
1. Assess and document signs and symptoms and reactions to treatment
2. Monitor skin, stool, and urine color
3. Promote balanced activity and rest periods
4. Maintain blood and body fluid precautions
5. Monitor IV therapy
6. Assess intake and output
7. Monitor vital signs at least q4h
8. Provide and encourage the prescribed diet
9. Support the resident and family
10. Administer prescribed medication and monitor for side effects
11. Monitor for bleeding tendencies
12. Educate resident concerning drug therapy, the prescribed diet, activity level, and monitoring for complications

CIRRHOSIS

A. Definition: cell degeneration occurring in the liver wherever scar tissue replaces normally functioning tissue
B. Cirrhosis is a complication of alcoholism, hepatitis, biliary disease, and certain metabolic disorders
C. Whatever the cause of the liver destruction, the course of cirrhosis is the same
1. Liver parenchyma dies and regenerates, and fibrous tissue (scarring) occurs
2. This alteration in structure progresses in the liver, causing problems in hepatic blood flow and normal liver function; in time the liver fails
D. Major complications of cirrhosis
1. Portal hypertension: hypertension resulting from the obstruction of normal blood flow through the portal system; the obstruction is caused by changes in the liver from the cirrhotic process
2. Esophageal varices
3. Ascites: the accumulation of fluid in the peritoneal or abdominal cavity, which is a later symptom in cirrhosis
4. Hepatic coma (encephalopathy): a condition of advanced liver disease; blood enters the general circulation without being properly detoxified by the liver
E. Signs and symptoms
1. Headache
2. Nausea and vomiting
3. Weight loss
4. Anorexia
5. Jaundice
6. Abdominal pain
7. Fatigue and weakness
8. Liver enlargement and fibrosis
9. Bleeding disorders caused by disruption in the manufacture of vitamin K–dependent factors
10. Edema
11. Telangiectasis (blood vessels develop a spiderlike appearance)
12. Ascites
13. Esophageal varices
14. Hepatic coma
F. Diagnostic tests/methods
1. Resident history and physical examination
2. Laboratory studies to assess liver function
3. Liver scan
4. Liver biopsy
G. Treatment
1. Rest with activity as tolerated
2. Nutritious diet with protein level determined by liver functioning
3. If ascites is present, restrict fluid and sodium, monitor weight, and monitor intake and output
4. Monitor for complications such as ascites, esophageal varices, and hepatic coma
5. Drug therapy to reduce ammonia levels, prevent bleeding, reduce edema, and provide comfort
H. Nursing intervention
1. Assess and document signs and symptoms and reactions to treatment
2. Administer prescribed medication and monitor for side effects
3. Provide and encourage the prescribed diet
4. Promote comfort
5. Monitor status of ascites
    a. Record weight
    b. Assess measurements of extremities and abnormal girth
    c. Monitor intake and output
6. Provide planned exercise and rest periods
7. Assist resident with activities of daily living
8. Monitor skin status and take measures to prevent skin breakdown
9. Protect against infection
10. Provide diversional activity
11. Offer emotional support
12. Provide ongoing assessment for evidence of hepatic encephalopathy

a. Monitor for symptoms of lethargy, confusion, twitching, tremors, sweetish breath odor, fever, and increasing somnolence
b. Eliminate dietary protein
c. Administer prescribed drugs and enemas to reduce ammonia levels
d. Monitor IV fluids
e. Give narcotics and sedatives cautiously

CANCER OF THE PANCREAS

A. Cancer of the pancreas can affect any portion of the pancreas, including the beta cells; metastasis readily occurs to adjacent structures
B. Cancerous tissue impairs normal pancreatic function, primarily by causing obstruction and hindering the flow of pancreatic secretions
C. Signs and symptoms
   1. Early symptoms may be vague
      a. Nausea and vomiting
      b. Anorexia
      c. Weight loss
      d. Weakness and fatigue
   2. Later symptoms
      a. Pain
      b. Jaundice
      c. Diabetes mellitus
D. Diagnostic tests/methods
   1. Resident history and physical examination
   2. Laboratory studies
   3. Pancreatic scan and sonography
   4. X-ray studies
   5. Visualization of the pancreatic duct
E. Treatment
   1. Supportive therapy
   2. Surgical excision: Whipple's procedure may be performed removing the head of the pancreas, lower portion of the common bile duct, distal portion of the stomach, and the duodenum
   3. Palliative surgery: to restore bile and pancreatic output
   4. Chemotherapy
F. Nursing intervention: see cancer of the stomach, p. 79

HERNIAS

A. Definition: a protrusion of an organ or structure through the wall of the containing cavity
B. Hernias may occur around the umbilical area, inguinal area, diaphragm, femoral ring, and at the site of an incision
C. Hernias are categorized as
   1. Reducible: can be returned to its normal position
   2. Irreducible: cannot be returned to the normal position
   3. Incarcerated: obstruction of intestinal flow
   4. Strangulated: blood supply is cut off (occluded)—surgical emergency
D. Causes
   1. Congenital weakness in the containing wall
   2. Weakness in containing wall is related to straining and the aging process
   3. Trauma
   4. Increased intraabdominal pressure (obesity)
E. Signs and symptoms
   1. Protrusion of a structure without symptoms
   2. Appearance of a protrusion when straining or lifting
   3. In certain instances there may be pain
   4. If the intestine is obstructed, there may be distention, pain, nausea, and vomiting
F. Diagnostic methods: resident history and physical examination
G. Treatment
   1. Surgery is the treatment of choice
      a. Herniorrhaphy: surgical repair of the hernia
      b. Hernioplasty: the surgical reinforcement of the weakened area
   2. Use of a truss (a support worn over the hernia to keep it in place)
H. Nursing interventions include educating the resident regarding activity restrictions and avoidance of constipation.

Review Questions

1. If a resident complains of cramping during a colostomy irrigation, the nurse should:
   ① Lower the container containing the fluid
   ② Discontinue the irrigation
   ③ Advance the catheter 2 more inches
   ④ Stop the flow until the cramping subsides

2. A resident has not had a bowel movement in 3 days. You can promote elimination by encouraging the resident to eat:
   ① Eggs and cheese toast
   ② Popsicles and oranges
   ③ Apples and carrot sticks
   ④ Chicken and whole grain cereal

3. A bowel-retraining program requires suppository insertion. The most appropriate time for the nurse to initiate this action would be:
   ① One hour before breakfast
   ② One hour after breakfast
   ③ One half hour before lunch
   ④ One half hour before supper

4. Nursing management of the resident with Crohn's disease includes monitoring the resident's diet. Which of the following diets would the physician most likely order for this resident?
   ① Full-liquid diet
   ② Clear liquid with potassium
   ③ Soft diet, no foods high in fiber
   ④ Soft diet with bulk-containing foods

5. A resident is diagnosed as having diverticulitis. Which one of the following menus would be most consistent with the resident's diet instructions?
   ① Turkey on whole wheat bread and an apple
   ② Ham omelet and ice cream
   ③ Cream of shrimp soup and canned pears
   ④ Strawberry yogurt and chocolate chip cookies

6. If a resident's problem was related to blockage of the bile duct by a stone, the nurse could anticipate the stool to appear:
   ① Tarry
   ② Very watery
   ③ Clay colored
   ④ Full of mucus

7. To prevent constipation in a cerebrovascular accident (CVA) residents, the nurse should encourage them to:
   ① Take daily enemas
   ② Use a daily laxative
   ③ Increase fruits and fluids in their diet
   ④ Plan a bowel movement for early morning

8. A resident has a duodenal ulcer. What foods would you suggest that the resident avoid?
   ① Refined cereals
   ② Protein foods
   ③ Raw foods
   ④ Broiled foods

9. The most important factor for a successful bowel-retraining program is:
   ① Establishing regular day(s) and time to assist the resident to the toilet
   ② Making sure the resident understands the purpose of the program
   ③ Regular administration of a mild laxative
   ④ Skipping a day in the program if the resident has had more than one bowel movement the day before

10. A resident has a diagnosis of ulcerative colitis. While teaching about the condition, the nurse informs the resident that the principal cause of ulcerative colitis is:
    ① Poor dietary habits
    ② Hypermotility of the large intestine
    ③ Bacterial infection of the intestines
    ④ Emotional stress

11. A resident with ulcerative colitis has been instructed to follow a low-residue diet. Which breakfast food selected by the resident would indicate the need for further instruction?
    ① Oatmeal, orange slices, and milk
    ② Soft-cooked egg, toast, and herb tea
    ③ Apple juice, English muffin, and jelly
    ④ Cream of rice cereal, white toast, and marmalade

12. A colostomy irrigation was ordered for a resident with a sigmoid colostomy. When doing an irrigation, the cone should be inserted into the stoma opening no more than:
    ① 2 inches
    ② 4 inches
    ③ 10 inches
    ④ 12 inches

13. Following surgery for a colostomy, the most effective way of helping a resident accept the colostomy would be to:
    ① Provide literature containing factual data about colostomies
    ② Point out the number of important people who have had colostomies
    ③ Begin to teach self-care of the colostomy immediately
    ④ Contact a member of Colostomies, Inc. to speak with the resident

ANSWERS AND RATIONALES FOR REVIEW QUESTIONS

1. **4** Cramping does occur when fluid is first introduced.
   1 The level of the container does not affect cramping.
   2 Cramping normally occurs, so there is no need to discontinue the procedure.
   3 This will not allow irrigation and will not change the cramping effect.

2. **2** Increasing fluids, cellulose, and bulk in the diet will facilitate bowel elimination.
   1 Not appropriate foods.
   3 Lack fluid, bulk and/or cellulose.
   4 Lack fluid, bulk and/or cellulose.

3. **2** Suppository insertion for bowel retraining is done 1 to 2 hours before the scheduled training time and after a meal.
   1,3,4 As indicated in answer choice 2, insertion is done after a meal, not before a meal, as with these responses.

4. **3** A soft diet of low-fiber, low-residue, bland foods that have a high protein and caloric content is ordered for residents with Crohn's disease.
   1 A full-liquid diet consists of only liquids and foods that liquefy at body temperature. There is no residue or fiber in this diet, which is usually ordered for residents unable to consume soft or semifluid foods after surgery.
   2 A clear liquid diet supplies fluids and provides minimal residue. The diet is nutritionally inadequate and is usually prescribed for a limited amount of time, such as 1 day, following surgery. Proteins are needed more than potassium.
   4 A soft diet is acceptable, but high-fiber foods are not permitted.

5. **1** The suggested diet for residents with diverticulitis is low-fat, no fried foods, and moderate fiber intake.
   2 This selection includes foods that are fried and high in fat.
   3 This selection includes foods with high fat content.
   4 Strawberry yogurt may be appropriate if it is low-fat, but the chocolate chip cookies are not.

6. **3** With blockage by a stone, little or no bile passes into the small intestines. Bile gives stool its classic color.
   1 May indicate upper GI bleeding or a normal change if the resident is on iron therapy.
   2 Not characteristic of a gallbladder dysfunction.
   4 Not characteristic of a gallbladder dysfunction.

7. **3** An increase in fruits in the diet will increase bulk in the intestines. Increasing bulk and fluids in the intestines will promote normal elimination.
   1 Not appropriate means of encouragement as a routine to follow.
   2 Not appropriate means of encouragement as a routine to follow.
   4 This may or may not be possible.

8. **3** A person with a duodenal ulcer is often advised to avoid all food that could be irritating to the intestinal mucosa. This would include all raw foods, which are generally high-residue and therefore more irritating.
   1 Refined cereals are lower in residue as a result of processing.
   2 Protein in most cases is not contraindicated.
   4 Broiling is an acceptable way to prepare foods for an ulcer resident.

9. **1** Pattern is essential with retraining.
   2 Not necessary for the resident to understand the program for the program to be successful.
   3 Laxatives never used with bowel retraining.
   4 Regular days and times must be strictly followed to establish a pattern.

10. **4** Psychosomatic factors may cause or aggravate the mucosa or submucosa of the colon.
    1 This is not a contributory factor.
    2 Increased motility of the intestine is not characteristic of the disease.
    3 In most cases it is a viral, not a bacterial, infection.

11. **1** Oatmeal and orange slices are high in fiber. Most ulcerative colitis residents have a lactose intolerance; milk should not be included.
    2 These are low-residue foods.
    3 These are low-residue foods.
    4 These are low-residue foods.

12. **2** This is adequate placement for the solution to reach the stool.
    1 This is not in far enough; solution will drain out.
    3 This is too far in for the solution to irrigate colon.
    4 This is too far in for the solution to irrigate colon.

13. **4** Residents who have radical changes in their body image as a result of surgery are usually best able to relate to someone who has faced the same stress and successfully adapted.
    1 Would provide information but do little to aid acceptance.
    2 Would do little to aid acceptance.
    3 The resident cannot learn to do colostomy care until he psychologically accepts its presence.

chapter *nine*

Nervous System Overview

The nervous system functions as a coordinated unit both structurally and functionally.

A. Functions
  1. Regulates system
  2. Controls communication among body parts
  3. Coordinates activities of body system
B. Divisions
  1. Central nervous system (CNS): brain and spinal cord; interprets incoming sensory information and sends out instruction based on past experiences
  2. Peripheral nervous system (PNS): cranial and spinal nerves extending out from brain and spinal cord; carries impulses to and from brain and spinal cord
    a. Autonomic nervous system: functional classification of the PNS; regulates involuntary activities
    b. Somatic nervous system: functional classification of the PNS; allows conscious or voluntary control of skeletal muscles
C. Structure and physiology
  1. Neurons or nerve cells: respond to a stimulus, connect it into a nerve impulse (irritability), and transmit the impulse to neurons, muscle, or glands (conductivity); consists of three main parts:
    a. Cell body
    b. Dendrites
    c. Axons
  2. Types of neurons
    a. Motor (efferent): conduct impulses from CNS to muscle and glands
    b. Sensory (afferent): conduct impulses toward CNS

    c. Connecting (interneuron): conduct impulses from sensory to motor neurons
  3. Synapse: chemical transmission of impulses from axon to dendrites
  4. Myelin sheath: protects and insulates the axon fibers; increases the rate of transmission of nerve impulses
  5. Neurilemma: sheath covering the myelin; found in PNS; function is regeneration of nerve fiber
  6. Neuroglia: connective or supporting tissue; important in reaction of nervous system to injury or infection
  7. Ganglia: clusters of nerve cells outside CNS
  8. White matter: bundles of myelinated nerve fibers; conducts impulses along fibers
  9. Gray matter: clusters of neuron cell bodies; fibers not covered with myelin; distributes impulses across selected synapses
D. Central nervous system
  1. Brain
    a. Cerebrum: largest part of brain; outer layer called cerebral cortex; cortex composed of dendrites and cell bodies; controls mental processes; highest level of functioning
    b. Cerebellum: controls muscle tone coordination and maintains equilibrium
    c. Diencephalon: consists of two major structures located between cerebrum and midbrain
      (1) Hypothalamus: regulates the autonomic nervous system, controls blood pressure, helps maintain normal body temperature and appetite, and controls water balance and sleep

(2) Thalamus acts as a relay station for incoming and outgoing nerve impulses; produces emotions of pleasantness and unpleasantness associated with sensations

d. Brainstem: connects the cerebrum with the spinal cord
   (1) Midbrain: relay center for eye and ear reflexes
   (2) Pons: connecting link between cerebellum and rest of nervous system
   (3) Medulla oblongata: contains center for respiration, heart rate, and vasomotor activity

2. Spinal cord
   a. Inner column composed of gray matter, shaped like an H, made up of dendrites and cell bodies; outer part composed of white matter, made up of bundles of axons called *tracts*
   b. Function: sensory tract conducts impulses to brain; motor tract conducts impulses from brain; center for all spinal cord reflexes

3. Protection for CNS
   a. Bone: vertebrae surround cord; skull surrounds brain
   b. Meninges: three connective tissue membranes that cover brain and spinal cord
      (1) Dura mater: white, fibrous tissue; outer layer
      (2) Arachnoid: delicate membrane, middle layer; contains subarachnoid fluid
      (3) Pia mater: inner layer; contains blood vessels
   c. Spaces
      (1) Epidural: between dura mater and vertebrae
      (2) Subdural space: between dura mater and arachnoid
      (3) Subarachnoid space: between arachnoid and pia mater; contains cerebrospinal fluid
   d. Cerebrospinal fluid: acts as a shock absorber; aids in exchange of nutrients and waste materials

E. Peripheral nervous system

1. Carries voluntary and involuntary impulses
2. Cranial nerves: 12 pairs; carry impulses to and from the brain
3. Spinal nerves: 31 pairs; conduct impulses necessary for sensation and voluntary movement; each group named for the corresponding part of the spinal column

F. Autonomic nervous system
1. Part of PNS; controls smooth muscle, cardiac muscle, and glands
2. Two divisions
   a. Sympathetic: "fight or flight" response; increases heart rate and blood pressure; dilates pupils
   b. Parasympathetic: dominates control under normal conditions; maintains homeostasis

The Neurologic System

Pathology of the CNS arises from injuries, new growths, vascular insufficiency, infections, and as complications secondary to other diseases; resident problems are related to interference with normal functioning of the affected tissue.

The following terms are used in describing the resident with a neurologic impairment:

anesthesia complete loss of sensation

aphasia loss of ability to use language

auditory/receptive aphasia loss of ability to understand

expressive aphasia loss of ability to use spoken or written words

ataxia uncoordinated movements

coma state of profound unconsciousness

convulsion involuntary contractions and relaxation of muscle

delirium mental state characterized by restlessness and disorientation

diplopia double vision

dyskinesia difficulty in voluntary movement

flaccid without tone—limp

neuralgia intermittent, intense pain along the course of a nerve

neuritis inflammation of a nerve or nerves

nuchal rigidity stiff neck

nystagmus involuntary, rapid movements of the eyeball

papilledema swelling of optic nerve head

paresthesia abnormal sensation without obvious cause, with numbness and tingling

spastic convulsive muscular contraction
stupor state of impaired consciousness with brief response only to vigorous and repeated stimulation
tic spasmodic, involuntary twitching of a muscle
vertigo dizziness

Nursing Assessment

A. Nursing observations
  1. Mental status: drowsiness or lethargy, ability to follow commands
  2. Level of consciousness (LOC): ability to be aroused in response to verbal and physical stimuli; ranges from awake and alert to "coma"; Glasgow Coma Scale is the usual guide for assessing and describing the degree of conscious impairment, based on three determinants:
     a. Eye opening
     b. Motor response
     c. Verbal response
  3. Orientation
     a. Time: knows month or year
     b. Place: has general knowledge of where resident is (e.g., hospital)
     c. Person: knows own name; able to name relative or friend
  4. Behavior: is it appropriate for the situation
  5. Emotional response: is it appropriate for the situation
  6. Memory: capability for early and recent recall
  7. Speech: presence of aphasia; appropriate speech; words distinct or slurred
  8. Vital signs: temperature, pulse, respirations, and blood pressure
  9. Ability to follow simple directions
  10. Eyes
     a. Pupillary reaction to light: the pupils are periodically assessed with a flashlight to evaluate and compare size, configuration, and reaction. Differences between both eyes and from previous assessments are compared for similarities and differences
     b. Movement of lids and pupils
  11. Motor function: coordination, gait, balance, posture, strength, and functioning
  12. Bladder and bowel control
  13. Ears for drainage
  14. Facial expression for symmetry
  15. Sensation for
     a. Pain
     b. Light
     c. Smell
     d. Temperature
B. Resident description (subjective data)
  1. History of head injury, loss of consciousness, vertigo, weakness, headache, sleep problems, paralysis, seizures, or diplopia
  2. Complaints of pain, numbness, problems with elimination, memory loss, difficulty concentrating, drowsiness, or visual problems
  3. Medications taken
C. History from family
  1. Medical
  2. Activities of daily living (ADLs)
  3. Behavior

Diagnostic Tests/Methods

A. Computed tomography (CT scan; CAT scan): computer analysis of tissues as x-rays pass through them; has replaced many of the usual tests; no special preparation or care after test
B. Lumbar puncture (spinal tap)
  1. Description: under local anesthesia a puncture is made at the junction of the third and fourth lumbar vertebrae to obtain a specimen of cerebrospinal fluid; cerebrospinal fluid pressure can be measured; this procedure is also used to inject medications (e.g., spinal anesthesia) and in diagnostic x-ray examination to inject air or dye (e.g., myelogram)
C. Cerebral angiography: intraarterial injection of radiopaque dye to obtain an x-ray film of cerebrovascular circulation
D. Electroencephalogram (EEG)
  1. Description: electrodes are placed on unshaven scalp with tiny needles and electrode jelly
  2. Nursing intervention
     a. Anticipate resident's fears about electrocution; do not give stimulants/depressants before test
     b. Wash hair and scalp after procedure to remove jelly
     c. Resident may resume all previous activities

E. Brain scan
  1. Description: after an IV injection of a radioisotope, abnormal brain tissue will absorb more rapidly than normal tissue; this can be detected with a Geiger counter to diagnose brain tumors
  2. Nursing intervention
     a. No observations
     b. Resident may resume all previous activities
F. Magnetic resonance imaging (MRI)
  1. Description: MRI uses a combination of radio waves and a strong magnetic field to view soft tissue (does not use x-rays or dyes); produces a computerized picture that depicts soft tissues in high-contrast color
  2. Nursing intervention
     a. Before the procedure, instruct the resident to remain perfectly still in the narrow, cylinder-shaped machine
     b. Inform the resident that there will be no pain or discomfort, but there is no room for movement during the MRI
     c. No specific care or observations are necessary after the procedure
G. Myelography
  1. Description: injection of a radiopaque dye into the subarachnoid space via a lumbar puncture; performed to locate lesions of the spinal column or ruptured vertebral disk
  2. Nursing intervention after the procedure
     a. Maintain bed rest
     b. Monitor vital signs
     c. Force fluids
     d. Observe for headache, pain in neck, and dizziness
H. Positron emission tomography (PET scan)
  1. The resident inhales or is injected with a radioactive substance
  2. The computer can diagnose and determine level of functioning of an organ
  3. Exposure to radiation is minimal and no special care is indicated
I. Skull x-ray examination: no preparation; no nursing care or observations indicated afterward

Common Resident Problems and Nursing Care

A. Impaired physical mobility related to progression of primary disease
  1. Give specific care and assessment as required
  2. Perform neurologic assessment q2-4h
  3. Initiate all nursing care measures to prevent complications of immobility
B. Risk for injury/infection related to "fixed eyes" (no blinking)
  1. Protect with eye shields
  2. If needed, remove dried exudate with warm saline solution and mineral oil
  3. Close eyes
  4. Inspect for inflammation
C. Ineffective breathing pattern related to neuromuscular impairment
  1. Maintain patent airway, suction as needed, and elevate head of bed 20 to 30 degrees
  2. Have tracheostomy set available (possible respiratory distress)
  3. Provide oxygen with humidity
  4. Monitor vital signs q2h
  5. Provide oral hygiene q2h
  6. Lubricate lips
D. Risk for altered body temperature related to neuromuscular impairment
  1. Assess rectal temperature q2h
  2. Use external heating and cooling as indicated by resident's temperature and status
E. Risk for aspiration related to neuromuscular impairment
  1. Maintain NPO
  2. Position resident on side; turn q2h
  3. Provide nasogastric tube feedings
  4. Monitor IV fluids
F. Risk for injury related to restlessness, involuntary motions, or seizures
  1. Maintain safety (e.g., padded side rails)
  2. Follow precautions, care, and observations for a resident with seizures
  3. Maintain plastic airway at bedside
G. Altered urinary elimination related to neuromuscular impairment
  1. Oliguria
     a. Provide indwelling catheter care
     b. Monitor intake and output qh
  2. Incontinence
     a. Wash, dry, and inspect skin as needed
     b. Implement measures to prevent decubitus ulcers
     c. Implement bladder training
H. Bowel incontinence/constipation related to neuromuscular impairment
  1. Bowel incontinence

a. Wash, dry, and inspect skin as needed
b. Implement measures to prevent decubitus ulcers
c. Provide bowel training
2. Constipation
   a. Record bowel movements
   b. Provide stool softeners, laxatives, and enemas as ordered
   c. Check for impaction; disimpact as needed
I. Fear/anxiety related to pain; complications; surgery; possible disfigurement, disability, or dependency; fatal prognosis
1. Explain everything (actions) carefully
2. Encourage resident to express feelings
3. Report to health care team

SPECIAL SITUATIONS

A. The resident in a coma
1. Unconscious state in which the resident is unresponsive to verbal or painful stimuli; this occurs with many primary diseases; the resident is dependent on the nurse for maintenance of all basic human needs, nourishment, bathing, elimination, respiration, prevention of complications, and assessment
2. Nursing intervention
   a. Include family in nursing care and care planning as much as possible
   b. Note LOC (see nursing assessment of the neurologic resident) every 15 minutes if LOC decreases; assess every 1, 2, or 4 hours as LOC improves
   c. Demonstrate respect in resident's presence
   d. Provide a quiet, restful, temperature controlled environment
   e. Speak to resident; use proper name; introduce self, and explain all care before starting (patient may be able to hear)
   f. Provide privacy and safety
B. The resident with paralysis
1. Paraplegia (tetraplegia): paralysis of the lower extremities from sudden injury (e.g., automobile accident) or progressive degenerative disease (e.g., multiple sclerosis) to the spinal cord; there may be no motion or sensory function or reflexes; there may be uncontrollable muscle spasms; perspiration ceases and then becomes profuse; there is a loss of bladder and bowel control; sexual dysfunction, anxiety, fear, depression, anger, and embarrassment are major resident problems; resident may be totally dependent
2. Quadriplegia (tetraplegia): paralysis of all four extremities from sudden injury (e.g., diving accident) or progressive degenerative disease (e.g., amyotrophic lateral sclerosis [ALS]); symptoms and resident problems include those encountered with paraplegia, as well as autonomic dysreflexia
3. Nursing intervention
   a. Take measures to prevent complications of immobility (contractures, renal calculi, pressure sores, constipation)
   b. Provide bowel and bladder training
   c. Prevent deformity: maintain joint mobility and correct alignment
   d. Force fluid intake
   e. Provide high-protein diet
   f. Encourage independence according to ability
   g. Communicate and work closely with the physiatrist, (a physician specializing in physical medicine and rehabilitations), physical therapist, occupational therapist, and other members of the rehabilitation team
   h. Include family in nursing care and planning

Major Medical Diagnoses
INCREASED INTRACRANIAL PRESSURE (IICP)

A. Description: fluid accumulation or a lesion takes up space in the cranial cavity, producing IICP; the brain is gradually compressed, or life-sustaining functions cease; may be sudden or progress slowly
B. Causes: tumors, hematoma, edema from trauma, and abscesses from infections
C. Signs and symptoms: related to primary diagnosis
1. Headache, restlessness, and anxiety
2. Vomiting: recurrent, projectile, and not related to nausea or meals
3. Change in pupil response to light
4. Seizures

5. Respiratory difficulty: irregular, Cheyne-Stokes, or Kussmaul's respiration
6. Blood pressure elevates, with wide pulse pressure
7. Pulse increases at first, then slows to 40 to 60 beats/min, regular and strong
8. Altered LOC: becomes lethargic, speech slows, becomes confused, and shows decreased level of response
9. Visual disturbances: diplopia and blurred vision and changes in size of pupil
10. Progressive weakness or paralysis
11. Loss of consciousness; coma; and death

D. Diagnostic tests/methods: neurologic assessment by physician and nurse
E. Treatment: depends on cause
   1. Surgical intervention (craniotomy)
   2. Steroids, anticonvulsants, mannitol, dexamethasone (Decadron), or urea to decrease edema
F. Nursing intervention
   1. Elevate head to semi-Fowler's position; never place in Trendelenburg's position
   2. Monitor vital signs every 15 minutes
   3. Prevent aspiration; place resident on side
   4. Maintain airway; O_2 therapy as necessary
   5. Observe pupillary response (usually unequal and may not react to light)
   6. Report any change in LOC immediately
   7. Provide special care and observation when a resident has a seizure
   8. Provide care and safety for an unconscious resident
   9. Monitor IV fluids closely to prevent over-hydration

CONVULSIVE DISORDERS

A. Description: frequently a convulsion or seizure is not a disease but a symptom of a neurologic disorder; epilepsy is a disease characterized by a disposition for seizures; the following are types of seizures:
   1. Generalized or grand mal: there may be a premonition or sign (aura); the individual cries out, loses consciousness, and enters a tonic phase (the body is rigid, and the jaw is clenched); then there is a clonic phase, with jerking movements of muscles, cessation of respirations, and fecal and urinary incontinence; lasts 1 to 2 minutes followed by a short period of unresponsiveness
   2. Partial or petit mal: loss of consciousness that lasts 5 to 30 seconds, during which time normal activities may or may not cease; there may be amnesia concerning this time
   3. Jacksonian (motor): a focal seizure that may be limited to jerky movements of one extremity; may precede a grand mal seizure

B. Causes
   1. May be secondary to another condition: cerebrovascular accident (CVA), head injury, brain tumor, markedly elevated temperature, toxins, or electrolyte imbalance
   2. Epilepsy may have no known cause; onset usually is in childhood, usually before 30 years of age

C. Resident problems
   1. Related to primary disease
   2. Fear of injury
   3. Anxiety related to a chronic, lifelong disease
   4. Embarrassment
   5. Fear of public rejection
   6. Side effects of drug therapy

D. Diagnostic tests/methods
   1. Specific tests to identify lesions
   2. EEG, CT scan, and MRI

E. Treatment
   1. Treat and remove cause, if known
   2. Anticonvulsant drugs

F. Nursing intervention
   1. Provide accurate observation and documentation, including aura, time of onset, whether seizure is general or focal, specific parts of body involved, eye movement, LOC, bowel and bladder control, condition after seizure, memory loss, weakness, and any injury caused by seizure
   2. Encourage resident to wear medical identification tag
   3. Have suction available
   4. Secure seizure stick and airway for easy accessibility
   5. During generalized (grand mal) seizure
      a. Insert seizure stick (padded tongue blade) between teeth before seizure (do not force)
      b. Maintain airway
      c. Prevent head injury

d. Place resident on side if possible
e. Protect extremities from injury by guiding movements
f. Do not restrain
g. Loosen clothing
h. Remove pillows
i. Maintain safety until fully conscious

TRANSIENT ISCHEMIC ATTACKS (TIAS)

Altered cerebral tissue perfusion related to a temporary neurologic disturbance
A. Manifested by sudden loss of motor or sensory function
B. Lasts for a few minutes to a few hours
C. Caused by a temporarily diminished blood supply to an area of the brain
D. Resident is at high risk for developing a stroke
E. Medical management is indicated (control of hypertension, low-sodium diet, possible anticoagulant therapy, stop smoking)
F. Nursing care would include close observation and assessment; specific care based on treatment

CEREBROVASCULAR ACCIDENT (CVA) (STROKE)

A. Description: decreased blood supply to a part of the brain caused by rupture, occlusion, or stenosis of the blood vessels; onset may be sudden or gradual; symptoms and resident problems depend on location and size of area of brain with reduced or absent blood supply (left CVA results in right-side involvement often associated with speech problems; right CVA results in left-side involvement often associated with safety/judgment problems)
B. Causes: increased incidence with aging
   1. Atherosclerosis
   2. Embolism
   3. Thrombosis
   4. Hemorrhage from a ruptured cerebral aneurysm
   5. Hypertension
C. Signs and symptoms
   1. Altered LOC
   2. Change in mental status: decreased attention span, decreased ability to think and reason, difficulty following simple directions
   3. Communication: motor or sensory aphasia; difficulty reading, writing, speaking, or understanding
   4. Bowel or bladder dysfunction: retention, impaction, or incontinence
   5. Seizures
   6. Limited motor function: paralysis, dysphagia, weakness, hemiplegia, loss of function, or contractures
   7. Loss of sensation/perception
   8. Headaches and syncope
   9. Loss of temperature regulation and elevated temperature, pulse, and blood pressure
   10. Absent gag reflex (aspiration)
   11. Unusual emotional responses: depression, anxiety, anger, verbal outbursts, and crying; emotional lability
   12. Problems related to immobility
D. Diagnostic tests/methods
   1. Physical assessment and resident or family history
   2. EEG, CT scan, lumbar puncture, or cerebral angiography
E. Treatment
   1. Remove cause, prevent complications, and maintain function; rehabilitation to restore function
   2. Provide antihypertensives, anticoagulants, and stool softeners
   3. Surgical removal of clot or repair of aneurysm
F. Nursing intervention
   1. Maintain bed rest; provide complete care; use turning sheet, foot board, firm mattress, pillows, and trochanter rolls to maintain proper body alignment; anticipate needs and leave things within reach (e.g., call bell)
   2. Reposition resident q2h; provide passive and active range of motion (ROM) exercises; place resident in chair as soon as allowed; use flotation mattress or sheepskin
   3. Provide bath, inspect, and provide nursing measures to prevent decubitus ulcers
   4. Provide oxygen with humidity; have resident cough and take deep breaths q2h if possible; maintain airway; suction as needed; prevent aspiration; keep head turned to side; place in semi-Fowler's position

5. Ensure adequate nutrition and fluid and electrolyte balance; provide nasogastric/gastrostomy tube feeding; maintain IV fluids; provide soft diet when tolerated; use total parenteral nutrition (TPN)
6. Establish means of communication: call bell, pad and pencil, and nonverbal gestures; use simple commands; speak slowly; explain all care; provide speech therapy
7. Be nonjudgmental about personality changes; encourage family participation; provide diversional activities; praise accomplishments realistically
8. Assess LOC; maintain safety in environment; use side rails; restrain only as necessary
9. Observe for IICP
10. Monitor vital signs q4h
11. Ensure elimination; check for impaction; monitor bowel movements; monitor intake and output; provide indwelling catheter care; then conduct bowel and bladder training
12. Provide care, safety, and precautions for a resident with seizures
13. Provide support for family
14. Schedule physical and occupational therapy as soon as possible
15. Provide nursing measures to prevent complications of immobility
16. Encourage self-care

BRAIN TUMOR

A. Description: a benign or malignant growth that grows and exerts pressure on vital centers of the brain, depressing function and causing increased pressure
B. Cause: unknown
C. Signs and symptoms: individual, depending on location and size
   1. Personality changes, fear, and anxiety
   2. Headaches, dizziness, and visual disturbance (e.g., double vision)
   3. Seizures
   4. Pituitary dysfunction
   5. Signs of IICP
   6. Local paresthesia or anesthesia
   7. Aphasia
   8. Problems with coordination
D. Diagnostic tests/methods

1. Resident history and physical examination
2. Neurologic assessment including EEG, CT scan, angiography, and MRI
E. Treatment: surgical removal if possible (craniotomy), frequently combined with radiotherapy and chemotherapy
F. Nursing intervention
   1. Perform neurologic assessment and documentation
   2. Provide safety and assist with care as needed
   3. Be nonjudgmental about personality changes; encourage the resident to express feelings

HEAD INJURIES

A. Description: trauma resulting in a fracture to the skull, either a simple break in the bone or bone fragmentation that penetrates the brain tissue; can also cause hemorrhage, concussion, or contusion
   1. Cerebral concussion: injury to the head; resident may be dazed or unconscious for a few minutes; some functions (e.g., memory) may be impaired for as long as several weeks
   2. Cerebral contusion: head injury causing bruising of brain tissue; person experiences stupor, confusion, or loss of consciousness; if severe, may go into coma
   3. Cerebral laceration: a break in continuity of brain tissue
B. Cause: blow to the head (e.g., from a fall or automobile accident)
C. Signs and symptoms: individual, according to location and extent of blow
   1. Nausea and vomiting
   2. Lethargy: increasing loss of consciousness to impending coma
   3. Disorientation
   4. Drainage of cerebrospinal fluid from ear or nose
   5. Convulsions
   6. Problems related to IICP
D. Diagnostic tests/methods
   1. Resident history and physical/neurologic assessment
   2. X-ray examination
   3. Angiography
   4. CT scan
   5. PET scan

E. Treatment
  1. Anticonvulsions
  2. Maintenance of fluid balance
  3. Surgery
F. Nursing intervention
  1. Neurologic assessment qh
  2. Maintain airway
  3. Give care as required for the unconscious resident if necessary
  4. Take precautions for a resident with seizures
  5. Observe for serous or bloody discharge from ears/nose

MULTIPLE SCLEROSIS

A. Description: a chronic, progressive disease of the brain and spinal cord; lesions cause degeneration of the myelin sheath and interfere with conduction of motor nerve impulses; there are periods of remissions and exacerbations; onset occurs in young adults; it has an unpredictable progression
B. Cause: unknown; exacerbates with stress
C. Signs and symptoms vary with individual
  1. Ataxia
  2. Paresthesia
  3. Weakness and loss of muscle tone
  4. Loss of sense of position
  5. Vertigo
  6. Blurred vision, diplopia, nystagmus, patchy blindness that may progress to total blindness
  7. Inappropriate emotions: euphoria/apathy/depression
  8. Dysphagia
  9. Slurred speech
  10. Bladder and bowel dysfunction: incontinence or retention
  11. Sexual dysfunction: impotence, diminished sensation
  12. Spasticity as disease progresses
D. Diagnostic tests/methods
  1. Resident history and physical/neurologic assessment
  2. CT scan
  3. MRI
  4. Examination of cerebrospinal fluid (CSF)
E. Treatment: symptomatic—corticosteroids during acute exacerbations
F. Nursing intervention
  1. Provide care to prevent complications of immobility

  2. Encourage resident to maintain independence
  3. Encourage resident to participate in care plan
  4. Encourage high-calorie, high-vitamin, high-protein diet; provide nutrition that can be swallowed easily
  5. Provide bowel and bladder training (may have indwelling catheter)
  6. Provide diversional activities
  7. Provide safety
  8. Allow time for residents to express concerns about disabilities and dependencies; be supportive
  9. Avoid precipitating factors that cause exacerbations (e.g., fatigue, cold, infections)
  10. Resident/family education

PARKINSON'S DISEASE

A. Definition: a progressive, degenerative disease causing destruction of nerve cells in the basal ganglia of the brain caused by a deficiency of dopamine; limbs become rigid, fingers have characteristic pill-rolling movement, and head has to-and-fro movement; the resident has a bent position and walks in short, shuffling steps; facial expression becomes blank, with wide eyes and infrequent blinking (Parkinson's mask); intelligence is not affected
B. Cause: unknown
C. Signs and symptoms
  1. Tremors
  2. Voluntary movement is slow and difficult; coordination is poor (ataxia)
  3. Impaired chewing and eating; excessive salivation and drooling
  4. Speech is slow and resident is soft spoken; written communication is difficult
  5. Excessive sweating
  6. Emotional changes: depression, paranoia, and eventually confusion
  7. Dependency
D. Diagnostic tests/methods
  1. Resident history and physical assessment
  2. Neurologic assessment
E. Treatment: many residents respond to drug therapy, and the disease is controlled with medication for the remainder of their lives; others have no response, and the disease progresses to a state of invalidism and immobility (usually treated with a combination of drugs)

F. Nursing intervention
1. Encourage resident to maintain independence as much as possible in hygiene and dressing; include resident in planning all aspects of care as much as possible
2. Encourage participation in previous work and social and diversional activities (avoid social withdrawal)
3. Help resident avoid embarrassment while eating; use straws, wipe drooling saliva, use bib, and keep clothing clean; use utensils with large handles for easy grip
4. Recommend a soft diet or one of a consistency the resident is able to chew
5. Provide diversional activity (resident may be highly intelligent)
6. Encourage daily exercises as tolerated, especially walking; take safety measures
7. Encourage resident to avoid fatigue
8. Help resident to avoid frustration; emphasize capabilities rather than limitations
9. Reinforce speech, physical, and occupational therapy treatment protocols
10. Administer stool softeners to avoid constipation
11. Provide bowel and bladder training
12. Be patient when resident is slow or clumsy
13. Establish a means of communication
14. Enhance cognitive skills (reorient frequently)
15. Prevent pneumonia; force fluids; turn resident when in bed and encourage resident to be out of bed as much as possible
16. Provide mouth care q4h
17. Encourage family participation in all aspects of rehabilitation

SPINAL CORD IMPAIRMENT

The vertebral column houses the spinal cord. A small cartilage disk acts as a cushion between the vertebrae. All sensory and motor nerves to the neck, trunk, and extremities branch out from the spinal cord. The degree of disability and resident problems are related to the location of the lesion in the body controlled by the injured or diseased nerves.

Herniated Intervertebral Disk

A. Description: a portion of the cartilage disk protrudes and compresses the nerves; continued pressure can cause degeneration

B. Causes
1. Straining
2. Lifting/pushing (poor body mechanics)
C. Signs and symptoms
1. Pain usually radiating over the buttock and down back of the leg
2. Weakness of ankle and knee; tingling; numbness
3. Complications of immobility
D. Diagnostic tests/methods
1. CT scan
2. X-ray examination
3. Myelogram (identifies level of herniation)
4. MRI
E. Treatment
1. Bed rest with traction
2. Muscle relaxants, antiinflammatory drugs, and narcotic analgesics
3. Brace
4. Surgery
   a. Laminectomy: with the resident under general anesthesia, first the lamina, or arch of the vertebra, is removed and then the disk; dangers include injury to motor roots, which can result in paralysis, and clot formation that will exert pressure on the spinal cord
   b. Spinal fusion (performed with laminectomy): a graft from the posterior iliac crest is taken and used as a bridge between the laminae; this supports the spinal column; after surgery the resident may be in a cast for immobilization to promote healing; recovery is slow (4 to 5 weeks)
F. Nursing intervention
1. Provide bed rest (may be in pelvic traction); give care as indicated to prevent complications of immobility (may be allowed to be out of traction at specific times [e.g., during meals or to use the bathroom])
2. Provide heat, either moist or dry, before surgery as ordered (patient may have decreased sensation)
3. Provide firm mattress; use bed board
4. Use fracture bedpan if bed rest is prescribed for resident
5. Anticipate and medicate for pain

Spinal Cord Lesion

A. Description: a growth compressing the spinal cord; may be benign or malignant; interferes with nerve function
B. Cause: unknown
C. Signs and symptoms: individual, according to area involved
D. Diagnostic tests/methods
   1. Resident history
   2. Myelography
   3. Neurologic assessment
E. Treatment: surgical removal
F. Nursing intervention: see care of a resident with a laminectomy (in preceding outline)

Spinal Cord Injuries

A. Description: complete or partial severing of the spinal cord; if severing is complete, there is permanent paralysis of body parts below site of injury; when there is partial damage, edema may cause a temporary paralysis
B. Cause: accident (e.g., automobile, shooting, or diving)
C. Signs and symptoms: individual, according to level of spinal cord involved
   1. Respiratory distress
   2. Paralysis
D. Diagnostic tests/methods: physical examination
E. Treatment
   1. Immobilization: Crutchfield tongs, halo traction, back brace, or body cast
   2. Surgery
F. Nursing intervention
   1. See care of a resident with paralysis (in preceding section)
   2. Maintain airway and respiratory function
   3. See emergency care of a resident with a spinal cord injury

AMYOTROPHIC LATERAL SCLEROSIS (ALS)

ALS is a progressively incapacitating and fatal disease of unknown cause in which there is degeneration of upper motor neurons (nerves leading from brain to medulla or to spinal cord) and to the lower motor neurons (nerves leading from spinal cord to muscles of body). There is loss of voluntary muscle function and subsequently the loss of functional capacity.

Clinical Manifestations

Depend on location of affected motor neurons, since specific neurons activate specific muscle fibers

A. Progressive weakness and wasting of muscles of arms, trunk, and/or legs from degeneration of anterior horn cells in various segments of spinal cord
B. Signs of spasticity, fasciculations (irregular twitching of muscles), and exaggerated reflexes
C. Progressive difficulty in speaking, swallowing, and ultimately breathing—as a consequence of degeneration of the motor cranial nerve nuclei in the lower brainstem (or bulb, hence the "bulbar" symptoms)
   1. Drooling; pseudoptyalism (accumulation of saliva in mouth)
   2. Regurgitation of liquids through nose
   3. Difficulty swallowing, with aspiration of food or fluid into trachea
   4. Nasal and unintelligible speech

Diagnostic Evaluation

A. Electromyography—demonstrates presence of denervation, muscle wasting, and atrophy
B. Nerve conduction study
C. Pulmonary function studies—to assess respiratory function
D. Barium swallow—to evaluate ability to achieve various phases of swallowing

Management

No specific treatment available at present time to arrest or alter course of disease. The supportive treatment, determined by functional loss, includes:
A. Baclofen—for spasticity
B. Diazepam—for fasciculations
C. Antidepressant medication
D. Anticholinergic medication (atropine)—to control saliva
E. Feeding gastrostomy—when resident can no longer eat without risk of aspiration
F. Mechanical ventilation

Complications

A. Respiratory failure
B. Cardiopulmonary arrest

Nursing Interventions

A. Establish techniques to cope with impaired physical mobility and lost function
   1. Encourage the resident to continue the usual activities as long as possible; avoid fatigue
   2. Work with physical therapist to teach resident and family exercises to strengthen unaffected muscles; carry out ROM exercises
   3. Encourage stretching exercises (stretch-hold-relax) to avoid contractures
   4. Give special attention to shoulder joint, as upper arm pain related to shoulder dysfunction is a major cause of discomfort
   5. Initiate referral to occupational therapist for instruction on use of orthoses (braces), splints, and supports for regions where weakness is disabling
   6. Instruct the resident to use energy-conservation and work-simplification methods
   7. Work cooperatively with occupational therapist to evaluate resident's needs and to advise on securing assistive devices (e.g., electrically powered wheelchair and bed, mechanical lift)
   8. Teach family the techniques of positioning, turning, and transfers
   9. Teach pressure sore prevention
B. Prevent aspiration and maintain nutritional status
   1. Observe resident swallowing fluids and look for regurgitation of fluid through nose—weakness of soft palate musculature prevents sealing off of nasopharynx during deglutition (swallowing)
   2. Examine oral cavity—dysfunction of tongue indicated by food debris on lingual surface of teeth
   3. Look for food spillage from oral cavity—from weakness of lips, buccal muscles, and tongue
   4. Control saliva buildup, as resident may be unable to move saliva to the back of his throat and swallow; use suctioning
   5. Encourage rest before meals to alleviate muscle fatigue
   6. Place resident in a bolt upright position with neck flexed (chin pointed toward the chest) to eat and drink—lessens risk of aspiration, as in this position the airway is partially blocked by the esophagus
   7. Use a soft cervical collar if resident has difficulty holding head up
   8. Give semisolid foods—tend to hold together in a bolus form and are generally easier to swallow
      a. Avoid easily aspirated, pureed foods and mucus-producing foods (milk)
      b. Offer very warm or very cold (not room temperature) food or drinks—makes use of temperature receptors in the mouth that are in part responsible for swallowing
      c. Use soft foods that hold together (casseroles, stews, food with gravy)
      d. Do not wash down solids with fluids—may cause choking and aspiration
   9. Instruct resident to take a breath before swallowing, hold breath, exhale or cough after the swallow, and then swallow again
      a. Turning the head to the side while swallowing may be helpful
      b. Avoid talking while eating
   10. Look for signs and symptoms of chronic dehydration: malaise, decreased urine output, dry mouth, thick mucus, decreased skin turgor
   11. Advise resident/family to keep intake and output record to ensure adequate fluid intake; liquid intake is compromised, as liquids fragment during swallowing and cause aspiration
      a. Offer cold, carbonated soft drinks—have more taste sensation than water
      b. Offer Jello, popsicles, fruit sherbets, and fruit ices—help with liquid ingestion
   12. Consider alternate feeding methods to maintain nutrition in residents with advanced dysphagia (nasogastric tube; feeding gastrostomy tube)
C. Monitor and manage potential respiratory failure
   1. Follow vital capacity measurements—vital capacity falling below 50% indicates considerable loss of muscular function
   2. Monitor for altered respiratory pattern during sleep: shallow respirations, fading in and out of sleep, nocturnal delirium, restlessness and anxiety—from chronic hypoxia

3. Be attentive to complaints of inordinate fatigue in the absence of physical exertion—may herald the onset of respiratory failure
4. Use techniques to enhance pulmonary function: upright position, suctioning of excessive secretions, chest physical therapy
5. Incentive spirometry may be helpful in exercising respiratory muscles and keeping lungs inflated

D. Enhance communication
   1. For residents with some speech abilities:
      a. Refer to speech-language pathologist to maximize remaining potential for speech
      b. Use mechanical speech aids; if possible, the system should be tried before it is essential
   2. When speech is lost:
      a. Communication board (ALS Association newsletter describes various communication devices, including eye-gaze communication boards)
      b. Use environmental control system—switch may be activated by slight movement of eyebrow, etc.
      c. Eye movement/eye blinks—may be the resident's only means of communication
      d. Understand that the resident is alert and retains vision, ocular movement, intelligence, and consciousness, but may be physically incapable of doing anything and cannot speak/swallow
   3. Have some type of signaling/alerting device. One possible source: National Association for Hearing and Speech Action, 10801 Rockville Pike, Rockville, MD 20852

E. Enhance coping abilities
   1. Understand that the resident may have involuntary outbursts of forced laughing/crying unrelated to mood/surroundings (pseudobulbar affect)
   2. Give the resident and family compassionate and caring support; problems are ever-changing
   3. Secure services of counselor, social worker, or ALS-experienced psychologist for family undergoing breakdown in communication

4. Advise the family of helping services of the ALS Association, 15300 Ventura Boulevard, Suite 315, Sherman Oaks, CA 91403 (pamphlets, newsletter, patient care tips); and Muscular Dystrophy Association, 810 Seventh Avenue, New York, NY 10019 (services and equipment)

HUNTINGTON'S DISEASE

A. Description: genetically transmitted autosomal dominant disease; affects both men and women; onset from age 35 to 45
B. Cause: involves the basal ganglia and extrapyramidal system. Involves a deficiency of the neurotransmitters ACH and γ-aminobutyric acid (GABA)
C. Clinical manifestations
   1. Abnormal and excessive involuntary movements (chorea)
   2. Writhing, twisting movements of face, limbs, and body
   3. Movements get worse as disease progresses
D. Complications
   1. Facial movements involving speech, chewing, and swallowing may cause aspiration and malnutrition
   2. Gait deteriorates and ambulation becomes impossible
   3. Mental deterioration includes intellectual decline, emotional lability, psychotic behavior
   4. Death usually occurs 10 to 20 years after onset
E. Treatment
   1. No known cure; treatment palliative
   2. Antipsychotic, antidepressant, antichorea medications sometimes helpful
F. Nursing Management goal
   1. Provide comfortable environment for resident and family
   2. Maintain physical safety
   3. Treat physical symptoms as they appear
   4. Provide emotional and psychologic support
   5. Be aware of resources for genetic counseling

MUSCULAR DYSTROPHY

A. Definition: a hereditary disease (recessive trait) characterized by gradual degeneration of muscle fibers that is evidenced by muscle wasting and weakness and increasing disability and deformity

B. Symptoms: gradual muscle weakness, including difficulty walking, standing up, a "waddle" gait, and mild mental retardation; most symptoms appear in children between 3 and 5 years of age

C. Diagnosis: based on the history of the symptoms, family history, muscle biopsy to determine muscle degeneration, and electromyogram (EMG)

D. Treatment/nursing interventions
   1. There is no cure for muscular dystrophy, so treatment is supportive
   2. Encouragement of the child is to be as active and to lead as normal a life as possible
   3. ROM exercises and physical therapy as ordered to prevent contractures
   4. Equipment as needed, such as walkers, crutches, braces, and wheelchairs (resident teaching important)
   5. Emotional support for the parents and child; this is a progressive disease, and the family requires ongoing support by the health care team
   6. Frequent medical checkups to observe for progressive symptoms such as respiratory distress
   7. Genetic counseling for the parents

Review Questions

1. When positioning a CVA resident on his back, the lower arm and hand of the affected side should be placed:
   ① Across the chest
   ② Parallel with the body, with the elbow extended
   ③ Elevated on a pillow beside his chest and trunk
   ④ Extended above the head

2. To promote retraining of the affected side and a faster return to independence, CVA residents should be encouraged to:
   ① Comb hair, wash face, brush teeth
   ② Participate actively in physical therapy
   ③ Perform daily push-ups
   ④ Use a pen with the affected hand

3. A person who has suffered damage to the cerebellum would most likely experience problems with:
   ① Breathing
   ② Hearing
   ③ Coordination of muscular activities
   ④ Visual and hearing disturbance

4. The resident who is immobilized because of spinal cord injuries should have a diet high in:
   ① Calories
   ② Carbohydrates
   ③ Fats
   ④ Proteins

5. As the nurse assesses a resident for IICP, the nurse would be concerned on observing:
   ① A change in LOC
   ② Anorexia and thirst
   ③ Increased pulse and respiration rates
   ④ Blurred vision and halos around lights

6. Nursing interventions for a resident with multiple sclerosis should be directed toward:
   ① Assisting the resident with social and occupational activities
   ② Encouraging the resident to seek treatment that promises a cure
   ③ Preventing pressure ulcers and contractures by use of proper supports
   ④ Providing complete bed rest and breathing exercises twice a day

7. The nurse notes that a resident exhibits the characteristic gait associated with Parkinson's disease. When recording on the resident's chart, the nurse should describe this gait as:
   ① Ataxic
   ② Spastic
   ③ Shuffling
   ④ Scissoring

8. A resident is admitted with a head injury and to rule out a subdural hematoma from being hit in the head with a baseball bat and then falling down 10 stairs. When assessing for the earliest sign of IICP, the nurse observes for changes in which of the following?
   ① LOC
   ② Intensity of a headache
   ③ Pupillary status
   ④ Vital signs

9. When assessing vital-sign changes in a resident with IICP, the nurse observes for which of the following?

① Bradycardia, hypertension, and subnormal temperature
② Fever and hypertension
③ Bradycardia, hypertension, and fever
④ Tachycardia and normal temperature

10. A resident recuperating from a spinal cord injury at the T4 level wants to use a wheelchair. In preparation for this activity the resident should be taught:
① Leg lifts to prevent hip contractures
② Push-ups to strengthen arm muscles
③ Balancing exercises to promote equilibrium
④ Quadriceps-setting exercises to maintain muscle tone

11. In planning nursing care for a resident with multiple sclerosis, the nurse should encourage the resident to:
① Remain as active as possible without becoming fatigued
② Exercise all joints several times a day
③ Adapt to complete bed rest and antibiotic therapy
④ Maintain a low-calorie, low-protein, and low-fat diet

12. While performing the history and physical examination of a resident with Parkinson's disease, the nurse should assess for:
① Frequent bouts of diarrhea
② Hyperextension of the neck
③ A low-pitched, monotonous voice
④ A recent increase in appetite and weight gain

13. A resident has recently suffered a CVA. In assisting the resident to improve cognitive skills, the nurse would:
① Provide memory aids and stimuli
② Provide ROM exercises
③ Initiate bowel and bladder training
④ Provide leisurely, recreational activities so he doesn't have to think

14. Long-term nursing measures for the resident with a cervical cord injury include:
① Meticulous skin care
② Weekly exercise programs
③ Taking vital signs q2h
④ Daily catheter care

15. The nurse is aware that autonomic dysreflexia is a complication associated with some spinal cord injuries. The nurse plans to observe for signs of this problem in a resident who sustained a spinal cord injury at the T2 level because:
① The injury has resulted in loss of all reflexes
② The injury is above the sixth thoracic vertebra
③ There has been a partial transection of the cord
④ There is a flaccid paralysis of the lower extremities

16. The nurse is aware that a resident with a spinal cord injury is developing autonomic dysreflexia when the resident has:
① Flaccid paralysis and numbness
② Absence of sweating and pyrexia
③ Escalating tachycardia and shock
④ Paroxysmal hypertension and bradycardia

17. A 17-month-old child has meningitis. In planning care for the child the nurse knows that symptoms will most likely include:
① Fever, stiff neck, and elevated WBCs in blood and spinal fluid
② Dyspnea, lethargy, and elevated pulse and blood pressure
③ Vomiting; diarrhea; dehydration; and red, raised rash
④ Red, raised rash; fever; diarrhea; and elevated WBCs in spinal fluid

ANSWERS AND RATIONALES FOR REVIEW QUESTIONS

1. **3** Elevation of the arm helps prevent edema and fibrosis, which will interfere with normal ROM.
   1 Inappropriate position that will promote, not prevent, edema/fibrosis.
   2 Inappropriate position that will promote, not prevent, edema/fibrosis.
   4 Inappropriate position that will promote, not prevent, edema/fibrosis.

2. **1** These activities will put the arm through ROM as the resident assumes some responsibility for personal care.
   2 Part of daily routine in rehabilitation.
   3 Inappropriate activity.
   4 Too fine a movement and one that does not allow full ROM.

3. **3** The cerebellum regulates coordination, balance, and muscle tone.
   1 Breathing is regulated by the medulla.
   2 Hearing is regulated by the midbrain.
   4 Vision and hearing are regulated by the midbrain.

4. **4** A diet high in proteins decreases the incidence of pressure ulcers.
   1 A diet high in calories is inappropriate for an immobilized resident.
   2 Necessary, but not in excessive amounts.
   3 Necessary, but not in excessive amounts.

5. **1** A change in LOC may be one of the first signs of IICP.
   2 Not associated; GI symptoms are nausea and vomiting.
   3 Pulse rate and respirations are decreased.
   4 Problems related to glaucoma.

6. **3** Proper supports and body alignment are important to prevent pressure ulcers and contractures that result from loss of muscle tone.
   1 The resident should be encouraged to maintain social activities as long as possible. Occupational activities may have to be changed if necessary. Appropriately trained persons would best meet these needs of the resident.
   2 The resident should be encouraged to avoid treatments that promise a cure, because there is no cure.
   4 The resident should avoid complete bed rest unless absolutely necessary. Encourage resident to be independent as long as possible.

7. **3** Steps are short and dragging; this is seen with basal ganglia defects.
   1 This is a staggering gait often associated with cerebellar disease.
   2 This is associated with unilateral upper motor neuron disease.
   4 This is associated with bilateral spastic paresis of the legs.

8. **1** Although all the answers are signs of IICP, change in LOC is the earliest sign.
   2,3,4 Presence or intensity of headache, changes in pupillary status, and changes in vital signs are late indicators of increased intracranial pressure.

9. **3** Vital-sign changes in IICP include elevated blood pressure; bradycardia; slow, irregular respirations; and elevated temperature.
   1 These are not indicative of vital-sign changes in IICP.
   2 These are not indicative of vital-sign changes in IICP.
   4 These are not indicative of vital-sign changes in IICP.

10. **2** Arm strength is necessary for transfers and ADLs and for the use of crutches or a wheelchair.
    1 The resident has no neurologic control of this activity.
    3 Equilibrium is not a problem.
    4 The resident has no neurologic control of this activity.

11. **1** The resident should remain active as long as possible and continue daily activities without becoming fatigued.
    2 This is recommended for Parkinson's disease.
    3 The resident is not to assume complete bed rest until complete loss of muscular function necessitates it. The drug therapy of choice is corticosteroids, which are antiinflammatory agents, not antibiotics.
    4 The diet recommended is high calorie, high vitamin, and high protein.

12. **3** Amplitude of the voice is reduced by neuromuscular involvement.
    1 Constipation is a common problem because of a weakness of muscles used in defecation.
    2 The tendency is for the head and neck to be drawn forward by loss of basal ganglia control.
    4 Usually loss of weight occurs because of the embarrassment caused by slowness and untidiness in eating.

13. **1** Weakened cognitive skills need stimulation.
    2 Unrelated to cognitive skill improvement.
    3 Unrelated to cognitive skill improvement.
    4 Contradictory to the goal of cognitive stimulation.
14. **1** Pressure ulcers form easily if proper care is not given.
    2 Not necessarily specific to spinal cord injury treatment.
    3 Not necessary.
    4 Not necessarily specific to spinal cord injury treatment.
15. **2** The T6 level is the sympathetic visceral outflow level, and any injury above this level results in autonomic dysreflexia.
    1 The reflex arc remains after spinal cord injury.
    3 The important point is not that the cord is totally transected but the level at which the injury occurs.
    4 This is not related to autonomic dysreflexia; all cord injuries result in flaccid paralysis during the period of spinal shock; as the inflammation subsides, spasticity gradually increases.

16. **4** These symptoms occur as a result of exaggerated autonomic responses, and if autonomic dysreflexia is identified, immediate intervention is necessary to prevent serious complications.
    1 Paralysis is related to transection, not dysreflexia; the resident will have no sensation below the injury.
    2 Profuse diaphoresis occurs.
    3 Bradycardia occurs.
17. **1** These are the most common symptoms of the disease, which also include severe headache and pain.
    2 Dyspnea and high blood pressure are not common to the disease.
    3 Red, raised rash is not common to the disease.
    4 Red, raised rash is not common to the disease.

chapter ten

Endocrine System Overview

A disturbance in one of the secreting glands may affect the regulation of another gland; therefore the resident may also experience multiple problems and needs. Some of these disturbances affect the resident's appearance, personality, and activity level. Because of this the nurse must be emotionally supportive to the resident and family. The nurse must also provide resident teaching because some residents must have lifelong hormonal drug therapy related to endocrine deficiencies.

Nursing Assessment

A. Nursing observations
  1. General appearance
  2. Vital signs
  3. Weight
  4. Skin
     a. Color
        (1) Pallor
        (2) Flushed
        (3) Yellow pigmentation
        (4) Bronze pigmentation
        (5) Purple striae over obese areas
     b. Temperature
     c. Dry
     d. Moist
     e. Excess diaphoresis
     f. Poor wound healing
  5. Hair
     a. Dry
     b. Brittle
     c. Thin
  6. Nails
     a. Dry
     b. Thin
     c. Thick
  7. Musculoskeletal
     a. Muscle mass distribution
     b. Fat distribution
     c. Change in height
     d. Changes in body proportions: enlarged ears, nose, jaws, hands, and feet
     e. Diminished muscle strength
  8. Central nervous system
     a. Personality changes
     b. Alterations in consciousness
        (1) Listlessness
        (2) Slowed cognitive ability
        (3) Stupor
        (4) Seizures
        (5) Confusion
        (6) Coma
     c. Slowed, hoarse speech
     d. Reflexes
        (1) Trousseau's sign: contraction of fingers and toes due to a decrease in calcium
        (2) Chvostek's sign: spasm of facial muscles due to a decrease in calcium
  9. Eyes
     a. Periorbital edema
     b. Protruding eyeball (exophthalmos)
     c. Drooping eyelids (ptosis)
  10. Gastrointestinal system
     a. Anorexia
     b. Polyphagia
     c. Polydipsia
     d. Constipation
     e. Diarrhea
     f. Nausea and vomiting
  11. Cardiovascular system
     a. Hypertension
     b. Hypotension
     c. Tachycardia
     d. Bradycardia
  12. Respiratory system
     a. Tachypnea

b. Acetone breath
c. Kussmaul-Kien respirations
13. Renal system
   a. Polyuria
   b. Oliguria
14. Reproductive system
   a. Menstrual disturbances
   b. Libido disturbances
   c. Galactorrhea (excess mammary gland secretion in females)
   d. Gynecomastia (increased breast tissue in males)

B. Resident description (subjective data)
1. Pain
   a. Headache
   b. Skeletal pain
   c. Back pain
   d. Muscle spasms
2. Appetite
   a. Anorexia
   b. Polyphagia
3. Weakness
4. Numbness
5. Tingling
6. Mood swings
7. Nausea
8. Intolerance to heat or cold
9. Polydipsia
10. Polyuria, nocturia, and dysuria
11. Decreased libido and impotence
12. Frequent infections

Common Resident Problems and Nursing Care
HYPERTHYROIDISM (GRAVES' DISEASE AND THYROTOXICOSIS)

A. Definition: overactivity of the thryoid gland with hypersecretion of thyroxine (T_4)
B. Pathology
1. Metabolic rate is increased, resulting in a high amount of energy and oxygen expenditure
2. May be caused by decreased production of thyroid-stimulating hormone (TSH) by malfunctioning pituitary gland, which results in high T_4 serum concentration
3. May be attributed to enlarged thyroid gland caused by decreased iodine intake
C. Signs and symptoms
1. Subjective

   a. Polyphagia
   b. Hyperexcitability/personality changes
   c. Heat intolerance
   d. Insomnia
   e. Amenorrhea
   f. Diarrhea/constipation
   g. Increased appetite
   h. Fatigue/weakness
2. Objective
   a. Weight loss
   b. Exophthalmos
   c. Excessive sweating
   d. Increased pulse rate
   e. Fine hand tremors
   f. Warm, flushed skin
   g. Elevated blood pressure
   h. Bruit over thyroid
D. Treatment
1. Medication to inhibit T_4 production
2. Radioactive iodine to destroy thyroid gland cells to decrease T_4 secretion
3. Drugs to control tachycardia and hyperexcitability
4. Subtotal or total thyroidectomy
E. Nursing intervention
1. Teach the resident and family signs and symptoms of hypothyroidism when resident is receiving thyroid-inhibiting drugs
   a. Increased body weight
   b. Sensitivity to cold
   c. Fatigue
   d. Dry skin, hair, and nails
   e. Slow, hoarse speech
   f. Constipation
2. Encourage adequate nutrition for increased energy expenditure
   a. High-calorie, high-vitamin, and high-carbohydrate intake
   b. Between-meal snacks
   c. Increased fluid intake
   d. Avoidance of caffeine
3. Plan undisturbed rest periods to restore energy: provide cool, quiet, nonstressful environment
4. Advise the resident to elevate the head of bed while recumbent to improve eye drainage
5. If the resident has undergone surgery
   a. Place resident on back in a low-Fowler's or semi-Fowler's position to avoid strain on sutures

b. Observe dressing for hemorrhage or constriction of the throat; examine back of neck for pooling
c. Keep tracheostomy set at bedside in event of respiratory obstruction caused by hemorrhage, edema of glottis, laryngeal nerve damage, or tetany
d. Encourage resident to cough and expectorate secretions from throat and bronchi
e. Observe for signs of thyroid storm (may occur as a result of gland manipulation during surgery): fever, tachycardia, and restlessness
f. Observe for signs of tetany (may occur if parathyroids are accidentally removed); numbness and tingling around mouth, carpopedal spasms, convulsions

DIABETIC COMA (KETOACIDOSIS)

A. Definition: excess glucose and acid (ketones) in the bloodstream
B. Pathology
   1. A response to insufficient insulin levels
   2. Fats are mobilized for energy; fatty acids are rejected by muscles, resulting in buildup of acids in the bloodstream
   3. Body's buffer system becomes exhausted
C. Signs and symptoms
   1. Subjective
      a. Weakness
      b. Polydipsia
      c. Abdominal pain
      d. Nausea
      e. Headache
      f. Polyphagia
   2. Objective
      a. Hot, dry, flushed skin
      b. Listlessness and drowsiness
      c. Kussmaul's respirations
      d. Sweet or acetone breath
      e. Hypotension
      f. Confusion
      g. Polyuria
      h. Nausea/vomiting
      i. Coma
D. Diagnostic tests
   1. Elevated serum glucose level
   2. Elevated serum and urinary ketones
   3. Lowered blood pH

E. Treatment
   1. Insulin replacement
   2. Correct electrolyte and pH imbalance
   3. Fluid replacement
F. Nursing intervention
   1. Give insulin as ordered; have another person check to prevent error
   2. Monitor and record vital signs and intake and output
   3. Test for glucose and acetone levels; record on diabetic flow sheet
   4. Position resident with head of bed elevated 30 degrees
   5. Maintain patent airway
   6. Give oral care q4h and when required (prn); keep lips and mouth moist
   7. Assess level of consciousness
   8. Observe resident for signs of hypoglycemia: pale, cool, clammy skin; lethargy; and hypotension
   9. Instruct resident and family on factors and signs of impending ketoacidosis
   10. Explain importance of balance among diet, exercise, and insulin
   11. Provide diabetic alert band

HYPOGLYCEMIA (INSULIN SHOCK)

A. Definition: abnormally low level of glucose in the bloodstream
B. Pathology
   1. Accelerated glucose is removed from the serum
   2. May be caused by overproduction or overdosage of insulin
   3. Omission of a meal or too little food eaten by a resident receiving insulin
   4. Too much exercise without extra food; rapid onset
C. Signs and symptoms
   1. Subjective
      a. Hunger
      b. Weakness
      c. Visual disturbances
      d. Tingling lips and tongue
      e. Nervousness
   2. Objective
      a. Pale, moist skin
      b. Tremors
      c. Tachycardia
      d. Hypotension
      e. Muscle weakness

f. Disorientation

g. Coma

D. Diagnostic test: lowered serum glucose level

E. Treatment

    1. Sweetened fluids or sugar given orally; oral glucose preparations

    2. Glucagon subcutaneously or intramuscularly (IM)

    3. Glucose IV

F. Nursing intervention

    1. Give medications as ordered

    2. Monitor and record vital signs and intake and output

    3. Resident teaching should include

        a. Always carry and ingest quick-acting carbohydrate when initial signs appear; fruit juices, sweetened sodas, granulated sugar, or hard candy

        b. Prevent medication error by having another person check dosage

        c. Record each administration of medication to avoid duplication

        d. Always wear medical identification tag

        e. Remember to eat a regular meal after raising glucose level to prevent a rebound effect

Review Questions

1. A resident has recently been diagnosed with diabetes. Which of the following symptoms should the nurse include in explaining insulin shock?

   ① Drowsiness, weakness, thirst, nausea and vomiting, dry skin, and flushed face

   ② Rapid pulse and respirations, restlessness, dizziness, headache, elevated temperature, and pain

   ③ Low blood pressure; rapid pulse; confusion; and pale, moist skin

   ④ Trembling, irritability, confusion, hunger, profuse perspiration, blurred or double vision, and poor concentration

Type	Product Name—Manufacturer	Appearance
Short Acting		
Onset 15 min to 1 hr	Regular (Lilly; Squibb-Novo)	Clear
Peak 2-4 hr	Actrapid (Squibb-Novo)	
Duration 5-7 hr	Velosulin (Nordisk)	
	Humulin R (Lilly)	
	Actrapid Human (Squibb-Novo)	
Intermediate Acting		
Onset 1-4 hr	Semilente (Lilly; Squibb-Novo)	Turbid
Peak 2-15 hr	Semitard (Squibb-Novo)	
Duration 12-28 hr	Protophane NPH (Squibb-Novo)	
	NPH (Lilly; Squibb-Novo)	
	Monotard (Squibb-Novo)	
	Insulatard (Nordisk)	
	Lente (Lilly; Squibb-Novo)	
	Lentard (Squibb-Novo)	
	Humulin N (Lilly)	
	Monotard Human (Squibb-Novo)	
Long Acting		
Onset 4-6 hr	PZI (Lilly; Squibb-Novo)	Turbid
Peak 10-30 hr	Ultralente (Lilly; Squibb-Novo)	
Duration 36+ hr	Ultratard (Squibb-Novo)	
	Mixtard (Nordisk)	

2. Which of the following descriptions of an injured area on a diabetic resident's right leg would be most appropriate to chart?
   ① Large excoriated area on anterior aspect of the shinbone
   ② Half-dollar size area on anterior aspect of lower leg with moderate amount of serous drainage
   ③ 5-cm abraised lesion with small amount of serous drainage noted on right lower leg
   ④ Severe injury with minimal amount of drainage noted on right lower leg

3. The nurse and a diabetic resident are reviewing exchange lists for meal planning. The resident shows an understanding of instructions by which of the following statements?
   ① "I should cut out desserts other than fresh fruit."
   ② "I should decrease my food intake during periods of heavy exercise."
   ③ "I should use only designated dietetic foods."
   ④ "I should schedule regular meals."

4. Elderly individuals with non–insulin-dependent diabetes mellitus (NIDDM):
   ① Seldom develop ketoacidosis
   ② Secrete no endogenous insulin
   ③ Have a lower incidence of chronic complications
   ④ Have a sudden and dramatic onset of symptoms

5. Symptoms of diabetic ketoacidosis are:
   ① Hypotension, hypoglycemia, and thirst
   ② Fasting blood sugar (FBS), 400 mg/dl; Kussmaul's respirations; fruity odor on breath
   ③ Tremors, sweating, and tachycardia
   ④ Hypertension, convulsions, and diaphoresis

6. The nurse would notify the physician immediately if which of the following findings were noted for a diabetic resident?
   ① Right pedal pulse was bounding; admission FBS, 168 mg/dl
   ② Right femoral pulse was difficult to palpate; right foot cooler than left foot
   ③ Right pedal pulse was not palpated; FBS, 320 mg/dl
   ④ Right pedal pulse was thready; right foot cooler than left foot

7. A diabetic resident's right lower leg is taut and shiny. This is significant because:
   ① These symptoms indicate the diabetes is worsening
   ② This indicates the circulation to this extremity may be compromised
   ③ Taut, shiny skin indicates edema of the extremity
   ④ These symptoms are consistent with a positive Homans' sign

8. The symptoms produced in insulin shock are caused by:
   ① Elevated blood sugar levels
   ② Abnormally low blood sugar levels
   ③ Insufficient insulin to metabolize glucose
   ④ Excessive food intake in relation to insulin dose

9. The nurse is teaching a resident the relationship between exercise and insulin requirements. Which of these statements made by the resident would indicate correct understanding of this relationship?
   ① "When I exercise, I may need less insulin."
   ② "When I exercise more, I need more insulin."
   ③ "There is no change in the insulin requirement when exercise is increased."
   ④ "If I eat enough, I don't need to exercise or adjust my insulin."

10. A resident with insulin-dependent diabetes mellitus of several years' duration takes 40 U of NPH and 20 U of regular insulin each morning. The resident's serum glucose level averages about 130 mg/dl. When the resident complains of symptoms of hypoglycemia, the nurse should suspect that the resident's serum glucose is:
    ① About 100 mg/dl
    ② Between 50 and 70 mg/dl
    ③ Between 100 and 120 mg/dl
    ④ At least 20 mg/dl below the norm

11. When planning care for a resident with diabetes mellitus, the nurse knows that this condition:
    ① Interferes with the absorption of minerals
    ② Interferes with the absorption of vitamins
    ③ Involves a disorder in carbohydrate metabolism
    ④ Involves the pituitary gland

12. The nurse should know that the two outstanding characteristic symptoms of diabetes mellitus are:
    ① Hypoglycemia and glycosuria
    ② Hyperglycemia and glycosuria
    ③ Hypoglycemia and hypokalemia
    ④ Hyperglycemia and glycogen

13. The nurse should teach a resident with diabetes that early symptoms of hypoglycemia include:
    ① Flushed face
    ② Diplopia
    ③ Slurred speech
    ④ Hunger

14. While caring for a diabetic resident, the nurse observes that the resident appears to be in a diabetic coma. Signs and symptoms of diabetic coma include:
    ① Cool, moist skin
    ② Rapid, shallow respirations
    ③ Increased blood pressure
    ④ Fruity odor to breath

15. When a resident is diagnosed with diabetes mellitus, the nurse should observe for symptoms of impending diabetic coma. These symptoms include:
    ① Skin moist and pale, and extreme thirst
    ② Skin dry and pale, and extreme hunger
    ③ Skin dry and flushed, and extreme thirst
    ④ Skin flushed and moist, and anorexia

ANSWERS AND RATIONALES FOR REVIEW QUESTIONS

1. **4** The fall in blood sugar decreases available glucose for cell metabolism, causing the motor and sensory symptoms; because the brain does not store glucose, a depletion of available glucose for metabolism affects the brain cells, rapidly causing the CNS symptoms: irritability, confusion, etc.
   1 Symptoms of hyperglycemia.
   2 Symptoms of thyrotoxicosis.
   3 Symptoms of hypovolemic shock.

2. **3** Size, location, and character of drainage should be noted on the chart; provides a reference for future evaluation of wound progress.
   1 Description lacks specific information about size, location, and character of drainage and wound.
   2 Description lacks specific information about exact location (which leg?).
   4 Description too subjective regarding the type of injury; also lacks size of and description of drainage.

3. **4** Regularly scheduled meals are part of the overall treatment plan. The timing of the meals and allowed snacks help prevent problems such as hypoglycemia and hyperglycemia.
   1 Desserts can be included in the diet as part of the daily caloric requirements. Desserts are not restricted to fresh fruit.
   2 Food may need to be increased during periods of heavy exercise.
   3 The exchange system allows for substitutions and flexibility in the diet. "Dietetic" foods do not have to be used. Often these foods are high in sodium and can be more costly.

4. **1** Lipolysis is not a common response to meeting the metabolic needs of those with NIDDM; therefore, ketones are not present in large enough amounts to cause ketoacidosis.
   2 Adults with NIDDM do secrete endogenous insulin, but secretion is slow and subnormal.
   3 The incidence of chronic complications is higher in those with NIDDM than those with insulin-dependent diabetes mellitus.
   4 The onset of NIDDM is usually slow, whereas in insulin-dependent diabetes mellitus it is sudden and dramatic.

5. **2** Diabetic ketoacidosis is manifested by elevated blood glucose levels; deep, blowing, rapid respirations (Kussmaul's respirations); and excessive protein and fat metabolism, which results in acidosis: fruity breath odor results when excessive acetones are excreted during respiration.
   1 Not correct symptoms for diabetic ketoacidosis.
   3 Not correct symptoms for diabetic ketoacidosis.
   4 Not correct symptoms for diabetic ketoacidosis.

6. **3** Absence of the pedal pulse on the affected leg indicates lack of circulation: FBS above 120 mg/dl is high and should be reported immediately to the physician.
   1 Situation should be noted but does not require immediate physician response; compromised circulation has been noted.
   2 Situation should be noted but does not require immediate physician response; compromised circulation has been noted.
   4 Situation should be noted but does not require immediate physician response; compromised circulation has been noted.

7. **2** Trophic change indicates circulation is poor.
   1 Not symptoms of diabetes.
   3 Edema may be present secondary to poor circulation.
   4 Incorrect symptoms for a positive Homans' sign.

8. **2** Insulin overdose, excessive exercise, illness, or insufficient food intake may cause insufficient glucose to be available, causing abnormally low blood sugar.
   1 Produces diabetic coma or acidosis.
   3 Excessive insulin causes shock.
   4 Produces diabetic acidosis.

9. **1** Exercise burns glucose; therefore, insulin needs may decrease.
   2, 3 Less insulin is required (see 1).
   4 Untrue statement. Food alone cannot control diabetes or affect insulin requirements. The combination of food, exercise, and insulin is needed.

10. **2** This is the point at which a resident is generally hypoglycemic, resulting in increased sympathetic nervous system activity and deprivation of CNS glucose supply.
   1 This is within the norm of 90 to 120 mg/dl.
   3 This is within the norm of 90 to 120 mg/dl.
   4 This is not a sufficient drop to cause hypoglycemia; hypoglycemia usually occurs at 50 to 70 mg/dl.

11. **3** There is a decreased production of insulin needed to metabolize carbohydrates.
    1 This condition does not interfere with the body's ability to absorb minerals.
    2 This condition does not interfere with the body's ability to absorb vitamins.
    4 Diabetes mellitus involves the pancreas and the lack of insulin secreted by the beta cells.

12. **2** An abnormally high glucose level in the blood and glucose in the urine are characteristic symptoms of diabetes mellitus.
    1 Hypoglycemia is an abnormally low glucose level in the blood, making this statement incorrect.
    3 Hypoglycemia is an abnormally low glucose level in the blood, and hypokalemia is an abnormally low potassium level in the blood.
    4 Hyperglycemia is correct, but glycogen is the product of the breakdown of carbohydrates and is stored in the liver and muscles.

13. **4** As blood glucose levels fall, the first symptom that develops is hunger.
    1 Flushed face may be a sign of hyperglycemia.
    2 Diplopia is not a symptom of hypoglycemia.
    3 Slurred speech is not an early symptom of hypoglycemia; it may be a sign of hyperglycemia.

14. **4** An increase of acetone in the body accounts for fruity-smelling breath and hot, dry skin.
    1 This is indicative of hypoglycemic reaction.
    2 This is indicative of hypoglycemic reaction.
    3 The systolic blood pressure drops and circulatory collapse may occur.

15. **3** The skin becomes dry and flushed and the resident usually complains of extreme thirst with diabetic acidosis (coma).
    1 The skin is not moist, but dry; not pale, but flushed. A gradual loss of appetite, not extreme hunger, occurs with diabetic acidosis.
    2 The skin is dry, but not pale. Extreme hunger makes this response wrong. The resident usually has a gradual loss of appetite.
    4 The skin is flushed and anorexia may be present. The skin is dry, not moist, with diabetic acidosis.

chapter *eleven*

Genitourinary System Overview

A. Organs
  1. Kidneys: bean shaped and reddish brown; lie against posterior abdominal wall; right kidney is slightly lower than left
     a. External structure
        (1) Hilus: concave notch; blood vessels, nerves, lymphatic vessels, and ureters enter the kidneys at this point
        (2) Renal capsule; protective fibrous tissue surrounding kidneys
     b. Internal structure
        (1) Cortex: outer portion; the greater portion of the nephron is located here
        (2) Medulla: inner portion; consists of 12 cone-shaped structures (pyramids); tip of pyramid points toward renal pelvis and drains waste and excess water into pelvis
        (3) Pelvis: funnel shaped; forms upper end of ureter and receives waste and water
     c. Nephron: basic unit of function; microscopic structure composed of capillaries; approximately 1 million per kidney; controls the processes of filtration, reabsorption, and secretion
        (1) Glomerulus: filtering unit; process of urine formation begins
        (2) Renal tubules: reabsorption occurs in the proximal convoluted tubules, through Henle's loops, and through the distal convoluted tubules; then the collecting tubules pass the final urine product into the pelvis
  2. Ureters: two long, narrow tubes; transport urine from kidney to bladder by peristalsis
  3. Bladder: elastic, muscular organ; capable of expansion; stores urine; assists in voiding (micturition: the release of urine or voiding)
  4. Urethra: narrow, short tube from bladder to exterior; exterior opening called the meatus
     a. Female: approximately $1^1/_4$ to 2 inches (3 to 5 cm) long; transports urine
     b. Male: approximately 8 inches (20 cm) long; transports urine and is a passageway for semen

B. Functions
  1. Excretion: nitrogen-containing waste (urea, uric acid, and creatinine) is excreted; normal daily output is 1200 to 1500 ml
  2. Maintenance of water balance: absorbs more or less water depending on intake; normally, intake is approximately equal to output
  3. Regulates acid balance; reabsorbs or actively secretes excess acids and bases produced by cell metabolism

C. Urine composition
  1. Clear, yellowish, slightly aromatic, and slightly acid
  2. Contains 95% water and 5% solids, which includes urea, uric acid, creatinine, ammonia, sodium, and potassium; specific gravity

(sp gr) indicates amount of the dissolved solids; normal range: 1.05 to 1.03 sp gr
   3. Abnormal substances: glucose, blood protein, RBCs, bile, and bacteria

Altered Urinary Elimination Incontinence

A. General information
   Urinary incontinence is the inability to control the release of urine. There are various types of urinary incontinence:
   1. Stress: weakness of supporting pelvic muscles that causes urine to be released through the bladder outlet when a person coughs, laughs, sneezes, or exercises
   2. Urge: spasm or irritated bladder walls that cause sudden need to void and involuntary passage of urine
   3. Reflex: lack of sensation of signal to void leading to involuntary loss of urine when a specific volume of urine fills bladder
   4. Overflow: excess accumulation of urine in bladder because of failure of bladder muscles to contract or lack of relaxation of periurethral muscles
   5. Total: constant loss of urine without any appreciable volume accumulating in the bladder and without sensation
   6. Functional: existence of factor that interferes with the ability to toilet and that is unrelated to disorders of the urinary tract
   Although not a normal outcome of aging, incontinence is more prevalent among older persons.
B. Causative/contributing factors
   1. Pelvic muscle weakness or relaxation secondary to multiple pregnancies; reduction in estrogen; obesity
   2. Urinary tract infection
   3. Dehydration (concentrated urine irritates bladder wall)
   4. Compression of urethra and bladder by prostatic hypertrophy, fecal impaction
   5. Bladder neck obstruction
   6. Neurologic disease (e.g., CVA, multiple sclerosis, Parkinson's disease)
   7. Impaired cognition; depression
   8. Confinement to bed
   9. Inaccessible bathroom
   10. Dependency on others for toileting
   11. Medications (e.g., anticholinergics, adrenergic antagonists, diuretics)
C. Clinical manifestations
   1. Involuntary loss of urine indicated by the following:
      a. Urine on floor
      b. Wet clothing, linens
      c. Urine odor
      d. Damp or stained clothing, furniture, floor
   2. Frequent toileting, reluctance to be far from bathroom
D. Assessment considerations
   1. Obtain history regarding the following:
      a. Date of onset
      b. Pattern (e.g., constant dribbling, sudden expulsion of large amounts)
      c. Frequency and occurrence (e.g., during night, only when sneezing)
      d. Precipitating factors (e.g., delay in voiding, laughing, diuretics)
      e. Related factors (e.g., weight gain, constipation, new medication)
      f. Intake and output
      g. Resident's reaction (e.g., unaware, embarrassed, socially isolated)
   2. Review of medications being taken for possible relationship
   3. Evaluation of functional status
   4. Inquiry about presence of other symptoms (e.g., abdominal pain, fever)
   5. Evaluation of neurologic and mental status
   6. Diagnostic tests
      a. Urinalysis
      b. Intravenous pyelogram (to determine renal function)
      c. Cystoscopy
      d. Cystometrogram (to determine pattern of bladder emptying)
      e. Cystometry (to determine motor and sensory function of bladder)
E. Goals
   1. Resident regains bladder continence
   2. Resident maintains or regains positive self-concept and dignity
   3. Resident is free from secondary problems such as skin breakdown, social isolation, and falls

F. Nursing interventions
1. Assist with identification and treatment of underlying cause; prepare resident for diagnostic tests as necessary
2. Record and monitor intake and output; estimate and record urine output when resident voids on clothing or linens (1 inch diameter = approximately 10 ml of urine)
3. Provide easily accessible toilet facilities; arrange for bedside commode, if necessary; move resident closer to bathroom

Urinary Tract Problems

A urinary tract infection is a bacterial invasion of the bladder or kidney. This is the most common infection in older persons. The most common causes of urinary tract infection are *Escherichia coli* in women and *Proteus bacilli* in men.

A. Causative/contributing factors
1. Obstructions of urinary flow; calculi
2. Diabetes mellitus
3. Neurologic disorders that promote postvoiding residual urine
4. Atrophic vaginal mucosa; senile vaginitis
5. Frequent catheterizations
6. Indwelling catheters
7. Poor hygiene or wiping techniques in women
8. Immunologic disease
B. Clinical manifestations
1. Frequency, urgency
2. Burning in urethra
3. Bladder, kidney, or suprapubic pain
4. Elevated temperature
5. Blood and/or pus in urine
6. Urinary incontinence
7. Confusion
C. Additional nursing interventions
1. Assist with identification and treatment of underlying cause
2. Encourage fluids (about 2000 ml daily unless contraindicated)
3. Observe quality of urine (e.g., color, odor) and pattern and frequency of urinary elimination; monitor intake and output
4. Prevent immobility and other sources of urinary stasis
5. Instruct resident on proper wiping and hygienic practices, if necessary
6. Use adult briefs and other alternatives to indwelling catheters if incontinence is a problem; the risk of urinary tract infection increases significantly in catheterized persons
7. Use proper techniques to care for indwelling catheters
D. Indwelling catheter care
1. Ensure indwelling catheters are used only when absolutely necessary for the clinical benefit of the resident
2. Adhere to strict aseptic technique during catheterization
3. Secure the catheter so that it is not pulled or dislodged
4. Keep the drainage system closed
5. Prevent urine from backflowing in the catheter; ensure collection unit is positioned below level of resident's bladder
6. Avoid and check for kinks in the tubing
7. Ensure resident is not sitting on tubing and that obstructions to drainage flow are not present
8. Do not irrigate the catheter unless obstruction is present
9. If a urine specimen must be obtained, withdraw from the system with a sterile needle; adhere to aseptic technique
10. Maintain regular and meticulous cleanliness of perineal area, meatus, and drainage system
11. Observe for and promptly report signs of urinary tract infection (e.g., cloudy urine, elevated temperature, altered mental status, hematuria)
E. Additional nursing interventions
1. Assist with diagnosis and treatment of underlying cause; treatment can include the following:
   a. Urinary antiseptics, if infection is present
   b. Prostatic massage to relieve congestion
   c. Medication to reduce benign prostatic hyperplasia
   d. Surgical intervention (transurethral resection, open prostatectomy)
2. Encourage good fluid intake during the day with reduced fluid intake at night
3. Monitor intake and output
4. Teach resident about condition:
   a. Most older men experience some degree of prostatic hypertrophy, most of which is benign

b. Medical evaluation every 6 months is important in detecting complications early; PSA (prostate-specific antigen) testing is advisable

c. Clarify misconceptions concerning relationship of prostate problems to sexual function

d. Reassure resident that most prostate surgeries do not result in impotency to ensure that resident will not be reluctant to have surgery for this reason

CYSTITIS

A. Definition: inflammation of the bladder mucosa; is difficult to cure; recurs and may be chronic

B. Pathology: is usually a bacterial infection
1. May be secondary to infection elsewhere in urinary system (e.g., urethritis)
2. Contamination during catheterization or instrumentation
3. An obstruction causing urinary stasis in the bladder (e.g., enlarged prostate or urethral stricture)

C. Signs and symptoms
1. Burning, dysuria, urgency, frequency, nocturia, hematuria, and pyuria
2. Low-back pain and bladder spasms
3. Elevation of temperature

D. Diagnostic tests/methods
1. Resident history and assessment
2. Urine culture

E. Treatment: systemic medications, urinary antiseptics, antibiotics, sulfonamides, and antispasmodics

F. Nursing intervention
1. Force fluids: 3000 ml daily over that of dietary intake unless contraindicated
2. Provide and supervise proper perineal care
3. Provide diet that acidifies urine (e.g., cranberry juice)
4. Monitor temperature and administer antipyretics as ordered
5. Provide sitz baths

URETHRITIS

A. Definition: inflammation of the urethra; may develop scar tissue and stricture, causing obstruction, cystitis, and nephritis

B. Pathology
1. Prostatitis: injury during instrumentation or catheterization

2. Gonococcus infection

C. Signs and symptoms
1. Urgency
2. Frequency
3. Dysuria
4. Burning on urination
5. Purulent discharge

D. Diagnostic tests/methods
1. Resident history and physical examination
2. Culture of discharge

E. Treatment
1. Antibiotics
2. Dilatation for stricture

F. Nursing intervention
1. Sitz baths
2. Isolation as indicated
3. Demonstrate and supervise thorough hand washing
4. Care of Foley catheter

PYELONEPHRITIS

A. Definition: infection of the kidney; may be acute or become chronic; kidney becomes edematous, mucosa is inflamed, and multiple abscesses may form; the kidney will become fibrotic, and uremia may develop

B. Pathology
1. Ascending infection from an infection lower in the genitourinary (GU) tract
2. Staphylococcal or streptococcal infection carried in the blood

C. Signs and symptoms
1. Markedly elevated temperature (102° to 105° F); shaking, chills
2. Nausea and vomiting
3. Dysuria, burning, frequency, pyuria, and hematuria
4. Flank pain and tenderness in kidney
5. Increased WBC count

D. Diagnostic tests/methods
1. Urine culture and sensitivity
2. Resident history and physical examination
3. Intravenous pyelogram (IVP)

E. Treatment: urinary antiseptics and specific antibiotics; follow-up care for at least 1 year

F. Nursing intervention
1. Prevent dehydration: force fluids and maintain IV therapy
2. Provide rest and conserve energy
3. Prevent chill; keep skin dry and clean
4. Provide mouth care q2h

5. Provide soft diet
6. Provide and assist with pericare; demonstrate proper technique and hand washing
7. Anticipate pain: administer analgesics and local heat
8. Administer antiemetic as needed
9. Control temperature: administer antipyretics and sponge baths as ordered

CALCULI (LITHIASIS)

A. Definition: formation of stones in the urinary tract caused by deposits of crystalline substance that normally remain in solution and are excreted in the urine; may be found in the kidney, ureters, or bladder; vary in size from renal calculi that can be as large as an orange or as small as grains of sand; can obstruct urine flow, causing chronic infection, backflow, hydronephrosis, and gradual destruction of kidney; many small stones pass spontaneously
B. Cause
   1. Infection
   2. Urinary stasis
   3. Dehydration and concentration of urine
   4. Metabolic diseases (e.g., gout)
   5. Immobility (see dangers of immobility)
   6. Familial tendency
C. Signs and symptoms
   1. Pain (can be extreme) radiates down flank to pubic area
   2. Frequency and urgency
   3. Hematuria and pyuria
   4. Diaphoresis, nausea, vomiting, and pallor (related to pain)
D. Diagnostic tests/methods: x-ray studies—kidney, ureter, and bladder (KUB); IVP; urine studies
E. Treatment: depends on location—stones are removed; normal urine production and elimination are restored; recurrence is prevented
   1. Cystoscopy and crushing of stones (litholapaxy)
   2. Dislodging ureteral stone by passing ureteral catheter
   3. Surgery to remove ureteral or kidney stone
      a. Pyelolithotomy: removal of stones from renal pelvis
      b. Nephrolithotomy: incision through kidney and removal of stone
      c. Ureterolithotomy: removal of ureteral calculus

d. Transcutaneous shock wave lithotripsy: ultrasonic waves used to disintegrate renal calculi
F. Nursing intervention
   1. Provide general preoperative and postoperative nursing care
   2. Supervise and explain diet restrictions as ordered according to type of stone
   3. Provide analgesics as ordered
   4. Observe, describe, and strain all urine
   5. Maintain gravity drainage: never clamp ureteral or nephrostomy catheters
   6. Observe patency of catheters: never irrigate renal or ureteral catheters
   7. Record output from each catheter separately; immediately report scanty output from one tube
   8. Force fluids (but keep NPO if there is nausea, vomiting, or abdominal distention)

HYDRONEPHROSIS

A. Definition: an accumulation of fluid in the renal pelvis; there is distention of the renal tubules, calyces, and pelvis; renal tissues are destroyed from pressure; leads to uremia (azotemia)
B. Pathology
   1. Congenital defective drainage; blockage from stones or scar tissues
   2. Reflux (backup) from obstructed bladder neck in benign prostatic hypertrophy
C. Signs and symptoms
   1. Related to cause
   2. Infection
   3. Flank tenderness and pain
D. Diagnostic tests/methods
   1. Resident history and physical examination
   2. Blood serum tests (urea/creatinine)
   3. Intravenous pyelogram (IVP)
E. Treatment
   1. Remove cause
   2. Provide for adequate urinary drainage (e.g., bladder catheter or nephrostomy tube)
   3. Antibiotics
F. Nursing intervention
   1. Provide rest
   2. Provide medication and care as needed for symptoms (e.g., elevation of temperature or pain)
   3. Assess for and provide care as indicated for resident with uremia

BLADDER TUMORS

A. Definition: benign or malignant lesions that ulcerate into the mucous membrane; bladder capacity is decreased; benign tumors tend to recur and become malignant
B. Pathology
  1. Related to cigarette smoking and exposure to dyes (industrial)
  2. Chronic bladder irritation (e.g., stones or infection)
  3. Related to aging
C. Signs and symptoms
  1. Painless, gross hematuria
  2. Anemia
  3. Signs of bladder infection: dysuria, frequency, urgency, and chills
D. Diagnostic tests/methods
  1. Resident history and physical examination
  2. X-ray studies: IVP
  3. Cystoscopy and biopsy examination
E. Treatment
  1. Removal of the tumor through cystoscopy if benign
  2. Surgery
    a. Partial cystectomy
    b. Cystectomy: total removal of the bladder and provision for urinary diversion (see the following outline)
    c. Radiation
    d. Chemotherapy
F. Nursing intervention: give according to method of treatment (see specific sections)

URINARY DIVERSION

A. Definition: surgical intervention to allow for urinary elimination; the bladder is removed; the procedure is permanent
  1. Ileal conduit (ileal passageway): a small segment of ilium is separated from the intestine and the distal end is brought out of the abdomen to form a stoma; the ureters are implanted into this ileal pouch; urine flows continuously from the renal pelvis through the ureters, into the ileal pouch, and into a collecting bag
  2. Ureterointestinal implant: the ureters are anastomosed into the sigmoid colon or rectum; urine is mixed with feces, and evacuation is controlled from the anal sphincter
  3. Cutaneous ureterostomies: the ureters are implanted on the abdomen, forming one or two stomas that drain urine continuously into drainage bags
B. Indication: cancer of the bladder
C. Resident problems (depends on procedure)
  1. Susceptibility to infection
  2. Anxiety or depression about diagnosis and change in body image
  3. Inability to control elimination
  4. Embarrassment
  5. Odor if urine leaks onto skin
D. Nursing intervention (varies with procedures)
  1. Provide time to listen to resident fears and anxieties
  2. Assess fluid and electrolyte imbalance
  3. Maintain integrity of the skin: clean, inspect, and change drainage bag as needed
  4. Prevent infection: maintain asepsis; force fluids; resident must know when to seek medical attention for pain or elevation of temperature
  5. Do not give resident laxatives or enemas (rectal implant)
  6. Elimination of odor in drainage bags; use weak solution of vinegar

KIDNEY TUMORS

A. Definition: most tumors of the kidney are malignant; no early symptoms are presented
B. Cause: unknown
C. Signs and symptoms (only in late stages)
  1. Hematuria with no pain
  2. Low-grade temperature
  3. Weight loss
  4. Anemia
  5. Symptoms related to metastasis (e.g., bone pain)
D. Diagnostic tests/methods
  1. Renal arteriogram: IVP
  2. Renal biopsy examination
  3. CT scan, MRI
E. Treatment
  1. Surgery: radical nephrectomy
  2. Radiation
  3. Chemotherapy
F. Nursing intervention
  1. Provide nursing care for individual symptoms

2. Provide general nursing care: before and after surgery, during radiation, and for a resident receiving chemotherapy

ACUTE RENAL FAILURE (RENAL SHUTDOWN)

A. Definition: sudden damage to the kidneys causing cessation of function and retention of toxins, fluids, and end products of metabolism; resident may recover, or disease may become chronic or be fatal
B. Causes: blood transfusion reaction, shock, toxins, burns, or trauma
C. Signs and symptoms
   1. Lethargy, headache, and drowsiness; convulsion; may go into coma
   2. Nausea, vomiting, and diarrhea
   3. Sudden oliguria or anuria
   4. Increased bleeding time
D. Diagnostic tests/methods
   1. Resident history and physical examination
   2. Blood serum tests
E. Treatment
   1. Removal of cause
   2. Peritoneal dialysis
   3. Hemodialysis
F. Nursing intervention
   1. Provide nursing observations and care as indicated for primary problem
   2. Provide care and observations as indicated for a resident with chronic renal failure
   3. Provide nursing care as indicated for a resident receiving peritoneal dialysis
   4. Provide nursing care as indicated for a resident receiving hemodialysis
   5. Offer emotional support

CHRONIC RENAL FAILURE (END-STAGE RENAL DISEASE)

A. Definition: progressive kidney damage; the nephron deteriorates; the kidneys stop functioning; this is the final stage of many chronic diseases (e.g., hypertension)
B. Causes
   1. Glomerulonephritis; pyelonephritis; polycystic kidney; or urinary tract obstruction, diabetes
   2. Essential hypertension
   3. Lupus erythematosus
C. Signs and symptoms
   1. Malaise

2. Nausea and vomiting
3. Anemia
4. Oliguria
5. Hyperkalemia
6. Twitching (from low serum calcium and increased phosphorus levels)
7. Hypertension (from fluid retention)
8. Very susceptible to infection: delayed wound healing and ulcers in the mouth
9. Bleeding tendency
10. Uremic frost: urea is excreted in perspiration onto the skin, and small crystals can be seen; this causes severe pruritus
11. Headaches and visual disturbances, disorientation, convulsions, coma, and death

D. Diagnostic tests/methods
   1. Resident history and physical examination
   2. Serum blood tests
   3. Kidney function tests; blood urea nitrogen (BUN); creatinine level
   4. X-ray studies
E. Treatment
   1. Remove (treat) cause
   2. Hemodialysis
   3. Peritoneal dialysis
   4. Kidney transplant
F. Nursing intervention
   1. Monitor fluid balance: weigh resident daily; record intake and output
   2. Maintain asepsis: provide catheter care, prevent infections, and encourage frequent hand washing; do not expose resident to staff or visitors with upper respiratory tract infections
   3. Conserve energy: provide care, maintain rest periods
   4. Relieve pruritus: wash resident frequently with tepid water; a weak solution of vinegar dissolves uric acid; handle skin gently; use skin lotion; cut nails; apply calamine lotion
   5. Assist with administration of transfusion
   6. Provide oral hygiene q1-2h; use cotton swabs and antiseptic mouthwash; apply mineral oil to lips
   7. Provide soft, high-carbohydrate, low-potassium, low-sodium, low-protein diet in small feedings
   8. Restrict fluids as ordered
   9. Anticipate cardiac arrest: monitor vital signs

10. Assess LOC: orient as necessary
11. Provide nursing care and precautions as indicated for a resident with seizures
12. Provide nursing measures to prevent dangers of immobility
13. Anticipate and prevent bleeding
    a. Observe stool, urine, sputum, and vomitus
    b. Monitor vital signs
    c. Use soft swab for mouth care
    d. Avoid injections if possible

Peritoneal Dialysis

A. Description: toxins, end-products of metabolism and fluids, are removed from the blood through the peritoneal membrane; a catheter is passed into the peritoneal cavity; dialyzing fluid, which is similar to plasma, is instilled by gravity into the abdominal cavity, and the catheter is clamped; toxins and electrolytes, which are in greater concentration in the blood vessels of the peritoneal membrane, pass into the dialyzing fluid; after 1 hour the catheter is unclamped, and the fluid drains out by gravity
B. Resident problems
   1. Risk for infection related to dialysis procedure
   2. Self-care deficit related to discomfort and immobility
C. Nursing intervention
   1. Record baseline vital signs; complete assessment; carefully measure fluid instilled/drained
   2. Maintain surgical asepsis; prevent peritonitis
   3. Assist resident with self-care activities
   4. Resident teaching to avoid complications from procedure

Hemodialysis

A. Description: blood leaves the resident through an arterial cannula and travels through coils placed in a solution; dialysis takes place, and the detoxified blood returns to the resident's venous circulation; a surgically created arteriovenous fistula (connection) is necessary for repeated dialysis
B. Resident problems
   1. Self-esteem disturbance related to threatened self-image
   2. Powerlessness related to dependency on machine
   3. Risk for infection related to the hemodialysis procedure
   4. Anxiety related to lifelong, life-threatening disease
C. Nursing intervention
   1. Maintain surgical asepsis
   2. Assess bruit patency
   3. Provide emotional support; alleviate anxiety
   4. Provide resident teaching with emphasis on diet, energy conservation, and signs and symptoms of complications

Male Reproductive System Overview
BENIGN PROSTATIC HYPERTROPHY (BPH)

A. Description: the prostate gland slowly enlarges (hypertrophies) and extends upward into the bladder; outflow of urine is obstructed; the urinary stream is smaller, and voiding is difficult; a pouch is formed in the bladder as the gland continues to enlarge; stasis of urine occurs; obstruction causes gradual dilatation of ureters and kidneys; may cause hydronephrosis; when obstruction is complete, there is acute urinary retention
B. Cause: unknown; increased incidence with age, usually over age 50; related to smoking
C. Signs and symptoms
   1. Dysuria, frequency, nocturia, urgency, retention, burning on urination, and decreased force of stream
   2. Urinary tract infection
   3. Acute urinary retention
D. Diagnostic tests/methods
   1. Resident history and assessment; palpation through rectal examination
   2. IVP, cystoscopy, and retrograde pyelography
   3. Urine culture
   4. BUN
   5. Serum creatinine
E. Treatment
   1. Immediate
      a. Bladder drainage with indwelling catheter
      b. Decompression
      c. Antibiotics as indicated

d. Suprapubic cystotomy and insertion of catheter for long-term drainage
2. Surgery: type depends on resident's age and size of enlargement
   a. Transurethral prostatic resection (TURP): an instrument is passed through the urethra to the prostate; under direct visualization, small pieces of the obstructing gland are removed with electric wire; the bleeding points are cauterized; there is no incision; bleeding is a common postoperative problem
   b. Suprapubic (transvesicle) prostatectomy: a low incision is made over the bladder; the bladder is opened, and the prostatic tissue is removed through an incision into the urethral mucosa; two drainage tubes are inserted (a cystotomy tube and a Foley catheter); these are connected to a continuous bladder irrigation setup
   c. Retropubic prostatectomy: a low abdominal incision is made; the bladder is not entered
   d. Perineal prostatectomy: the gland is removed through an incision in the perineum; the entire gland and capsule are removed
   e. Bilateral vasectomy may be performed with a prostatectomy to reduce risk of epididymitis

HYDROCELE

A. Definition: a cystic mass filled with fluid that forms around the testicle
B. Causes
   1. Infection
   2. Trauma
C. Signs and symptoms
   1. Swelling of testicle
   2. Discomfort in sitting and walking
D. Diagnostic tests/methods: assessment
E. Treatment: aspiration (usually only in children)

CANCER OF THE PROSTATE

A. Definition: a malignant tumor; it has no symptoms until it has become large or metastasized
B. Cause: unknown; increased incidence with age (all men over age 40 should have rectal examinations yearly)

C. Signs and symptoms
   1. Early tumor has no symptoms
   2. Frequency, nocturia, and dysuria
   3. Back pain
   4. Symptoms from metastasis
D. Diagnostic tests/methods
   1. Rectal examination
   2. Biopsy examination
   3. Acid phosphatase
E. Treatment: surgery
   1. Radical perineal prostatectomy (removal of prostate, capsule, and seminal vesicles)
   2. Bilateral orchiectomy (removal of both testicles)
   3. TURP
   4. Estrogen therapy
F. Nursing intervention
   1. See nursing intervention for a resident with BPH
   2. Be supportive as concerns are expressed about a malignancy and feminization from estrogens; answer questions; refer problems to physician

Female Reproductive System Overview

A. External genitals
   1. Vulva
      a. Labia majora: two long folds of skin on each side of the vaginal orifice outside of the labia minora
      b. Labia minora: two flat, thin, delicate folds of skin that are highly sensitive to manipulation and trauma; enclose the region called the vestibule, which contains the clitoris, the urethral orifice, and the vaginal orifice
      c. Clitoris: very sensitive erectile tissue; becomes swollen with blood during sexual excitement
      d. Vaginal orifice: opening into vagina; hymen, fold of mucosa, partially closes orifice and generally is ruptured during first sexual intercourse
      e. Bartholin's glands: located on each side of vaginal orifice; secrete lubrication fluid
   2. Perineum: between vaginal orifice and anus; forms pelvic floor
B. Internal organs
   1. Ovaries: main sex glands

a. Located on either side in pelvic cavity
b. Produce ova, which form in the graafian follicles
c. Graafian follicle produces estrogen
d. Rupture of a follicle releases an ovum (ovulation)
e. Ruptured follicle becomes glandular mass called corpus luteum
f. Corpus luteum secretes estrogen, but mainly progesterone

2. Fallopian tubes
a. Extend from point near ovaries to uterus; no direct connection between ovaries and tubes
b. Fimbriae: fingerlike extensions on tubes; pick up ova and transport into fallopian tubes
c. Fertilization occurs in outer third of the fallopian tubes

3. Uterus
a. Upper portion rests on upper surface of bladder; the lower portion is embedded in pelvic floor between the bladder and the rectum
b. Pear-shaped, hollow organ that expands tremendously to accommodate a fetus
c. Divisions
(1) Body: upper main part
(2) Fundus: bulging upper surface of the body
(3) Cervix: neck of the uterus
d. Endometrium: uterine lining; sloughs off during menstruation
e. Functions
(1) Menstruation
(2) Pregnancy
(3) Labor

4. Vagina
a. Located between rectum and urethra
b. Structure: wrinkled mucous membrane (rugae); capable of great distention
c. Functions
(1) Lower part of birth canal
(2) Receives semen from male
(3) Passageway for menstrual flow

C. Breasts (mammary glands)
1. Located over pectoral muscles
2. Size depends on adipose tissue rather than glandular tissue
3. Consists of lobes, lobules, and milk-secreting cells (acini)
4. Ducts lead to the opening called the nipple
5. Areola: pigmented area surrounding the nipple

D. Function
1. Reproduction
2. Production of estrogen and progesterone

E. Menstrual cycle
1. Phases: regulated primarily by the hormonal control of pituitary gland, ovaries, and uterus
a. One ovum discharged each month from an ovary; ripens in the graafian follicle; follicle-stimulating hormone (FSH) from anterior lobe of pituitary stimulates the formation of the follicle
b. Estrogen produced by the follicle builds up the endometrium in expectation of a fertilized ovum
c. Ovum is discharged into the fallopian tube by luteinizing hormone (LH) from the anterior lobe pituitary; follicle is converted into the corpus luteum
d. Postovulation: corpus luteum secretes progesterone and estrogen for final preparation of the endometrium
e. Premenstrual: the gradual drop in progesterone and estrogen leads to menses
2. Length of cycle: usually 28 days; highly variable; ovulation occurs midway
3. Menopause (climacteric): gradual cessation of the menstrual cycle; the ability to bear children ends; occurs at approximately age 45
a. Ovaries lose their ability to respond to hormones
b. Decrease in levels of estrogen and progesterone
(1) Failure to ovulate
(2) Monthly flow is less, irregular, and gradually ceases
(3) Reproductive organs atrophy

VAGINITIS

A. Definition: inflammation of the vaginal mucosa
B. Pathology
1. Invasion of virulent organisms permitted by changes in normal flora; pH becomes alkaline

2. Four classifications
   a. Trichomoniasis: parasitic organism
   b. *Candida albicans* (moniliasis): fungal organism
   c. Atrophic (senile): occurs in post-menopausal women because of atrophy of vaginal mucosa
   d. Simple: invasion by staphylococci, streptococci, or *Escherichia coli*
C. Signs and symptoms
   1. Trichomoniasis: thick, white or yellow, frothy, malodorous discharge causing itching, burning, and excoriation of vulva
   2. Monilial: thick or watery, white or yellow, curdlike discharge; mucosa becomes reddened
   3. Atrophic: blood-flecked discharge with burning and itching of the vagina and dyspareunia
   4. Simple: profuse, yellow mucoid discharge with irritation to vulva and urethra
D. Diagnostic tests/methods: culture and sensitivity
E. Treatment
   1. Trichomoniasis: metronidazole (Flagyl), Floraquin tablets administered vaginally, and carbarsone suppositories administered rectally
   2. Candidiasis: nystatin (Mycostatin) and gentian violet applied to vaginal mucosa
   3. Atrophic: antibiotics and estrogen therapy
   4. Simple: antibiotics and sulfonamide creams
   5. Acetic acid douches
F. Nursing intervention
   1. Reassure resident during vaginal examination to decrease anxiety
   2. Instruct resident on perineal hygiene: cleansing from front to back
   3. Advise resident that gentian violet causes staining of clothes; resident may wish to use perineal pads

UTERINE CANCER (ENDOMETRIUM)

A. Definition: new growth of abnormal cells in the uterine lining
B. Pathology
   1. Spreads to cervix, fallopian tubes, ovaries, bladder, and rectum
   2. Associated factors are women over age 50, obesity, diabetes, and hypertension
   3. Prognosis is good if identified in early stages
C. Signs and symptoms
   1. Subjective
      a. Postmenopausal bleeding
      b. Bleeding between cycles
      c. Bleeding after intercourse
      d. Watery vaginal discharge
   2. Objective
      a. Uterine enlargement
      b. Suspicious Pap test results
D. Diagnostic tests/methods
   1. D & C
   2. Tissue biopsy examination
E. Treatment
   1. Surgical intervention
      a. Panhysterectomy (removal of uterus and cervix)
      b. Oophorectomy (removal of ovaries)
      c. Salpingectomy (removal of fallopian tubes)
   2. Chemotherapy
   3. Radiation
F. Nursing intervention: refer to section on cancer of the cervix

UTERINE FIBROID TUMORS

A. Definition: a benign tumor located in the uterus
B. Pathology
   1. Develops slowly; symptoms occur only in relation to size, location, and number of tumors present
   2. Occurs in 25% of women over age 35
C. Signs and symptoms
   1. Subjective
      a. Menstrual disturbances
      b. Backache
      c. Frequent urination
      d. Constipation
   2. Objective; uterine enlargement
D. Diagnostic tests/methods
   1. Pelvic examination
   2. Laparoscopy
E. Treatment: Observation; possible surgical intervention

VAGINAL FISTULA

A. Definition: tubelike opening between two internal organs
B. Pathology

1. Causes include radiation therapy, gynecologic surgery, or traumatic childbirth
2. Results in impaired blood supply and sloughing of tissue, leading to abnormal opening
3. Three types affect female reproductive organs
   a. Ureterovaginal: between ureter and vagina; urine leaks into vagina
   b. Vesicovaginal: between bladder and vagina; urine leaks into vagina
   c. Rectovaginal: between rectum and vagina; flatus and fecal matter leak into vagina

C. Signs and symptoms
   1. Subjective
      a. Leakage of urine, flatus, and fecal matter
      b. Pain in affected area
   2. Objective
      a. Excoriation
      b. Malodor

D. Diagnostic methods
   1. Symptoms and physical examination
   2. History of radiation therapy

E. Treatment
   1. Small fistula may heal spontaneously
   2. Surgical excision
   3. Temporary colostomy for rectovaginal fistula

F. Nursing intervention
   1. Provide psychologic support: offer reassurance and acceptance
   2. Encourage verbalization of feelings and express empathy
   3. Observe vaginal discharge and record
   4. Change perineal pad q4h and prn
   5. Give instruction on perineal hygiene
   6. Provide sitz bath and irrigation solutions for hygiene if ordered

PROLAPSED UTERUS

A. Definition: downward displacement of the uterus through the vaginal orifice

B. Pathology
   1. A result of weakened supporting muscles and ligaments of the pelvis
   2. Causes include childbirth injuries, repeated pregnancies with short intervals between, menopausal atrophy, and congenital weakness

C. Signs and symptoms
   1. Subjective
      a. Pain in lower abdomen
      b. Feeling of pressure within pelvis
      c. Stress incontinence
      d. Dyspareunia
      e. Backache
   2. Objective
      a. Urinary stasis
      b. Elongated cervix

D. Diagnostic methods
   1. Signs and symptoms
   2. Pelvic examination

E. Treatment
   1. Placement of a pessary in the vagina to support uterus
   2. Surgical suspension of the uterus
   3. Hysterectomy if condition is postmenopausal

F. Nursing intervention
   1. Approach unhurriedly, demonstrate calmness, and encourage expression of feelings to decrease anxiety
   2. Explain all procedures

CYSTOCELE AND RECTOCELE

A. Definition
   1. Cystocele: abnormal protrusion of the bladder against the vaginal wall
   2. Rectocele: abnormal protrusion of part of the rectum against the vaginal wall

B. Pathology
   1. Result of weakened supporting muscles and ligaments of the pelvis
   2. Causes include childbirth injuries, repeated pregnancies with short intervals between, menopausal atrophy, and congenital weakness

C. Signs and symptoms
   1. Subjective
      a. Pelvic pressure
      b. Stress incontinence and dysuria (cystocele)
      c. Constipation or incontinence of feces and flatus (rectocele)
   2. Objective
      a. Residual urine after voiding (cystocele)
      b. Hemorrhoids (rectocele)

D. Diagnostic methods
   1. Signs and symptoms

2. Pelvic examination
E. Treatment
   1. Anterior colporrhaphy to adjust cystocele
   2. Posterior colporrhaphy to adjust rectocele
F. Nursing intervention
   1. Administer catheter care twice a day (bid) and prn
   2. Splint abdomen when coughing
   3. Place in low-Fowler's position or flat in bed to avoid pressure on suture line
   4. Explain to resident that she should respond to bowel stimuli to avoid suture strain
   5. After each bowel movement, clean perineum with warm water and soap; pat dry from front to back
   6. Apply heat lamp, anesthetic spray, or ice packs if ordered to relieve discomfort
   7. Resident teaching: heavy lifting and prolonged standing, walking, and sitting are contraindicated

OVARIAN TUMORS

A. Definition: a mass of tissue growing on the ovary; is usually asymptomatic until large enough to cause pressure
B. Pathology: two classifications
   1. Ovarian cyst: a benign condition but may transform to a malignancy; may be small, containing clear fluid, or may be filled with a thick yellow fluid; size varies
   2. Malignant tumors: usually a cancerous cell travels from another organ, and a secondary malignant site is established
C. Signs and symptoms
   1. Subjective
      a. Pelvic pain
      b. Menstrual disturbances
      c. Abdominal distention
      d. Constipation
      e. Dyspareunia
   2. Objective: palpable mass
D. Diagnostic tests/methods
   1. Culdoscopy
   2. Ultrasonography
   3. Biopsy examination
E. Treatment
   1. Cyst may be observed for regression in size
   2. Oophorectomy (removal of ovaries)
   3. Removal of all reproductive organs

4. Estrogen replacement therapy

CANCER OF THE CERVIX

A. Definition: new growth of abnormal cells in the neck of the uterus
B. Pathology
   1. Early stage is confined to epithelial cervical layer
   2. Will continue to invade surrounding area such as bladder and rectum
   3. Metastasizes to lungs, bones, and liver
C. Signs and symptoms
   1. Subjective
      a. Asymptomatic in early stage
      b. Menstrual disturbances
      c. Postmenopausal bleeding
      d. Bleeding after intercourse
      e. Watery discharge
   2. Suspicious Pap test result
D. Diagnostic tests/methods
   1. Cervical biopsy examination
   2. Colposcopy
   3. Schiller's test
   4. Conization
E. Treatment
   1. Panhysterectomy (excision of uterus and cervix)
   2. Radiation in advanced case
   3. Chemotherapy
F. Nursing intervention
   1. Reassure resident and family that adjustment to illness can be slow
   2. Acknowledge that resident must adapt to illness according to her age, developmental stage, and past life experiences

BARTHOLIN'S CYSTS

A. Definition: a tumorlike capsule formed of retained secretions
B. Pathology
   1. May develop as a consequence of an earlier bacterial infection of these structures
   2. Formation of these cysts is due to obstruction in the outlet of these glands
C. Signs and symptoms
   1. Subjective
      a. Pain on walking
      b. Dyspareunia
   2. Objective: mobile nodule
D. Diagnostic methods

1. Pelvic examination
2. Palpable nodule
E. Treatment
   1. Incision and drainage
   2. Antiseptic wound packing
F. Nursing intervention
   1. Reassure the resident that normal function of the gland will be regained after the procedure
   2. After surgery provide a sterile perineal pad q4h and PRN
   3. Provide sterile wound care as ordered
   4. Instruct on perineal hygiene
   5. Provide sitz baths for increased circulation and comfort

CANCER OF THE BREAST

A. Definition: small, painless, fixed lump most frequently located in the upper, outer portion of the breast
B. Pathology
   1. High-risk factors include women age 30 to 50, those who have not nursed, women with fibrocystic breast disease, those with a positive family history, those with early menarche and prolonged menstrual history, and women whose first pregnancy was after age 25 or who have never had children
   2. Sites of metastasis are lymph nodes, lungs, liver, brain, and bones
C. Signs and symptoms
   1. Subjective: nontender nodule
   2. Objective
      a. Enlarged axillary nodes
      b. Nipple retraction or elevation
      c. Skin dimpling
      d. Nipple discharge
D. Diagnostic tests/methods
   1. Mammography
   2. Thermography
   3. Xerography
E. Treatment
   1. Lumpectomy: removal of the lump and partial breast tissue; indicated for early onset
   2. Mastectomy
      a. Simple mastectomy: removal of breast
      b. Modified radical mastectomy: removal of breast, pectoralis minor, and some adjacent lymph nodes
      c. Radical mastectomy: removal of the breast, pectoral muscles, pectoral fascia, and nodes
   3. Oophorectomy, adrenalectomy, or hypophysectomy to remove source of estrogen and those hormones that stimulate the breast
   4. Radiation therapy to destroy malignant tissue
   5. Chemotherapeutic agents to shrink and retard cancer growth
   6. Corticosteroids, androgens, and antiestrogens to alter cancer that is dependent on hormonal environment
F. Nursing intervention
   1. Provide atmosphere of acceptance, frequent resident contact, and encouragement in illness adjustment
   2. Encourage grooming activities (e.g., hair, nails, teeth, skin)
   3. Arrange attractive environment
   4. If the resident is receiving radiation or chemotherapy, explain and assist her with potential side effects
      a. Nausea and vomiting
      b. Anorexia
      c. Diarrhea
      d. Stomatitis
      e. Malaise
      f. Itching
      g. Hair loss

Review Questions

1. Fluids and electrolytes are carefully monitored in residents with renal disease. A priority concern would be an elevation of:
   ① Sodium
   ② Potassium
   ③ Chloride
   ④ Calcium

2. Methenamine hippurate (Urex) 1 g qid is prescribed for a resident with a urinary tract infection. Which of the following statements by the resident indicates an understanding of the instructions given by the nurse about this medication?
   ① "I will expect my urine to be a red-orange color from the medication."

② "I should reduce the amount of fluids I take so that the medication will remain in the bladder longer."

③ "My urine may appear pink or slightly bloody as a result of the cleansing action of this medication."

④ "My urine will appear to have a blue or blue-green coloration."

3. A resident has been treated with antibiotics for an upper respiratory tract infection for the past few months and is now complaining of a white, cheesy vaginal discharge with severe itching. The resident's symptoms are suggestive of:
① Trichomonas vaginitis
② Monilial vaginitis
③ Simple vaginitis
④ Gonorrhea

4. A resident is scheduled to have hemodialysis. An external shunt is inserted into the left forearm. The nurse should assess the resident for which of the following to ensure proper functioning of the external shunt?
① There is no bleeding at the site
② The arm is not edematous
③ A radial pulse is palpable
④ A bruit is audible

5. The nurse teaches a resident with renal failure about a low-protein diet. The resident would demonstrate an understanding of the protein content of food if which of these desserts were selected?
① Baked custard with caramel sugar
② Yogurt with fruit
③ Applesauce with raisins
④ Gelatin with whipped cream

6. The best means of preventing a urinary tract infection (UTI) is:
① High fluid intake and clean, intermittent catheterizations
② High fluid intake and continuous bladder irrigations
③ Lower fluid intake and indwelling catheterizations
④ Lower fluid intake and continuous bladder irrigations

7. Which of the following is an accurate statement about diuretics?
① Diuretics act by increasing sodium reabsorption
② Osmotics are often used before eye surgery to increase intraocular pressure
③ Diuretics should be scheduled early in the morning or no later than 5 PM if possible
④ Carbonic anhydrase inhibitors are strong and frequently used to lower blood pressure

8. An important nursing consideration in the administration of diuretics is to:
① Limit the resident's intake of fluids
② Withhold the diuretic if pulse rate is below 80 beats/min
③ Give in the early morning if ordered daily
④ Delay the administration if BP is below 110/80

9. A resident who has repeated episodes of cystitis is scheduled for a cystoscopy to determine the possibility of urinary abnormalities. In answer to the resident's questions about the procedure the nurse describes the procedure as:
① A computerized scan that clearly outlines the bladder and surrounding tissue
② An x-ray film of the abdomen, kidneys, ureters, and bladder after administration of dye
③ The visualization of the urinary tract through ureteral catheterization using a radiopaque material
④ The visualization of the inside of the bladder with an instrument connected to a source of illumination

10. A resident with a history of BPH mentions that he has heard cranberry juice prevents bladder infection. The nurse replies that cranberry juice may be helpful because it:
① Increases the acidity of the urine
② Soothes the irritated bladder walls
③ Improves the glomerular filtration rate
④ Destroys microorganisms in the urinary tract

11. A resident with acute renal failure complains of nausea, pain in the abdomen, diarrhea, and muscular weakness. The nurse notes an irregularity in pulse and signs of pulmonary edema. These are probably manifestations of:
    1. Calcium deficiency
    2. Calcium excess
    3. Sodium deficiency
    4. Potassium excess

12. To control uremia in a resident with renal failure, the nurse should teach the resident to limit the intake of:
    1. Potassium
    2. Fluid
    3. Sodium
    4. Protein

ANSWERS AND RATIONALES FOR REVIEW QUESTIONS

1. **2** Potassium affects muscle tissue, specifically cardiac muscle.
   1 Imbalance not as life threatening.
   3 Imbalance not as life threatening.
   4 Imbalance not as life threatening.

2. **4** Methenamine will make the urine a blue or blue-green color.
   1 Nitrofurantoin, not methenamine, will make the urine a red-orange color.
   2 A resident with an infection or bladder inflammation should increase the amount of fluids taken.
   3 Urine that appears pink or bloody should be reported to the physician because it is not caused by the medication.

3. **2** Correct; drainage is white or yellow and curd-like.
   1 Discharge is white or yellow, frothy, and malodorous.
   3 Discharge is profuse, yellow, and mucoid.
   4 Discharge, if noted at all, is puslike and yellow.

4. **4** Hearing a bruit indicates that blood is rushing through the shunt and the shunt is functioning properly.
   1, 2, 3 It is not conclusive that the shunt is patent.

5. **3** Applesauce and raisins contain no protein.
   1 Custard is made with milk and eggs, which contain protein.
   2 Yogurt is made with milk.
   4 Gelatin contains protein, and cream also has a small amount of protein.

6. **1** High fluid intake and intermittent catheterizations keep the kidneys active and initiate voiding.
   2 Not the best way to keep kidneys active, because of continuous irrigations.
   3, 4 Low fluid intake and continuous bladder irrigations or indwelling catheters are conducive to UTIs because of decreased urinary output from decreased fluid intake, as well as from preventing the bladder from functioning on its own due to the indwelling catheter or continuous bladder irrigation.

7. **3** Diuretics given after 5 PM may work effectively but may keep the resident up all night. Scheduling the drugs early in the morning would allow the action to occur during waking hours.
   1 The action of diuretics is to decrease sodium reabsorption.

2 Osmotics are used to decrease intraocular pressure.
   4 Carbonic anhydrase inhibitors are weak and infrequently used today.

8. **3** To allow for diuresis during resident's normal waking hours.
   1 Fluids are not usually limited when a resident is on diuretics although they may be on intake and output.
   2,4 Change in pulse rate or BP is not a consideration when administering a diuretic.

9. **4** This answers the resident's question and provides an accurate description of a cystoscopy.
   1 This is not a computerized examination.
   2 This procedure does not involve x-ray films or dye.
   3 Radiopaque material is not used and the catheter is inserted via the urethra, not the ureters.

10. **1** An acid-ash diet, including cranberries, lowers the pH of the urine and discourages pathogenic growth.
   2 Acid urine does not soothe bladder walls.
   3 The glomerular filtration rate is not affected.
   4 An acid medium will discourage further growth but will not kill existing organisms.

11. **4** Hyperkalemia occurs in renal failure. Because the kidneys are damaged, the body does not excrete K+.
   1 Calcium deficiency would be manifested by tingling of the nose, ears, and fingertips, along with muscle spasms and tetany.
   2 Calcium excess would produce renal calculi and pathologic fractures.
   3 Hyponatremia would cause headache, muscle weakness, apathy, and abdominal cramps.

12. **4** The waste products of protein metabolism are the main cause of uremia. The degree of protein restriction is determined by the severity of the disease.
   1 Potassium is restricted to prevent hyperkalemia, not uremia.
   2 Fluid restriction may be necessary to prevent edema, congestive heart failure, or hypertension; fluid does not directly influence uremia.
   3 Sodium is often restricted to control fluid retention, not uremia.

chapter *twelve*

Integumentary System Overview

A. The skin is the largest organ of the body
B. Composed of three layers:
   1. Epidermis
      a. Outermost layer
      b. Main function is to protect body against invasion by environmental substances
      c. Restricts water loss
      d. Synthesizes keratin cells
   2. Dermis: contains blood vessels and nerve elements
   3. Subcutaneous layer
      a. Composed of loose connective tissue and fat cells
      b. Main function:
         (1) Provides heat
         (2) Insulates
         (3) Caloric reserves
         (4) Acts as shock absorber

Problems
PRESSURE ULCERS

A. Definition: localized ulceration of the skin or deeper structures that occurs when pressure greater than normal capillary pressure is applied to the skin for a prolonged period of time
B. Stages of pressure ulcers
   1. Stage I
      a. Epidermis remains intact
      b. Erythema not resolving within 30 minutes
   2. Stage II: partial loss of skin layer thickness involving the epidermis but not penetrating into the dermis
   3. Stage III: full thickness tissue loss extending through dermis to involve subcutaneous tissue
   4. Stage IV: deep tissue destruction extending through subcutaneous tissue to fascia and may involve connective tissue, bone or muscle
C. Causative factors
   1. Impaired circulation
   2. Anemia
   3. Immobility
   4. Incontinence
   5. Malnutrition
   6. Decreased immune response
D. Interventions/prevention
   1. Turn resident every 2 hours
   2. Inspect skin for breakdown
   3. Control incontinence
   4. Eliminate shearing
   5. Provide optimal nutrition
   6. Utilize pressure relief devices

Collaborative Management of Pressure Ulcers

A. Debriding enzymes—to soften and remove necrotic tissue
B. Dressings
   1. To provide debridement
   2. Keep healthy tissue moist
   3. Applied with an antiinfective agent
C. Hydrophilic agents—to remove contaminants and excess moisture
D. Hydrotherapy—to soften and remove debris mechanically

E. Diet —adequate protein and calories to promote positive state for rapid wound healing
F. Supplemental vitamins and minerals as needed
G. Surgical debridement: removal of devitalized tissue with a scapel to reduce the amount of debris and fibrotic tissue
H. Tissue flaps: to provide wound care closure with its own blood supply

CONTACT DERMATITIS

A. Definition: an inflammatory response of the skin with redness, edema, thickening of the skin, and frequent scaling; there may be vesicles and papules
B. Cause: an allergic reaction or unusual sensitivity when a substance comes in direct contact with the skin (e.g., poison ivy, soaps, cleaning agents, fabrics)
C. Symptoms: pruritus; erythema
D. Diagnostic tests/methods
   1. Allergy testing
   2. Resident history and assessment
E. Treatment
   1. Systemic medication: antihistamines, antipruritics, and corticosteroids
   2. Topical medication: corticosteroids
   3. Remove cause
F. Nursing intervention
   1. Prevent scratching
   2. Give tepid baths
   3. Cut nails
   4. Administer prn medications as soon as possible

WOUNDS CLOSED BY PRIMARY INTENTION

A. Definition: clean, surgical, or traumatic wounds whose edges are closed with suture clips or sterile tape strips
B. Impairments of healing
   1. Dehiscence
   2. Evisceration
   3. Infection
C. High risk for complications
   1. Obese residents
   2. Diabetic residents
   3. Older residents
   4. Malnourished residents

5. Residents receiving steroids
6. Residents undergoing chemotherapy or radiation
D. Surgical or traumatic wounds healing by secondary intention. Wounds with tissue loss or heavy contamination that form granulation tissue and contract in order to heal
E. Impairment to healing
   1. Contamination
   2. Impairment of perfusion
   3. Diabetic residents
   4. Malnourished residents
   5. Older residents
   6. Residents receiving steroids
   7. Residents receiving chemotherapy—radiation

HERPES ZOSTER (SHINGLES)

A. Definition: crops of vesicles and erythema following sensory nerves on face and trunk; higher incidence in older residents
B. Cause: varicella-zoster virus (chickenpox)
C. Signs and symptoms
   1. Severe pain
   2. Elevation of temperature
   3. Malaise
   4. Anorexia
   5. Pruritus
D. Diagnostic methods: physical examination; vesicles follow sensory nerve paths
E. Treatment: no specific treatment (symptomatic only); analgesics may be used for pain; usually subsides in 3 weeks (pain may last for months); antivirals, corticosteroids, antibiotics
F. Nursing intervention
   1. Keep resident in isolation while vesicles are present
   2. Apply topical lotions to lesions for itching
   3. Give baths or compresses for cooling and soothing
   4. Prevent scratching and secondary infection
   5. Anticipate pain: medicate as needed
   6. Provide small, frequent, well-balanced meals

Review Questions

1. While bathing a resident, the nurse notices a reddened area on the right hip. The appropriate nursing action is to:
   ① Massage the area every 2 hours and keep the resident off his right side
   ② Clean with alcohol and apply a sterile dressing
   ③ Apply warm, moist compresses intermittently
   ④ Apply lotion and powder before turning the resident on the right side

2. When teaching older residents how to limit the itching that results from dry skin, the nurse should instruct them to:
   ① Take hot tub baths
   ② Wear warm clothes
   ③ Use a moisturizer
   ④ Expose skin to the air

3. Impetigo is:
   ① A streptococcal or staphylococcal infection of the skin
   ② The same as pinworms
   ③ Dermatitis caused by an allergic reaction
   ④ Infestation of lice on the scalp

4. The nurse is aware that the most common secondary infection to head lice (pediculosis capitis) is:
   ① Eczema
   ② Cellulitis
   ③ Impetigo
   ④ Tinea capitis

5. To protect a diabetic resident's affected extremity from further injury you would:
   ① Promote mobility and apply antiembolism stockings
   ② Administer anticoagulants and apply warm, moist compresses
   ③ Wrap the leg tightly with an elastic bandage and administer antibiotics
   ④ Apply a bed cradle and heel protectors

6. The nurse should question residents with basal cell carcinoma about:
   ① Their dietary patterns
   ② Familial tendencies
   ③ Ultraviolet radiation exposure
   ④ Their smoking history

7. The nurse should explain to the resident with psoriasis that treatment usually involves:
   ① Avoiding exposure to the sun
   ② Potassium permanganate baths
   ③ Topical application of steroids
   ④ Debridement of necrotic plaques

8. The nurse must help the resident with pemphigus vulgaris deal with the resulting:
   ① Impaired digestion
   ② Infertility
   ③ Paralysis
   ④ Skin lesions

9. The assessment that is most indicative of systemic lupus erythematosus (SLE) is:
   ① A butterfly rash
   ② An inflammation of small arteries
   ③ Muscle mass degeneration
   ④ Firm skin fixed to tissue

10. Although no cause has been determined for scleroderma, it is thought to be a defect in:
    ① Amino acid metabolism
    ② Sebaceous gland formation
    ③ Autoimmunity
    ④ Ocular motility

11. The nurse should assess a resident with psoriasis for:
    ① Shiny, scaly lesions
    ② Pruritic lesions
    ③ Multiple petechiae
    ④ Erythematous macules

ANSWERS AND RATIONALES FOR REVIEW QUESTIONS

1. **1** Massaging the area and avoiding repeated pressure will enhance circulation.
   2 Inappropriate nursing action for pressure areas.
   3 Inappropriate nursing action for pressure areas.
   4 Inappropriate nursing action for pressure areas.

2. **3** Lubricating the skin with a moisturizer effectively relieves the dryness and thus the pruritus.
   1 Warm or cool, not hot, tub baths would decrease the itching.
   2 This would do nothing to lubricate the skin or relieve the pruritus.
   4 Exposing the skin to air causes further drying and would not relieve the pruritus.

3. **1** Impetigo can be caused by streptococcal or staphylococcal infections.
   2 It is not the same as pinworms.
   3 Impetigo is not caused by an allergic reaction.
   4 This is called pediculosis.

4. **3** Impetigo may develop as a secondary bacterial infection because of breaks in the skin from scratching.
   1 Eczema is an allergic response, not an infection.
   2 This is an extended inflammation that is not commonly found in children with pediculosis.
   4 This is a fungal infection of the scalp; it usually occurs by itself, not as a secondary infection to pediculosis.

5. **4** Appropriate nursing intervention; bed cradle to prevent sheets from irritating injured area and heel protectors to prevent friction from sheets and eventual heel breakdown.
   1,2,3 Inappropriate nursing interventions for this resident because each action noted could possibly increase chances of injury, such as wrapping the leg tightly with elastic bandage or autiembolism stockings, which decrease circulation; administering anticoagulants and/or antibiotics may not be part of the resident's treatment and may not prevent injury to the affected extremity.

6. **3** Basal cell carcinoma, the most common type of skin cancer, is most closely linked to solar ultraviolet radiation.
   1 Diet is not a risk factor.

2 While skin type is a genetically determined risk factor, it cannot be altered, and it is influenced by solar ultraviolet radiation.
4 Smoking is not a risk factor.

7. **3** Steroids are applied locally and are usually covered with plastic (or Saran Wrap) at night to reverse the inflammatory process.
   1 Solar rays are used in the treatment of psoriasis.
   2 Potassium permanganate is an antiseptic astringent used on infected, draining, or vesicular lesions.
   4 The plaques are not necrotic and therefore do not require debriding.

8. **4** Pemphigus is primarily a serious disease characterized by large vesicles called bullae. Although potentially fatal, it has been relatively controlled by steroid therapy.
   1 Pemphigus is a disease of the skin.
   2 Pemphigus is a disease of the skin.
   3 Pemphigus is a disease of the skin.

9. **1** The connective tissue degeneration of SLE leads to involvement of the basal cell layer, producing a butterfly rash over the bridge of the nose and in the malar region.
   2 This occurs in polyarteritis nodosa, a collagen disease affecting the arteries and nervous system.
   3 This occurs in muscular dystrophy, which is characterized by muscle wasting and weakness.
   4 This occurs in scleroderma and may advance until the resident has the appearance of a living mummy.

10. **3** Scleroderma is an immunologic disorder characterized by inflammatory, fibrotic, and degenerative changes.
    1 This is not involved in development of scleroderma.
    2 This is not involved in development of scleroderma.
    4 This is not involved in development of scleroderma.

11. **1** Psoriasis is characterized by dry, scaly lesions that occur most frequently on the elbows, knees, scalp, and torso.
    2 Pruritis, if present at all, is generally mild.
    3 Petechiae are not characteristic.
    4 Erythematous flat spots on the skin as in measles; no scales are present.

chapter *thirteen*

Sensory Disorders Overview

Impaired Verbal Communication

Speech and language problems include disorders that interfere with the production, comprehension, or expression of words. Speech and language are not synonymous. Speech is the mechanics of producing words; language is the comprehension and expression of ideas. People can have speech problems, language problems, or a combination of both. Effective nursing care depends on knowing the specific cause of the speech or language problem. Early rehabilitative measures can decrease psychologic trauma and promote normal function and independence.

CAUSATIVE/CONTRIBUTING FACTORS

A. Anatomic defects
B. Motor disorders that interfere with word formation
C. Neurologic disturbances that limit comprehension, expression
D. Altered cerebral circulation

CLINICAL MANIFESTATION

A. Aphasia—loss of language function, usually within the central nervous system
   1. Types of aphasia
      a. Expressive—inability to communicate thoughts verbally or in writing because of a motor problem
      b. Receptive—inability to comprehend language because of a sensory problem
      c. Mixed—combination of expressive and receptive
B. Dysphasia—impaired use of words
   1. Types
      a. Receptive—inability to understand words
      b. Expressive—inability to organize words correctly or use the right name for person or object
C. Dysarthria—resident will use correct word but have difficulty pronouncing it because of poor motor control of:
   1. Lips
   2. Tongue
   3. Pharynx
D. Paraphasia—mild form of aphasia in which one word is substituted for another (e.g., *clock* for *watch*)

ASSESSMENT CONSIDERATIONS

A. Lip and tongue motion
B. Soft palate symmetry and rise
C. Vocal cord movement
D. Gag reflex, swallowing
E. Respiration
F. Articulation (speed and quality)
G. Appropriateness of language
H. Hearing
I. Simple tests of language difficulty
   1. Show five everyday objects and ask the name of each (e.g., pen, cup, book, comb, paper clip)
   2. Put the objects aside and then have resident point to each as you name it
   3. Ask resident to repeat several simple sentences
   4. State an expression or truism and ask the resident to explain its meaning (e.g., "People in glass houses shouldn't throw stones.").
   5. Have resident repeat "ma, ma, ma" (tests motor control of lips); "la, la, la" (tests tongue); "ga, ga, ga" (tests pharynx); note distortions and slurring

GOALS

A. Resident is able to communicate needs and comprehend what is being said
B. Resident communicates in a clear and appropriate manner

NURSING INTERVENTIONS

A. Refer to speech therapist; support speech therapy plan
B. Determine the resident's actual deficits and capabilities
C. Describe the speech or language impairment to the resident (if possible), the family, and all care givers
D. Treat the resident like an intelligent adult; realize that an inability to form words does not necessitate shouting or talking as if to a child
E. Keep resident oriented by describing current events, introducing care givers, and explaining activities
F. Maximize existing strengths by using visual cues and assistive devices such as flash cards and communication boards containing common words for the resident to point to pen and paper, synthesizers, and other assistive devices as recommended by the therapist
G. Be patient and accepting of the resident's impairment; allow the resident time to process words
H. Promote socialization and diversion; encourage family to visit; talk to resident during care activities
I. Refer to support groups (e.g., Lost Chord Club) as appropriate

EVALUATION

A. Resident communicates effectively
B. Resident participates in activities of daily living to maximum degree possible

POSSIBLE RELATED NURSING DIAGNOSES

A. Anxiety
B. Self-esteem disturbance
C. Fear
D. Risk for injury

Hearing
OVERVIEW OF THE EAR

A. External ear
  1. Components
    a. Pinna
    b. Auricle
  2. Purpose: gathers sound and sends it into the auditory canal
B. Middle ear
  1. Contains three small bones
    a. Ossicles
    b. Malleus
    c. Incus
  2. Bones are mobile, vibrate; conduct sound waves
  3. The eustachian tube extends into nasopharynx and equalizes the pressure in the middle ear
C. Internal ear (labyrinth) vestibule
  1. Cochlea, snail-shaped bony tube
  2. Contains organ of Corti (organ of hearing)
  3. Semicircular canals are receptors for equilibrium and head movement
D. Function
  1. Transmission of sound waves; result is hearing
  2. Maintenance of equilibrium

Nursing Assessment

A. Nursing observations
  1. Difficulty hearing or understanding verbal communication
  2. Not responding to loud or sudden noises
  3. Use of hearing aid, lip reading, or sign language
  4. Drainage, dried secretion, or deformities of the ear
B. Resident description (subjective data)
  1. Earache or headache
  2. Difficulty hearing (or lack of hearing) in one or both ears
  3. Itching, drainage, pressure, or full feeling
  4. Ringing, buzzing, popping, or echoes
  5. Vertigo
  6. Medications taken
C. Note history of:
  1. Ear infections
  2. Ear surgery
  3. Head injury
  4. Medication taken

Diagnostic Tests/Methods

A. Audiometry: a hearing test to determine ability to discriminate sounds, voices, and degrees of loudness and pitch

B. Otoscopy: visual examination of the ear canal and tympanic membrane
C. Weber's test: a tuning fork is struck and placed midline on the resident's forehead; the resident is asked where the sound is heard; in this test of conduction, sounds should be heard equally well in both ears
D. Rinne's test: the tuning fork is struck and placed on the mastoid process of the skull behind the ear; the fork is removed, and the resident indicates when the sound can no longer be heard; the still-vibrating fork is then placed near the external ear canal; normally the sound will be heard longer through air conduction than through bone

THE RESIDENT WITH IMPAIRED HEARING

A. Definition
  1. Conductive hearing loss occurs when injury or disease interferes with the conduction of sound waves to the inner ear (e.g., cerumen in canal)
  2. Sensory hearing loss occurs when there is malfunction of the inner ear, auditory nerve, or auditory center in the brain (e.g., toxic effect to eighth cranial nerve from drugs [aspirin])
B. Resident problems
  1. Inability to communicate
  2. Inability to hear hazards in the environment (e.g., automobiles)
  3. Frustration, anxiety, anger, and insecurity
  4. Misinterpretation of communication
C. Treatment: according to cause; frequently none

HEARING DEFICIENCIES/INTERVENTIONS

A. Older residents usually do poorly on hearing tests because of their cautious responsiveness
B. Reduce distractions
C. Do not fatigue with unnecessary noise and talk
D. Speak in a normal tone of voice; shouting is misinterpreted by those who have normal hearing
E. Observe for signs of developing hearing loss
  1. Leaning forward
  2. Inappropriate responses
  3. Cupping ear when listening
  4. Loud speaking voice
  5. Requests to repeat what has been said
F. Reduce background noise before speaking (e.g., television and radio)

G. Hearing deficits increase social isolation, suspiciousness, and fear
H. Speak toward the better ear
I. Be sure to have the person's attention before speaking
J. Use resources and aids for the hearing impaired (e.g., television and telephone amplifiers, sound lamps, and alarm clocks that shake the bed)
K. Remove cerumen accumulation if present; soften wax with ceruminolytic agent
L. Irrigate with body-temperature water under low pressure
M. Avoid using cotton-tip applicators (they push cerumen farther into canal and cause impaction)
N. Use a loud but low-pitched voice: raising the voice in a yelling manner will raise the high-frequency sounds even higher and cause the resident to hear less of the intended speech
O. Supplement words with exaggerated facial movements and body language
P. Give the resident the opportunity to ask for clarification or repetition

PRESBYCUSIS

Presbycusis is a sensorineural hearing loss experienced with age and is a common problem of older residents
A. Characterized by:
  1. Loss of the ability to hear high-pitched sounds
  2. As condition progresses, middle-low frequency sounds are difficult to hear
  3. Affects the ability to hear consonants more than vowels

CARE OF THE HEARING AID

A. Assessment:
  1. Assess resident's knowledge of and routines for cleansing and caring for hearing aid
  2. Determine whether resident can hear clearly with use of aid by talking slowly and clearly in normal voice tone
  3. Assess whether hearing aid is working by removing it from resident's ear. Close battery case and turn volume slowly to high. Cup hand over hearing aid. If squealing or a whistling sound (feedback) is heard, it is working. If no sound is heard, replace batteries and test again

4. Check ear mold for cracked or rough edges
5. Check for accumulation of cerumen around aid and plugging of opening in aid

Major Medical Diagnosis
MÉNIÈRE'S SYNDROME

A. Definition: a chronic disease with sudden attacks of vertigo and tinnitus (ringing in the ear) with progressive hearing loss; attacks last a few minutes to a few weeks; usually occurs in women over age 50
B. Cause: unknown; related to fluid in cochlea—either increased production or decreased absorption
C. Signs and symptoms
   1. Vertigo
   2. Nausea and vomiting
   3. Ringing in the ears and hearing loss
D. Diagnostic tests/methods: resident history
E. Treatment
   1. Diuretics, low-sodium diet, and dimenhydrinate (Dramamine)
   2. Surgery: destruction of the labyrinth as a last resort
F. Nursing intervention
   1. Bed rest; position of comfort
   2. Maintain quiet and safety
   3. Low-sodium diet
   4. Provide specific nursing care as that for resident with limited hearing
   5. Provide general preoperative and postoperative care
   6. Provide nursing care for resident after ear surgery

MASTOIDITIS

A. Definition: infection of the mastoid process; may be acute or chronic
B. Cause: extension of middle ear infection that was inadequately treated
C. Signs and symptoms
   1. Elevation of temperature
   2. Headache, ear pain, and tenderness over mastoid process
   3. Drainage from ear
D. Treatment
   1. Antibiotics
   2. Surgery
      a. Simple mastoidectomy: removal of infected cells
      b. Radical mastoidectomy: more extensive excision resulting in some degree of hearing loss
E. Nursing intervention
   1. Provide general preoperative and postoperative care
   2. Provide nursing care for resident after ear surgery

OTOSCLEROSIS

A. Definition: a progressive formation of new bone tissue around the stapes, preventing transmission of vibrations to the inner ear
B. Cause: unknown
C. Signs and symptoms
   1. Loss of hearing
   2. Ringing or buzzing (tinnitus)
D. Treatment
   1. Hearing aid
   2. Surgery; stapedectomy (removal of diseased bone and replacement with prosthetic implant)
E. Nursing intervention
   1. Provide general care for resident who is hearing impaired
   2. Give general preoperative and postoperative care
   3. Follow specific orders from physician
   4. Provide general nursing care for resident after ear surgery

Vision
OVERVIEW OF THE EYE

A. Lies in a protective bony orbit in the skull
B. Eyebrows, eyelids, and lashes also protect the eye
C. Sphere consists of three layers of tissue
   1. Sclera: thick, white, fibrous tissue (white of eye); a transparent section over the front of the eyeball, the cornea, permits light rays to enter
   2. Choroid: the middle vascular area: brings oxygen and nutrients to the eye: choroid extends to ciliary body (two smooth muscle structures), which helps control shape of the lens; the front is a pigmented section (iris), which gives the eye color; in the center of the iris is the pupil, the "window of the eye" (allows light to pass to lens and retina)

3. Retina: inner layer; physiology of vision takes place; contains receptors of optic nerve; neurons are shaped like rods and cones; cones permit perception of color, and rods permit perception of light and shade

D. Chambers
   1. Anterior: contains aqueous humor; maintains slight forward curve in cornea
   2. Posterior: contains vitreous humor: maintains spherical shape of eyeball

E. Conjunctiva: mucous membrane that covers eyeball and eyelid; keeps eyeball moist

F. Lens: transparent structure behind iris; focuses light rays on retina

G. Lacrimal apparatus: gland located in upper, outer part of eye; produces tears to lubricate and cleanse; nasolacrimal duct is located in nasal corner (tears drain into nose)

H. Function: vision

VISION INTERVENTIONS

A. Bright, diffused light is best
B. Place items on better-vision side
C. Avoid glare
D. Strips on stairs improve depth perception
E. Glasses should be kept clean (older residents frequently forget or ignore this)
F. Use colors that increase visual acuity, (i.e., red, orange, and yellow)
G. Avoid night driving
H. Use resources and aids for visually impaired
I. Preserve independence
J. Visual losses increase susceptibility to illusions, disorientation, confusion, and isolation
K. Place objects directly in front of individual with decreased peripheral vision
L. Stimulate other senses

NURSING INTERVENTIONS FOR VISION DEFICITS

A. Always identify yourself when approaching resident
B. Help strangers recognize resident's visual deficit by providing resident with a white cane or placing a sign on the door (may vary according to facility)
C. Make a special effort to keep the resident oriented
   1. Read newspapers and books to the resident; read mail if resident desires and approves
   2. Describe colors and layout of surroundings
   3. Have a radio available; use clocks that chime

D. Assist the resident with mobility and transfers
   1. Have resident hold your arm above the elbow rather than you holding the resident; walk naturally.

E. Warn resident when approaching stairs or curbs; describe depth and number

F. When seating resident, describe where seat is; place resident's hand on back of seat for orientation

G. Ensure safety of environment
   1. Keep doors completely open or closed
   2. Remove cords, furniture, buckets, and other obstacles from resident's path.
   3. Keep bed cranks in and slippers out of the way

H. Place resident's belongings and items on food tray in same location at all times to facilitate independent functioning

I. Explore with occupational therapist or local service agencies the use of assistive devices

J. Support resident's independence and involvement in social and life activities

Glaucoma

A. Definition: intraocular pressure increases because of a disturbance in the circulation of aqueous humor; there is an imbalance between production and drainage as the angle of drainage closes
   1. Acute (closed-angle) glaucoma: dramatic onset of symptoms; immediate treatment is required, usually surgery
   2. Chronic (open-angle) glaucoma: symptoms progress slowly and are frequently ignored; if disease is not detected early, it may lead to permanent loss of vision

B. Pathology
   1. Familial tendency
   2. Related to age; incidence increases over age 40
   3. Secondary to injuries and infections

C. Signs and symptoms
   1. Loss of peripheral vision, halos around lights, and permanent loss of vision (a leading cause of blindness)
   2. Pain, malaise, nausea, and vomiting
   3. Pupils fixed and dilated

D. Diagnostic tests/methods
  1. History of symptoms
  2. Measurement of visual fields
  3. Measurement of intraocular pressure

E. Treatment
  1. Miotics to decrease intraocular pressure
  2. Surgery: iridectomy (an incision through the cornea to remove part of the iris to allow for drainage); laser trabeculoplasty (relieves excess intraocular pressure)
  3. Continued medical supervision

F. Nursing intervention
  1. Encourage resident to wear medical identification tag
  2. Administer eye medications on schedule
  3. Inform the resident to avoid drugs with atropine; discourage straining and lifting
  4. Give preoperative and postoperative care according to that for a resident with a cataract; pay careful attention to specifics in physician's orders

Detached Retina

A. Definition: the sensory layer of the retina pulls away from the pigmented layer; vitreous humor may leak into the space occupying the position the retina normally assumes

B. Cause: usually unknown and spontaneous; may be related to sudden blow to the head or follow eye surgery (e.g., removal of cataract)

C. Signs and symptoms
  1. Loss of vision in affected area (may be complete loss)
  2. Visual disturbance (blurring)
  3. Spots and flashes of light

D. Diagnostic tests/methods
  1. Resident history and physical assessment
  2. Retinal examination with ophthalmoscope

E. Treatment: depends on area of detachment
  1. Bed rest
  2. Prevention of extension of detachment
  3. Mydriatics
  4. Surgical intervention

F. Nursing intervention
  1. Provide individual care according to location of detachment; physician's orders will be specific
  2. Maintain absolute rest; restrict activity; patch eye to limit eye movement

  3. Prepare resident for postoperative care: inform resident that both eyes may be patched and he may be unable to see
  4. Postoperative care: position resident exactly as ordered; maintain eye patch(es); have resident deep breathe and avoid coughing; administer medication for pain; provide care as needed for a person with limited sight

Conjunctivitis

A. Definition: infection or inflammation of the conjunctiva

B. Causes: bacteria, usually *Staphylococcus*, and allergens

C. Resident problems
  1. Very contagious (especially in young children)
  2. Purulent drainage and itching

D. Diagnostic method: physical assessment

E. Treatment: ophthalmic antibiotics

F. Nursing intervention
  1. Prevent transmission to others: encourage frequent hand washing
  2. Provide warm compresses; cleanse eyelids; remove crusts before administering ophthalmic medications
    a. Discourage rubbing of eyes
    b. Isolate personal items (towels, washcloths, and pillowcases)

Cataract

A. Definition: the crystalline lens becomes clouded and opaque (not transparent)

B. Causes
  1. Trauma
  2. Congenital
  3. Related to diabetes
  4. High incidence in older persons (senile cataracts)
  5. Heredity
  6. Infections
  7. Longtime exposure to the sun

C. Signs and symptoms
  1. Loss of vision
  2. Progressive blurring
  3. Haziness with eventual complete loss of sight

D. Diagnostic tests/methods
  1. Examination with ophthalmoscope

2. Resident history

E. Treatment: surgical removal of opaque lens, usually on an outpatient basis; after surgery, corrective lenses are necessary (glasses, contact lenses, or surgical implantation of an artificial lens)

F. Nursing intervention

1. Give general preoperative care
2. Provide nursing care as for the resident with low vision
3. Postoperative management depends on surgical procedure; be careful to adhere to physician's order
4. Caution resident to avoid:
   a. Coughing, sneezing, and aggressive nose blowing
   b. Strenuous exercise
   c. Constipation; straining during defecation
   d. Emotional stress
   e. Assess extent of visual deficits and assist resident with activities of daily living as needed
   f. Counsel resident to use eyes in moderation and prevent overuse or strain

Review Questions

1. A resident cannot close the left eye completely because of a recent injury. Nursing measures to protect the eye include:
   ① Irrigating the eye daily with sterile water
   ② Keeping the lights dim in the room
   ③ Instilling artificial tears and covering eye with a patch
   ④ Applying an antibiotic ointment to the lower eyelid

2. The nurse observes that a resident has sustained a contusion to the left eye from a recent fall. The nurse's initial intervention should be to:
   ① Apply a sterile patch immediately
   ② Apply an ice pack immediately
   ③ Apply warm compresses immediately
   ④ Irrigate the eye with saline solution

3. A resident asks for an explanation about glaucoma. The nurse explains that with glaucoma there is:
   ① An increase in the pressure within the eyeball

② An opacity of the crystalline lens or its capsule
③ A curvature of the cornea that becomes unequal
④ A separation of the neural retina from the pigment retina

4. When assisting the family to help an aphasic member to regain as much speech as possible, the nurse should instruct them primarily to:
   ① Speak louder than usual to the resident during visits
   ② Tell the resident to use the correct words when speaking
   ③ Give positive reinforcement for correct communication
   ④ Encourage the resident to speak, while being patient with all attempts

5. The nurse should identify glaucoma as the physiologic result of a(n):
   ① Increase in the vitreous humor fluid
   ② Increase in the intraocular pressure
   ③ Decrease in the aqueous fluid
   ④ Decrease in the intraocular pressure

6. The resident with glaucoma should not receive:
   ① Atropine sulfate
   ② Morphine sulfate
   ③ Meperidine hydrochloride (Demerol)
   ④ Hydroxyzine hydrochloride (Vistaril)

7. A resident has difficulty communicating because of expressive aphasia following a cerebral vascular accident. When the nurse asks the resident how he is feeling, his wife answers for him. The nurse should:
   ① Ask the wife how she knows how the resident feels
   ② Instruct the wife to let the resident answer for himself
   ③ Acknowledge the wife but look at the resident for a response
   ④ Return later to speak to the resident after the wife has gone home

8. When a mydriatic eye medication has been administered, the nurse should observe for:
   ① Decreased drainage
   ② Constriction of the pupil
   ③ Dilatation of the pupil
   ④ Decreased intraocular pressure

9. When assessing a resident with Ménière's disease, the nurse should expect the resident to experience:
   ① Nystagmus
   ② An increase in temperature
   ③ Diarrhea
   ④ A decrease in pulse rate

10. An air-conduction hearing aid increases hearing sensitivity in instances of:
    ① Diminished sensitivity of the cochlea
    ② Perforation of the tympanic membrane
    ③ Immobilization of the auditory ossicles
    ④ Destruction of the auditory nerve

11. When caring for a resident with angle-closure glaucoma, the nurse should understand that the goal of therapy is:
    ① Controlling intraocular pressure
    ② Dilating the pupil to allow for an increase in visual field
    ③ Resting the eye to reduce pressure
    ④ Preventing secondary infections that can add to the visual problem

ANSWERS AND RATIONALES FOR REVIEW QUESTIONS

1. **3** Artificial tears and a patch will protect the cornea from drying, trauma, and ulceration.
   1 Will not protect cornea over long period of time.
   2 Will not protect cornea over long period of time.
   4 Will not protect cornea over long period of time.

2. **2** Prevents edema, facilitates vasoconstriction, increases blood viscosity, and acts as local anesthetic.
   1 No indication for an eye patch.
   3 Inappropriate to promote vasodilation and reduce blood viscosity at this time.
   4 No indication for irrigation.

3. **1** An increase in intraocular pressure (IOP) results from a resistance of aqueous humor outflow; open-angle glaucoma, the most common type of glaucoma, results from increased resistance to aqueous humor outflow through the trabecular meshwork, Schlemm's canal, and the episcleral venous system.
   2 This is the description of a cataract.
   3 This is the description of astigmatism.
   4 This is the description of a detached retina.

4. **4** In addition to the extent of injury, a factor in relearning speech is the resident's motivation and effort; the more the resident attempts to talk, the more likely speech will progress to its optimal level; relearning is a slow process.
   1 Resident with aphasia are not deaf.
   2 This will cause frustration and anger in the resident.
   3 Although the nurse should instruct the family to approve and support every effort by the resident to communicate, their action would provide external rather than internal motivation and is therefore not as effective.

5. **2** Increased intraocular pressure is a result of a blockage of the aqueous humor fluid in the anterior chamber of the eye.
   1 The vitreous humor is in the posterior chamber of the eye.
   3 An increase, not a decrease, of aqueous fluid causes glaucoma.
   4 In glaucoma there is an increase, not a decrease, in the intraocular pressure.

6. **1** Dilates the pupil and increases intraocular pressure.
   2 Morphine sulfate is a sedative and is not usually contraindicated for a resident with glaucoma.
   3 Meperidine hydrochloride is a narcotic analgesic and is not usually contraindicated for a resident with glaucoma.
   4 Hydroxyzine hydrochloride is a mild sedative and minor tranquilizer and is usually not contraindicated for use in a resident with glaucoma.

7. **3** The opportunity must be provided for the resident to practice language skills; family participation must be accepted and recognized.
   1 This demeans the spouse and cuts off communication.
   2 This demeans the spouse and cuts off communication.
   4 The spouse should be included and involved in the resident's care.

8. **3** Mydriatic action.
   1 Antiinfective action.
   2 Miotic action.
   4 Osmotic action.

9. **1** Jerky lateral eye movement, particularly toward the involved ear.
   2 Not usually associated with Ménière's disease.
   3 Not usually associated with Ménière's disease.
   4 Not usually associated with Ménière's disease.

10. **1** Since air-conduction hearing aids utilize the person's own middle ear, they increase hearing acuity in cases of diminished sensitivity of the cochlea. The amplified signal from the hearing aid gives the cochlea greater stimulation and promotes hearing.
    2 Perforation of the tympanic membrane prevents ossicular conduction, which involves transmission of resonant vibrations from the tympanic membrane to the ossicles of the cochlea; hearing aids will not correct this.
    3 Immobilization of the ossicles prevents conduction of resonant vibrations from the tympanic membrane to the cochlea; air-conduction hearing aids will not correct this problem.
    4 Destruction of the auditory nerve results in deafness, because impulses cannot be transmitted to the brain's auditory center.

11. **1** Glaucoma is a disease in which there is increased intraocular pressure resulting from narrowing of the aqueous outflow channel (Schlemm's canal). This can lead to blindness caused by compression of the nutritive blood vessels supplying the rods and cones.
    2 Pupil dilatation increases intraocular pressure because it narrows Schlemm's canal.
    3 Intraocular pressure is not affected by activity of the eye.
    4 Increased intraocular pressure can result in blindness and therefore must be reduced; although secondary infections are not desirable, the priority is to maintain vision.

Pharmacology

Principles of Drug Action
MECHANISMS OF DRUG THERAPY

A. Dissolution: disintegration of dosage form; dissolution of an active substance

B. Absorption: the process that occurs between the time a substance enters the body and the time it enters the bloodstream

C. Distribution: the transport of drug molecules within the body

D. Metabolism: biotransformation—the way in which drugs are inactivated by the body

E. Excretion: elimination of a drug from the body

VARIABLES THAT AFFECT DRUG ACTION

A. Dosage

B. Route of administration

C. Drug-diet interactions: food slows absorption of drugs; some foods containing certain substances react with certain drugs

D. Drug-drug interactions
  1. Additive effect: occurs when two drugs with similar actions are taken together
  2. Synergism (potentiation): a total effect of two similar drugs that is greater than the sum of the effects if each is taken separately
  3. Interference: occurs when one drug interferes with the metabolism or elimination of a second drug, resulting in intensification of the second drug
  4. Displacement: occurs when one drug is displaced from a plasma protein-binding site by a second, causing an increased effect of the displaced drug
  5. Antagonism: a decrease in the effects of drugs caused by the action of one on the other

E. Age
  1. Children: depends on age and developmental stage
  2. Older adults: physiologic changes may alter a drug's actions in the body
     a. **Pharmacokinetics in Older Adults**

(1) Absorption	↑ Gastric pH or acidity
	↓ Intestinal blood flow
(2) Distribution	↓ Lean body mass
	↑ Adipose (fat) stores
	↓ Total body water
	↓ Serum albumin
(3) Metabolism	↓ Liver size
	↓ Liver blood flow
	↓ Liver functions (microsomal enzyme activity)
(4) Excretion	↓ Kidney function

F. Body weight: affects drug action mainly in relation to dosage

G. Pathologic conditions: disease processes are capable of altering drug mechanisms (e.g., residents with kidney disease have increased risk of drug toxicity)

H. Psychologic considerations: attitudes and expectations influence resident response (e.g., anxiety can decrease effect of analgesics)

ADVERSE REACTIONS TO DRUGS

A. Idiosyncratic reaction: unusual, unexpected reaction usually the first time a drug is taken

B. Allergic reactions: stimulate antibody reactions from the immune system of body
  1. Urticaria (hives)
  2. Anaphylaxis: severe allergic reaction involving cardiovascular and respiratory systems; may be life-threatening

C. Gastrointestinal effects
   1. Anorexia
   2. Nausea, vomiting
   3. Constipation
   4. Diarrhea
   5. Abdominal distention
D. Hematologic effects
   1. Blood dyscrasia
   2. Bone marrow depression
   3. Blood coagulation disorders
E. Hepatotoxicity
   1. Hepatitis
   2. Biliary tract obstruction or spasms
F. Nephrotoxicity: renal insufficiency or failure; kidney stones
G. Drug dependence
   1. Physiologic: physical need to relieve shaking; pain
   2. Psychologic: need to relieve feeling of anxiety; stress
H. Teratogenicity: ability of a drug to cause abnormal fetal development

TOLERANCE AND CROSS TOLERANCE

A. Tolerance: acclimation of the body to a drug over a period of time so that larger doses must be given to achieve the same effect
B. Cross tolerance: tolerance to pharmacologically related drugs

FACTORS THAT MAY COMPLICATE DRUG THERAPY IN OLDER ADULTS

Older adults:
A. Are living longer
B. Have one or more chronic diseases
C. Receive prescriptions from two or more prescribing physicians
D. Undergo physiologic changes that may result in
   1. Altered pharmacokinetics
   2. Altered pharmacodynamics
E. Limited income may affect continuity of drug therapy
F. Average use of prescription and OTC drugs much higher than general population
G. Polypharmacy has resulted in increased reports of drug interactions, side effects, and adverse reactions
H. Cognitive impairment, sensory-perceptual alterations, and impaired mobility may contribute to problems with self-administration of medications

I. **Selected Problem Medications in Older Adults**

Medication	Response
1. digoxin, digitalis preparations	Visual disorders, nausea, diarrhea, cardiac arrhythmias, hallucinations
2. anticholinergics (antispasmodics)	Blurred vision, dry mouth, constipation, confusion, urinary retention, tachycardia
3. phenothiazines	Hypotension, tremors, extrapyramidal side effects, restlessness
4. analgesics, opioid	Confusion, constipation, urinary retention, nausea, vomiting, respiratory depression, addiction
5. analgesics, non-narcotic (aspirin)	Tinnitus, gastric distress, GI bleeding
6. anticoagulant (heparin, warfarin)	Bleeding episodes, hemorrhage
7. antihypertensives (e.g., methyldopa)	Nausea, hypotension, diarrhea, bradycardia, heart failure
8. antiarthritics (e.g., ibuprofen)	Edema, nausea, abdominal distress, gastric ulceration, and/or bleeding
9. thiazide diuretics	Electrolyte imbalance (hypokalemia), rashes, fatigue, leg cramps, dehydration
10. hypnotic-sedatives	Confusion, daytime sedation and ataxia, lethargy, increased forgetfulness

PREVENTING AND REPORTING ERRORS

To prevent medication administration errors, the following guidelines should be observed:
A. Question the calculations or order if it appears that multiple tablets or several vials are necessary to prepare a single dose.
B. Carefully read all labels for all the "Five Rights," including the drug's name—the pharmacist can make a mistake too, by sending the wrong medication.
C. Be wary about ambiguous orders or drug names, or drug names that include numerals. Consult with the prescriber if in doubt.
D. Be alert to unusually large dosages or excessive increases in dosages ordered.

E. When in doubt, check the order with the prescriber, a pharmacist, and the literature. Check even simple calculations with a peer.

F. Double-check with a resident with known allergies as new drugs are added to the treatment plan.

G. Routinely refer to drug interaction charts. Commit common interactive drugs to memory.

H. Question the use of nonstandard abbreviations and symbols; do not use them yourself.

I. Read the package insert carefully for specific instructions when giving a drug for the first time.

J. Do not use slang names or colloquialisms that may be unfamiliar to others.

K. Do not decipher illegible orders or make assumptions. Do not accept incomplete orders. Obtain a clear copy from the prescriber.

L. Do not accept verbal or telephone orders except in an emergency.

M. Question a drug form used in an unfamiliar way (e.g., suspensions are usually given orally; an intravenous [IV] drug form ordered to be administered by feeding tube).

N. Question an unusual single order containing more than one drug.

INTRAVENOUS INFUSIONS

Administration of a large amount of fluid into a vein

A. Purposes
   1. To restore or maintain electrolyte balance
   2. To supply drugs for immediate effect
   3. To replace nutrients and vitamins
   4. To replace blood loss

B. Calculation of Drip Rate for Intravenous Infusion
   1. Information that must be known
      a. Volume of solution to be infused
      b. Length of time over which this volume is to be infused
      c. Number of drops per milliliter delivered by the administration set being used
   2. The drip rate may be calculated as follows:
      a. Find the volume of fluid to be administered per hour

$$\frac{\text{Milliliters of fluid to be infused}}{\text{Number of hours for infusion}} =$$

Milliliters of fluid per hour

      b. Find the volume of fluid to be administered per minute

$$\frac{\text{Milliliters of fluid per hour}}{60 \text{ min/hr}} =$$

Milliliters to run per minute

      c. Multiply the milliliters of fluid to run per minute by the number of drops per milliliter delivered by the infusion set; this gives the number of drops that should fall in the drip chamber per minute

Milliliters per minute ×

drops per milliliter =

Drops per minute

EXAMPLE: Administer 1000 ml of dextrose 5% in water (D_5W) over 8 hours using an infusion set that delivers 10 gtt per minute

$$\frac{1000 \text{ ml}}{8 \text{ hr}} = 125 \text{ ml/hr}$$

$$\frac{125 \text{ ml/hr}}{60 \text{ min/hr}} = 2.1 \text{ ml/min}$$

2.1 ml/min × 10 gtt ml = 21 gtt/min

      d. If the administration rate has been ordered as milliliters per hour, step 1 above is omitted

      e. Alternate formula to calculate drip rate

$$\frac{\text{Milliliters to administer} \times \text{Drops per milliliter}}{\text{Hours to run} \times 60 \text{ min/hr}} =$$

Drops per minute

EXAMPLE: Administer 1000 ml of D_5W over 8 hours using an infusion set that delivers 10 gtt/min

$$\frac{1000 \text{ ml} \times \text{gtt/ml}}{8 \text{ hr} \times 60 \text{ min/hr}} = 21 \text{ gtt/min}$$

f. Adjust the flow rate to the number of drops per minute as calculated; assess the fluid volume at hourly intervals to see that the fluid is being administered at the desired rate; the calculated drip rate is an approximation of the actual flow rate; the type of solution, additives, position of the resident or infusion tubing, height of the reservoir, and volume of fluid in the container can influence the actual drip rate; the nurse should verify computations with another knowledgeable nurse before readjusting the drip rate to ensure volume delivery for the prescribed time

C. Intravenous fluids
   1. Dextrose solution: contains 2.5%, 5%, 10%, 20%, 40%, 50%, 60%, and 70% dextrose; the 20% to 50% solutions are used for calories in total parenteral nutrition (TPN) and administered through a central or subclavian catheter
   2. Dextrose and sodium chloride solution: most commonly used concentrations are 5% dextrose in 0.25% or 0.45% sodium chloride
   3. Amino acid solution (Aminosyn): contains essential and nonessential amino acids; most often used with dextrose in TPN
   4. Liposyn, Intralipid: concentrated calories and essential fatty acids; most often used as part of TPN

D. Fluid and electrolyte imbalance
   1. Signs and symptoms
      a. Muscle twitching
      b. Convulsions
      c. Vital sign changes
      d. Diarrhea
      e. Oliguria
      f. Restlessness, weakness, delirium
      g. Flat or distended neck veins
      h. Decreased skin turgor
      i. Thirst
      j. Anorexia, nausea, vomiting
      k. Pitting edema
      l. Pulmonary crackles

E. Monitor rate of flow
F. Monitor site for pain, tenderness, redness, or swelling
G. Change site dressing and IV tubing per facility policy
H. Document interventions
I. Electronic flow-rate regulators
   1. Monitor function
   2. Follow manufacturer's directions
   3. Double check flow rate
   4. Explain purpose and alarm system to resident

J. Complications
   1. Infiltration
   2. Thrombophlebitis
   3. Bacteremia
   4. Circulatory overload
   5. Air embolism
   6. Mechanical failure

K. Blood transfusion: infusion of whole blood from a healthy person into a recipient's vein
   1. Blood is typed and cross matched before administration to determine compatibility
   2. Nurse's responsibility for blood transfusion
      a. Check and double-check
        (1) The labels (indicate type and product)
        (2) The numbers (cross-referenced with laboratory documentation)
        (3) The Rh factor
        (4) Compatibility
      b. Stay with resident for at least the first 5 minutes after transfusion is started
      c. Monitor rate of transfusion frequently
      d. Assess resident for signs of adverse reactions frequently
        (1) Hemolytic reaction: stop transfusion immediately, keep vein open with slow drip normal saline solution, and notify physician immediately; indications include
          (a) Headache
          (b) Sensations of tingling
          (c) Difficulty in breathing
          (d) Pain in lumbar region or legs
        (2) Allergic reactions: stop transfusion immediately and notify physician; indications include
          (a) Pruritus
          (b) Hives (urticaria)
          (c) Difficulty in breathing
        (3) Febrile reactions resulting from contaminant in the blood: usually occurs late in the transfusion or after it is completed; indications include

(a) Flushed skin
(b) Elevated temperature
(c) General malaise
(d) Signs of systemic infection
(4) Circulatory overload can lead to pulmonary edema; indications include
(a) Increased pulse rate
(b) Dyspnea
(c) Respiratory distress
(d) Moist coughing
(e) Expectoration of blood-tinged mucus
(5) Anticoagulant reaction: indications include
(a) Tingling in the fingers
(b) Muscular cramping
(c) Convulsions
3. Blood extracts: specific components of whole blood that meet specific needs of the resident
a. Packed red blood cells (RBCs)
b. Plasma
c. Human albumin
d. Fibrinogen
e. Gamma globulin

Central Nervous System
DEPRESSANTS

A. Characteristics of drug-induced central nervous system (CNS) depression
1. Mild: disinterest in surroundings, inability to focus on a topic or to initiate talking or movement, slowed pulse and respirations
2. Moderate or progressive: drowsiness or sleep, decreased muscle tone and ability to move, diminished acuity of all sensations—touch, vision, hearing, heat, cold, or pain
3. Severe: unconsciousness or coma, loss of reflexes, respiratory failure, death
B. Analgesics: drugs used to relieve pain
1. Narcotic analgesics (opioids: morphine, prototype)
a. Actions
(1) Raises pain perception threshold
(2) Reduces fear and anxiety
(3) Induces sleep
(4) Depresses respiratory and cough centers in medulla

(5) Inhibits gastric, biliary, and pancreatic secretions; depressing gastrointestinal tract
(6) Stimulates release of antidiuretic hormone, resulting in decreased urine volume
(7) Induces hypotension
(8) Slows heart rate
(9) Causes pupillary constriction
2. Agents

Examples	Comments
Alphaprodine hydrochloride (Nisentil)	Not given orally; schedule II drug
Anileridine hydrochloride (Leritine)	Schedule II drug
Butorphanol tartrate (Stadol)	Currently not classified as a controlled drug
Codeine sulfate	Schedule II drug
Codeine phosphate	
Hydromorphone hydrochloride (Dilaudid)	Schedule II drug
Levorphanol tartrate (Levo-Dromoran)	Schedule II drug
Meperidine hydrochloride (Demerol)	Schedule II drug
Methadone hydrochloride (Dolophine, Methadose)	Also used as a replacement drug for opiate dependence or to ease withdrawal; schedule II drug
Morphine sulfate	Poor oral absorption; schedule II drug
Nalbuphine hydrochloride (Nubain)	Currently not classified as a controlled drug
Oxycodone hydrochloride (Percodan)	Schedule II drug
Oxymorphone hydrochloride (Numorphan)	Schedule II drug
Pentazocine hydrochloride (Talwin)	Schedule IV drug; oral preparation
Pentazocine lactate (Talwin)	Schedule IV drug; parenteral preparation
Propoxyphene hydrochloride (Darvon)	Schedule IV drug
Propoxyphene napsylate (Darvon-N)	Schedule IV drug

c. Adverse reactions and contraindications
   (1) Nausea and vomiting
   (2) Constipation
   (3) Urinary retention
   (4) Pruritus
   (5) Hypotension
   (6) Morphine can cause respiratory depression, so it is used cautiously for residents with impaired respiratory function; it is not used for residents with head injury as it will obscure CNS evaluation
d. Dependency: develops rapidly
   (1) There is a distinct physical reaction when the drug is suddenly stopped and the body readjusts to functioning in the absence of the drug (abstinence syndrome); symptoms include
      (a) Runny nose
      (b) Goose flesh
      (c) Tearing
      (d) Yawning
      (e) Muscle twitching and abdominal cramping
      (f) Insomnia
      (g) Nausea and vomiting
      (h) Diarrhea
   (2) Methadone hydrochloride is used for detoxification and maintenance
e. Acute toxicity: usual cause of death is respiratory depression; treated with support to respiration and with a narcotic antagonist such as levallorphan tartrate (Lorfan), nalorphine hydrochloride (Nalline), or naloxone hydrochloride (Narcan)

2. Nonnarcotic analgesics/antiinflammatory analgesics
   a. Action: sensitization of peripheral pain receptor
   b. Agents
      (1) Acetylsalicylic acid (aspirin): effective in management of low-intensity pain
         (a) Adverse reactions
            ■ Gastric irritation
            ■ Ulceration and gastric bleeding
            ■ Intoxication (salicylism): tinnitus, reversible hearing loss, hyperventilation, fever, metabolic acidosis, vomiting, hypokalemia, convulsions, coma, and death
         (b) Drug interactions with aspirin
            ■ Anticoagulants: increase likelihood of bleeding
            ■ Alcohol: increases likelihood of gastrointestinal irritation and bleeding
      (2) Acetaminophen (Datril, Tylenol): effective in management of low-intensity pain; does not produce gastric irritation or alter platelet function and bleeding times as does aspirin; does not interact with oral anticoagulants; prolonged use or frequent high doses can cause liver and kidney damage
      (3) Nonsteroidal antiinflammatory drugs (NSAIDs): effective in treatment of osteoarthritis, degenerative joint disease, rheumatic diseases
         (a) Adverse reactions
            ■ Heartburn/indigestion
            ■ Nausea/vomiting
            ■ Constipation or diarrhea
            ■ Fluid retention
            ■ Hypertension
            ■ Dizziness
            ■ Blurred vision
            ■ Skin rash
         (b) Drug interactions vary because of the chemical makeup of the various NSAIDs
         (c) Agents: the following are examples: Ibuprofen (Motrin, Nuprin, Advil); Indomethacin (Indocin); Meclofenamate sodium (Meclomen); Phenylbutazone (Azolid); Piroxicam (Feldene)

3. Nursing assessment: determine character, location, onset, contributing factors, duration of pain, time of last dose
4. Nursing management
   a. Determine the most effective way to manage the pain: drug versus nondrug measure (e.g., repositioning, turning, massage, visual imagery)
   b. Obtain vital signs
      (1) Be alert to hypotension/hypertension
      (2) Analyze rate and character of respiration
      (3) Withhold drug and notify physician in presence of respiratory depression: respiratory rate of 10 or less respirations per minute or a decrease of 8 or more respirations per minute from baseline data
   c. Advise resident to remain quiet after drug administration to decrease possible nausea and vomiting
   d. Implement safety measures: use side rails and advise resident to remain in bed if there are changes in mental status: alterations in judgment or unsteadiness
   e. Initiate intake and output records to determine effectiveness of bladder function
   f. Determine efficacy of bowel activity
   g. Resident instruction concerning:
      (1) How to take the drug
      (2) Safe storage in the home
      (3) Avoidance of driving
      (4) Danger of simultaneous administration of alcohol or other CNS depressant with narcotics
5. Nursing evaluation
   a. Subjective interviewing: ask if resident is comfortable
   b. Objective observations
      (1) Decreased restlessness and anxiety
      (2) Ability to function
C. Anesthetics: provide a pain-free experience during an operative procedure along with a relaxed state of mind and sense of security

1. General anesthetics: provide loss of pain sensation, loss of consciousness, loss of memory, and loss of voluntary and some involuntary muscle activity
   a. Inhalation agents: the following are examples

Cyclopropane	Methoxyflurane
Ether	(Penthrane)
Halothane	Nitrous oxide

   b. Intravenous agents: the following are examples

Droperidol	Methohexital
(Inapsine)	sodium
	(Brevital)
Droperidol–Fentanyl	Thiamylal
citrate (Innovar)	sodium
	(Surital)
Ketamine hydro-	Thiopental
chloride	sodium
	(Pentothal)

2. Regional anesthetics: provide loss of sensation and motor activity in localized areas of the body
   a. Types
      (1) Topical
      (2) Infiltration
      (3) Peripheral nerve blocks
      (4) Spinal
      (5) Epidural
      (6) Caudal
   b. Agents: the following are examples
      (1) Carbocaine
      (2) Novocain
      (3) Nupercaine
      (4) Pontocaine
      (5) Xylocaine
3. Nursing assessment
   a. Preoperative: obtain health history including allergies, psychologic status, physiologic baseline data
   b. Postoperative: determine vital signs and respiratory function
4. Nursing management
   a. Preoperative: prepare resident physically and psychologically; initiate measures to prevent complications: deep breathing and bed exercises; administer preoperative medications; initiate safety measures and provide quiet environment

b. Postoperative: preserve quiet atmosphere; maintain airway, control pain using careful nursing judgment; prevent complications by encouraging deep breathing, coughing

5. Nursing evaluation
   a. Preoperative: effects of preoperative medication
   b. Postoperative: concerned with pulmonary complications, thrombophlebitis, infection, or other complications

D. Anticonvulsants: drugs used to control seizures

1. Action: not completely understood; thought to depress neuron excitability and to modify the ability of brain tissue to respond to stimuli that initiate seizure activity

2. Agents

Examples	Adverse reactions
a. Long-acting barbiturates Mephobarbital (Mebaral) Phenobarbital (Luminal) Primidone (Mysoline)	Sedation, drowsiness, tolerance, nystagmus, ataxia, anemia, congenital malformations in fetus; sudden withdrawal can induce convulsions
b. Hydantoins Ethotoin (Peganone) Mephenytoin (Mesantoin) Phenytoin (Dilantin)	Nystagmus, ataxia, slurred speech, tremors, nervousness, drowsiness, fatigue, overgrowth of the gums (gingival hyperplasia), occasional folic acid or vitamin D deficiency; congenital malformations in fetus
c. Succinimides Ethosuximide (Zarontin) Methsuximide (Celontin) Phensuximide (Milontin)	Gastrointestinal irritation, dizziness, drowsiness, headache, fatigue

2. Agents—cont'd

Examples	Adverse reactions
d. Oxazolidinediones Trimethadione (Tridione)	Serious allergic dermatitis, kidney and liver damage, vertigo, photophobia, spontaneous abortion, congenital malformations
e. Benzodiazepines Clonazepam (Klonopin) Diazepam (Valium)	Drowsiness, ataxia, personality changes
f. Miscellaneous Acetazolamide (Diamox)	Loss of apetite, drowsiness, confusion
Carbamazepine (Tegretol)	Drowsiness, dizziness, ataxia, double vision, gastrointestinal upset
Lidocaine hydrochloride (Xylocaine)	Depressed heart action
Paraldehyde	Bronchopulmonary irritation, thrombophlebitis at intravenous injection site
Valproic acid (Depakene)	Gastrointestinal distress, sedation

3. Nursing assessment: observe course of the seizure; assist in case finding; assess baseline data with concentration on areas known to be affected by the drug, e.g., phenytoin (Dilantin): assess mouth, teeth, and gums for development of gingival hyperplasia

4. Nursing management: instruct resident concerning
   a. Drug characteristics
   b. Importance of taking medication even when resident is seizure free; awareness that reaching a therapeutic level may take time
   c. Wearing or carrying identification indicating seizure activity and drugs and dosages being taken
   d. Reducing gastric irritation by taking drug with meals
   e. Good gum massage

5. Nursing evaluation: continued medical follow-up; blood level tests at regular intervals

E. Skeletal muscle relaxants: drugs used to treat muscle spasticity

    1. Action: thought to restore some inhibitory tone in neural pathways from the brain or spinal cord or by acting within the muscle itself by interfering with the intracellular release of calcium necessary to initiate contraction

    2. Agents

Examples	Adverse reactions
a. Drugs to treat spasticity	Drowsiness, incoordination, gastrointesintal upset
Baclofen (Lioresal)	
Dantrolene sodium (Dantrium)	Liver damage
Diazepam (Valium)	Drowsiness, incoordination
b. Drugs to treat muscle spasm	Drowsiness, dizziness
Carisoprodol (Rela, Soma)	
Chlorphenesin carbamate (Maolate)	
Chlorzoxazone (Paraflex)	
Cyclobenzaprine hydrochloride (Flexeril)	
Dantrolene (Dantrium)	
Diazepam (Valium)	
Meprobamate (Miltown, Equanil)	
Methocarbamol (Delaxin, Robaxin)	
Orphenadrine citrate (Flexon, Norflex)	

    3. Nursing assessment: obtain baseline data, focusing on spasticity, including degree, aggravating factors, associated pain, and interference with activities of daily living (ADLs); observe baseline liver function studies

    4. Nursing management: monitor for drug effectiveness and side effects; institute safety measures if drowsiness occurs

5. Nursing evaluation: at regular intervals, assess the continuing degree of spasticity

F. Antiparkinsonian drugs: drugs used in the management of Parkinson's disease

    1. Action: restores action of the neurotransmitter dopamine to the basal ganglia of the brain or blocks the effects of excessive action of acetylcholine

    2. Agents

Examples	Adverse reactions
a. Anticholinergics	Dry mouth, constipation, urinary retention, blurred vision; impairment of recent memory, confusion, insomnia, and restlessness
Benztropine mesylate (Cogentin)	
Biperiden (Akineton)	
Cycrimine hydrochloride (Pagitane hydrochloride)	
Ethopropazine hydrochloride (Parsidol)	
Procyclidine hydrochloride (Kemadrin)	
Trihexyphenidyl hydrochloride (Artane, Pipanol, Tremin)	
b. Antihistamines	Sedation
Chlorphenoxamine hydrochloride (Phenoxene)	
Diphenhydramine hydrochloride (Benadryl)	
Orphenadrine citrate (Disipal)	
c. Other drugs	
Amantadine hydrochloride (Symmetrel)	Dry mouth, constipation, urinary retention, blurred vision
Levodopa (Dopar, Larodopa)	Nausea, vomiting, anorexia, orthostatic hypotension, GI bleeding, cough, hoarseness, dyspnea, blurred vision, increased sex drive
Carbidopa-levodopa (Sinemet)	Same as Levodopa

G. Sedatives, hypnotics, antianxiety drugs
   1. Sedatives: small dose to calm an anxious resident
   2. Hypnotics: larger dose to induce sleep
   3. Antianxiety drugs (minor tranquilizers): drugs used to treat anxiety
   4. Barbiturates: classified according to duration of action: ultra short-acting, short-acting, intermediate-acting, and long-acting
      a. Action: produce CNS depression ranging from sedation to anesthesia
      b. Adverse reactions
         (1) Mild withdrawal symptoms: rebound REM sleep, nightmares, daytime agitation, and a "shaky" feeling
         (2) Acute overdose: depression of medullary centers regulating respiration and cardiovascular system—tachycardia, hypotension, loss of reflexes, marked depression of respiration
      c. Agents: the following are examples
         (1) Amobarbital (Amytal, Tuinal)
         (2) Butabarbital sodium (Butalan, Butisol Sodium)
         (3) Pentobarbital (Nembutal)
         (4) Phenobarbital (Luminal)
         (5) Secobarbital (Seconal)
   5. Benzodiazepines
      a. Action: produce CNS depression
      b. Adverse reactions: daytime sedation, motor incoordination, dizziness, headaches; schedule IV substances
      c. Agents: the following are examples
         (1) Chlordiazepoxide hydrochloride (Librium)
         (2) Clorazepate dipotassium (Tranxene)
         (3) Diazepam (Valium)
         (4) Flurazepam hydrochloride (Dalmane)
         (5) Lorazepam (Ativan)
         (6) Oxazepam (Serax)
         (7) Prazepam (Verstran, Centrax)
   6. Miscellaneous
      a. Action: produce CNS depression; generally short acting
      b. Agents

Examples	Adverse reactions
Chloral betaine (Beta-Chlor)	Gastric irritation; schedule IV substance
Chloral hydrate (Noctec)	Gastric irritation; schedule IV substance
Ethchlorvynol (Placidyl)	Muscular weakness, schedule IV substance
Glutethimide (Doriden)	Dilated pupils, dry mouth; schedule III substance
Hydroxyzine hydrochloride (Vistaril)	Dry mouth, hypotension, blurred vision, urinary retention
Meprobamate (Equanil, Miltown)	Schedule IV substance
Methaqualone (Quaalude, Sopor, Parest)	Paresthesia, peripheral neuropathy; schedule II substance
Methyprylon (Noludar)	Schedule II substance

   7. Nursing assessment: give special attention to vital signs, level of consciousness, sleep patterns
   8. Nursing management: observe for signs of CNS depression; identify nondrug solutions to sleep problems; monitor safety aspects of care; instruct resident concerning self-medication, medical follow-up, and drug-dependence potential
   9. Nursing evaluation: review purpose for which drug is given and observe effectiveness

H. Alcohol
   1. Action: produces CNS depression: sedation, disinhibition, sleep, anesthesia; vasodilation; gastric irritation
   2. Effects of an acute overdose: death, accidents, hangover: upset stomach, thirst, fatigue, headache, depression, anxiety; chronic toxicity can lead to liver, esophagastrointestinal, and cardiovascular disorders
   3. Withdrawal symptoms after chronic use: tremors, anxiety, tachycardia, increased blood pressure, diaphoresis, anorexia, nausea, vomiting, insomnia, hallucinations, seizures, delirium tremens

4. Treatment of withdrawal: one of the benzodiazepines; restoration of normal metabolic functions, and vitamin B_1, B_{12}, and folic acid
5. Aversion therapy: disulfiram (Antabuse) given to detoxified individuals who wish to avoid drinking again; produces unpleasant reaction in presence of alcohol: flushing, throbbing in head and neck, respiratory difficulty, nausea, copious vomiting, diaphoresis, fainting, dizziness, blurred vision, confusion

PSYCHOTHERAPEUTIC AGENTS

A. Antidepressants: characteristic of drug-induced prevention or relief of depression
   1. Tricyclic antidepressants
      a. Action: primarily used to relieve symptoms of endogenous depression; also used to treat mild exogenous depression
      b. Agents: the following are examples
         (1) Amitriptyline hydrochloride (Elavil)
         (2) Clomipramine hydrochloride (Anafranil)
         (3) Doxepin hydrochloride (Adapin, Sinequan)
         (4) Imipramine hydrochloride (Tofranil)
         (5) Nortriptyline hydrochloride (Aventyl Hydrochloride, Pamelor)
   2. Monoamine oxidase (MAO) inhibitors
      a. Action: relieve symptoms of severe reactive or endogenous depression that has not responded to tricyclic antidepressant therapy, electroconvulsive therapy, or other modes of psychotherapy
      b. Agents: the following are examples
         (1) Isocarboxazid (Marplan)
         (2) Phenelzine sulfate (Nardil)
         (3) Tranylcypromine sulfate (Parnate)
   3. Nursing assessment: obtain complete health history, history of insomnia, fatigue, or loss of motivation; observe motor movements, facial expression and posture; assess for any feelings of suicide
   4. Nursing management: administer medication with food to avoid gastric distress

5. Nursing evaluation: observe for adverse effects such as drowsiness
6. Education: stress compliance of taking medication as ordered; instruct resident to avoid using alcohol with sleeping pills and hay fever or cold medications because doing so increases the effects of these medications; caution resident regarding drug/food interactions

B. Antipsychotic drugs
   1. Phenothiazines/thioxanthenes
      a. Action: primarily to reduce or relieve symptoms of acute and chronic psychoses, including schizophrenia, schizoaffective disorders, and involutional psychoses
      b. Agents: the following are examples
         (1) Chlorpromazine (Thorazine)
         (2) Promazine hydrochloride (Sparine)
         (3) Thioridazine hydrochloride (Mellaril)
         (4) Trifluoperazine hydrochloride (Stelazine)
         (5) Triflupromazine hydrochloride (Vesprin)
   2. Nursing assessment: obtain complete health history, current use of medications, and possibility of pregnancy; obtain history of emotional unrest, agitation, paranoid ideation, delusions, and inability to cope with reality
   3. Nursing management: administer medication with food or milk to avoid or reduce gastric distress
   4. Nursing evaluation: observe for adverse effects such as urinary retention, change in vision, sore throat with fever, muscle spasms, trembling, or shaking of hands, skin rash, yellow tinge to skin or eyes, uncontrollable movements of the tongue

C. Antimanic drugs: used to treat manic-depressive psychoses in the acute manic phase; also used to prevent recurrent episodes of mania in the manic-depressive patient
   1. Agent: lithium carbonate (Lithane, Carbolith)
   2. Nursing assessment: obtain complete health history, possibility of pregnancy, and medications currently being taken; observe for restlessness, hyperactivity, aggressiveness

3. Nursing management: ensure adequate fluid and electrolyte balance
4. Nursing evaluation: monitor serum lithium levels to avoid drug toxicity and reduce side effects
5. Education: stress compliance of taking medication as ordered; instruct resident to wear medical identification tag

D. Neuroleptic extrapyramidal adverse effects

1. Tardive dyskinesia (TD)
   a. A potentially irreversible neurologic disorder that primarily involves the buccolingual and masticatory muscles.
   b. This adverse effect to the antipsychotic agents may occur within a few months or years of treatment or after these agents have been discontinued.
   c. The risk of inducing TD increases with total dosage of the drug given and the length of the treatment period.
   d. Incidence: although 0.5% to 65% of the treated population may develop this syndrome, recent reports place the percentage of residents at risk as 10% to 20%.
   e. Presenting features:
      (1) Facial: grimacing or scowl expression, facial tics, arching of the eyebrows
      (2) Ocular: blinking, eyelid spasms (blepharospasm)
      (3) Oral/buccal: lip smacking, lower lip thrusting, sucking, puffing of the cheeks, chewing of the cheeks (the inside of the mouth should be checked for this)
      (4) Lingual/masticatory: lateral jaw movements, tongue protrusion or thrusting such as "fly catching movements," tongue in lip or cheek, resulting in an observable bulge in the specific area
      (5) Systemic effects: foot tapping; rocking from side to side; arms, hands, and fingers may display a jerking and/or a writhing motion (choreoathetoid motion); pelvic thrusting motions
   f. Treatment: prevention only. Early assessment and diagnosis is crucial in preventing the development of an irreversible disorder. Decreasing or discontinuing the antipsychotic agent if possible is the recommended procedure. At present, there is no known effective treatment for TD.

2. Akathisia
   a. Description:
      (1) Motor restlessness; person unable to sit or stand still, feels urgent need to move, pace, rock, or tap foot.
      (2) May also present as apprehension, irritability, and general uneasiness and may be mistaken for agitation.
   b. Incidence
      (1) More common in women than in men; usually occurs in 5 to 30 days (up to 90 days) of starting drug therapy.
   c. Treatment: lower dose of neuroleptic agent, switch to a different drug, or administer an antiparkinson drug, such as benztropine

3. Dystonia
   a. Description:
      (1) Acute reaction requiring immediate intervention. Resident exhibits muscle spasms of face, tongue, neck, jaw, and/or back. Hypertension of neck and trunk and arching of back.
      (2) Tongue may protrude; facial grimaces; exaggerated posturing of head, neck, or jaw; difficulty swallowing and/or talking. Person may have a fixed upward gaze and/or eye muscle spasms. May be accompanied by excessive salivation.
   b. Commonly occurs after large doses of neuroleptics, usually within an hour up to a week of drug therapy. Occurs more often in men than women.
   c. Treatment: depending on the severity of reaction, one or more of the following may be necessary; lower neuroleptic dose, administer benztropine IM or IV, or diphenhydramine

4. Drug-induced Parkinson

a. Description:
  (1) Symptoms similar to Parkinson's disease; shuffling gait, drooling, tremors, increased rigidity (cogwheel). Bradykinesia (slow movements) and akinesia (immobility) also reported.
b. Treatment:
  (1) Add antiparkinson drug, such as benztropine or diphenhydramine
  (2) Physician may switch to a neuroleptic less likely to induce this effect, such as thioridazine
5. Nursing assessment: regular schedule of assessment for abnormal movements. Commonly used scales included Abnormal Involuntary Movement Scale (AIMS) and Dyskinesia Identification System Condensed User Scale (DISCUS).

STIMULANTS

Stimulants are medically accepted only for treatment of narcolepsy, hyperkinetic behavior in children, and obesity. Occasionally, they are used for depression in older adults and to reverse respiratory depression from CNS depressants.

A. Amphetamines
  1. Action: increase the release and effectiveness of catecholamine neurotransmitters in the brain and peripheral nerves and create increased alertness and sensitivity to stimuli
  2. Adverse reactions
    a. Gastrointestinal system: vomiting, diarrhea, abdominal cramps, dry mouth, anorexia
    b. CNS: restless behavior, tremor, irritability, talkativeness, insomnia, mood changes, excessive aggressiveness, confusion, panic, increased libido
    c. Autonomic nervous system: headache, chilliness, palpitation, pallor or facial flushing
    d. Children: growth retardation
  3. Agents: the following are examples
    (1) Amphetamine sulfate
    (2) Dextroamphetamine sulfate (Dexedrine, Ferndex)
    (3) Methamphetamine hydrochloride (Desoxyn)
    (4) Methylphenidate (Ritalin)
    (5) Pemoline (Cylert)
  4. Nursing assessment: obtain thorough history of resident's presenting problem; obtain vital signs, weight, and height in children
  5. Nursing management: monitor height, weight, and vital signs; inquire about relief of subjective symptoms such as insomnia, agitation, headache, and irritability; begin preparation of resident and family for long-term management
  6. Nursing evaluation: success of goals of therapy evaluated
    a. Hyperkinesis: less hyperactivity and a more normal attention span
    b. Narcolepsy: ability to remain awake and alert during specified appropriate time periods

B. Appetite suppressants: used to help control obesity
  1. Action: exert an anorectic effect on the appetite-control center in the brain
  2. Agents

Examples	Adverse reactions
Amphetamine sulfate (Benzedrine)	See Amphetamines
Benzphetamine (Didrex)	See Amphetamines
Caffeine	Nervousness, jitteriness, gastrointestinal bleeding, nausea, vomiting, excessive CNS stimulation, and convulsions
Caffeine sodium benzoate injection	Same as caffeine
Dextroamphetamine sulfate (Dexedrine)	See Amphetamines
Diethylpropion hydrochloride (Propion, Tenuate)	Dry mouth, constipation; schedule IV drug
Doxapram hydrochloride (Dopram)	Dizziness, apprehension, disorientation
Fenfluramine hydrochloride (Pondimin)	Sedation and depression; schedule IV drug
Mazindol (Sanorex)	Insomnia, dizziness, agitation; schedule III drug
Methamphetamine hydrochloride (Desoxyn, Obedrin-LA)	See Amphetamines

2. Agents—cont'd

Examples	**Adverse reactions**
Nikethamide (Coramine)	Hypertension, tachycardia, tremors, flushing, increased body temperature, convulsion
Phendimetrazine tartrate (Bacarate)	Gastrointestinal distress; schedule III drug
Phenmetrazine hydrochloride (Preludin)	Schedule II drug; see Amphetamines
Phentermine hydrochloride (Adipex-P, Fastin, Tora)	Insomnia; schedule IV drug
Phenylpropanolamine hydrochloride (Acutrim, Control, Diadax, Dexatrim)	Blood pressure increases
Theophylline	Increased heart rate, nervousness, jitteriness, nausea, vomiting, excessive CNS stimulation, and convulsions

3. Nursing assessment: obtain vital signs and weight, discuss usual eating habits, and establish reasonable goals for losing weight
4. Nursing management: promote weight reduction, monitor for adverse reactions, offer support
5. Nursing evaluation: instruct resident concerning medication and its potential for drug abuse; assess achievement of goal—weight loss

C. Respiratory stimulants (analeptics): used to stimulate respiration when it has been depressed by drugs, asphyxiation, or electric shock
  1. Action: stimulates CNS medullary centers controlling respiration, vasomotor tone, and vagal tone
  2. Agents: see Amphetamines, p. 154
  3. Nursing assessments: check respiratory rate and depth of respirations; may measure vital capacity and arterial blood gas levels

4. Nursing management: monitor vital signs with focus on respirations; keep suction machine at bedside
5. Nursing evaluation: observe whether resident is breathing at a rate and depth nearing normal and whether short-term hospitalization is necessary

Autonomic Nervous System
CHOLINESTERASE INHIBITORS (CHOLINERGIC AGENTS)

A. Description: drugs that produce a physiologic response similar to that of acetylcholine released on nerve stimulation
B. Action
  1. Direct-acting cholinergic stimulants: mimic the action of acetylcholine
  2. Indirect-acting cholinergic stimulants: inhibit the enzyme cholinesterase, which acts to limit acetylcholine action
C. Effects
  1. Vasodilation
  2. Lowered blood pressure
  3. Slowing of heart rate
  4. Salivation
  5. Perspiring
  6. Increased tone and movement in the gastrointestinal and genitourinary systems
  7. Increased tone and contractility in striated muscles
D. Adverse reactions: heart block, arrhythmias, hypotension, hypertension, nausea, vomiting, cramps, diarrhea, heartburn, muscle weakness, increase in intraocular pressure
E. Agents: the following are examples
  1. Ambenonium chloride (Mytelase Chloride, Mysuran)
  2. Demecarium bromide (Humorsol)
  3. Echothiophate iodide (Phospholine iodide)
  4. Edrophonium chloride (Tensilon)
  5. Isoflurophate (Floropryl)
  6. Neostigmine bromide (Prostigmin)
  7. Pyridostigmine bromide (Mestinon)
F. Nursing assessment: history of lung disease, hyperthyroidism
G. Nursing management: monitor vital signs; insert rectal tube to relieve flatus
H. Nursing evaluation: observe for adverse reactions, bowel activity, intake and output records

PARASYMPATHETIC BLOCKING AGENTS (PARASYMPATHOLYTIC OR CHOLINERGIC BLOCKING AGENTS)

A. Action: prevent acetylcholine released by nerve stimulation from exerting its effects
B. Effects:
  1. Gastrointestinal: slows peristalsis
  2. Heart: increases rate
  3. Secretions: depresses all body secretions including perspiration and respiratory, salivary, pancreatic, and gastric secretions
  4. Eye: dilates pupils (mydriasis); paralyzes ciliary muscles; increases intraocular pressure
C. Adverse reactions: dry skin, delirium, convulsions, tachycardia, convulsions, mydriasis, hypertension, dry mouth, urinary retention
D. Agents

Examples	Clinical uses
Atropine sulfate	Adjunct to anesthesia, antispasmodic, cardiac stimulant
Cyclopentolate hydrochloride (Cyclogyl)	Mydriatic, cycloplegic
Homatropine hydrobromide	Mydriatic, cycloplegic
Scopolamine hydrobromide (Hyoscine)	Sedative-hypnotic, adjunct to anesthesia, antiemetic, mydriatic, cycloplegic
Isopropamide iodide (Darbid)	Antispasmodic
Methantheline bromide (Banthine)	Antispasmodic
Propantheline bromide (Pro-Banthine)	Antispasmodic
Benztropine mesylate (Cogentin)	Antiparkinsonian agent
Procyclidine hydrochloride (Kemadrin)	Antiparkinsonian agent
Trihexyphenidyl hydrochloride (Artane)	Antiparkinsonian agent

E. Nursing assessment: monitor vital signs; tachycardia; bowel functions; stimulation or depression of central nervous system; elevation in temperature; respiratory status; history of urinary difficulty; familial history of glaucoma
F. Nursing management: maintain oral hygiene for dry mouth; initiate methods to prevent abdominal distention, and constipation and safety measures in presence of blurred vision
G. Nursing evaluation: establish intake and output records when these drugs are given to elderly males; observe for effectiveness of drug

NEUROMUSCULAR BLOCKING AGENTS

A. Action: act at the striated neuromuscular junction to produce paralysis of the voluntary muscles
B. Effects
  1. Produce muscular relaxation for insertion of endotracheal tubes during surgical interventions
  2. Protect against violent thrashing that occurs with electroconvulsive therapy
  3. Alleviate spasms that accompany tetanus
C. Adverse reactions: paralysis of respiration, which may be reversed with neostigmine or Tensilon
D. Agents: the following are examples
  1. Decamethonium bromide (Syncurine)
  2. Pancuronium bromide (Pavulon)
  3. Succinylcholine chloride (Anectine)
  4. Tubocurarine chloride (Tubarine)
E. Nursing assessment: elicit medical history: asthma, myasthenia gravis remission; potassium blood levels
F. Nursing management: cardiopulmonary resuscitation skills—have resuscitative equipment available; monitor vital signs
G. Nursing evaluation: observe for early signs of flaccid paralysis in muscles of face, neck, eyes

SYMPATHOMIMETIC DRUGS: ADRENERGIC STIMULANTS

A. Actions
  1. Act directly on adrenergic receptors to produce either excitation or inhibition of a particular effector organ
  2. Act indirectly by releasing the stored catecholamines, norepinephrine, and epinephrine
B. Major effects
  1. Excitation of the heart, both its rate and force of contraction
  2. Excitation and constriction of smooth muscle in blood vessels
  3. Inhibition and relaxation of smooth muscles in bronchi, gastrointestinal tract, and skeletal muscle blood vessels

4. Metabolism: release of fatty acids from adipose tissue and increased gluconeogenesis in muscle and liver
5. Excitation of functions controlled by CNS (e.g., respiration)
6. Suppression of appetite
7. Lessening of fatigue

C. Adverse reactions: anxiety, apprehension, headache, arrhythmias, cerebral hemorrhage, heart failure, pulmonary edema

D. Agents

Examples	Clinical indications
Dopamine hydrochloride (Intropin)	Hypotension
Ephedrine hydrochloride (Bronkotabs)	Bronchospasms, nasal decongestion, allergy
Epinephrine bitartrate (Medihaler-Epi)	Acute or chronic bronchial asthma, allergic disorders, acute hypersensitivity to drugs
Epinephrine hydrochloride (Adrenalin Chloride)	Cardiac arrest, heart block, acute asthma, adjunct to local anesthesia, acute hypersensitivity to drugs Ophthalmic use: control hemorrhage, decrease intraocular pressure
Isoproterenol hydrochloride (Isuprel)	Bronchodilation, cardiac stimulant
Isoproterenol sulfate (Medihaler-Iso)	Bronchodilation
Mephentermine sulfate (Wyamine)	Maintain blood pressure during anesthesia
Metaraminol bitartrate (Aramine)	Hypotension
Naphazoline hydrochloride (Privine)	Nasal decongestion
Norepinephrine bitartrate (Levophed, Noradrenalin)	Shock, cardiac arrest
Nylidrin hydrochloride (Arlidin)	Peripheral vascular disease

E. Nursing assessment: obtain history of hyperthyroidism, diabetes, hypertension, emotional lability, heart disease

F. Nursing management: monitor vital signs; check infusion rate often; observe for infusion infiltration; record bowel and urinary activity

G. Nursing evaluation: monitor effect on blood pressure, pulse rate, and regularity of heart rate; observe for therapeutic and adverse effects

ADRENERGIC RECEPTOR BLOCKERS AND NEURON BLOCKERS

A. Action: interfere with peripheral adrenergic activity by blocking alpha and beta receptors, by depleting peripheral neural stores of norepinephrine, and by inhibiting peripheral sympathetic activity through an action on the CNS

B. Adverse reactions: postural hypotension, miosis, inhibition of ejaculation, headache, intense vasoconstriction, diarrhea, nausea, disturbances of vision, insomnia, depression

C. Agents

Examples	Clinical indications
Clonidine (Catapres-TTS)	Chronic hypertension
Ergoloid mesylate (Hydergine)	Mental and emotional complaints of the elderly
Guanethidine monosulfate (Ismelin)	Hypertension
Methyldopa (Aldomet)	Hypertension
Metoprolol tartrate (Lopressor)	Chronic hypertension, angina prophylaxis
Nadolol (Corgard)	Chronic hypertension, angina prophylaxis
Phenoxybenzamine hydrochloride (Dibenzyline)	Peripheral vascular disease
Phentolamine mesylate (Regitine)	Hypertension secondary to pheochromocytoma, adrenal tumor surgery
Prazosin hydrochloride (Minipress)	Chronic hypertension
Propranolol hydrochloride (Inderal)	Chronic hypertension, angina prophylaxis, cardiac dysrhythmias, migraine headaches

C. Agents—cont'd

Examples	Clinical indications
Reserpine (Serpasil)	Chronic hypertension
Timolol maleate (Timoptic)	Glaucoma
Tolazoline hydrochloride (Priscoline)	Peripheral vascular disease

D. Nursing assessment: ascertain if resident has history of ulcer disease, diabetes, ulcerative colitis, emotional depression, renal problems, coronary heart disease, predisposition to asthma, or congestive heart failure

E. Nursing management: aim instruction toward resident compliance; administer medications with meals or milk; maintain safety measures in presence of postural hypotension; monitor vital signs

F. Nursing evaluation: observe for therapeutic and adverse reactions; observe for changes in sleep patterns and appetite and depression or suicidal tendencies

GANGLIONIC AGENTS

A. Action: reduces sympathetic tone, particularly in the cardiovascular system

B. Adverse reactions: postural hypotension, pupillary dilation, blurring vision, dry mouth, constipation

C. Agents

Examples	Clinical indications
Mecamylamine hydrochloride (Inversine)	Hypertensive crisis, chronic hypertension
Pentolinium (Ansolysen) tartrate	Hypertensive crisis, chronic hypertension
Trimethaphan camsylate (Arfonad)	Hypertensive crisis

D. Nursing assessment: obtain baseline vital signs; assess factors contributing to hypertension such as diet, weight, exercise, and lifestyle

E. Nursing management: instruction aimed at resident compliance

F. Nursing evaluation: observe for therapeutic effects and adverse reactions

Respiratory System
ANTIHISTAMINES

A. Action: blocks histamine effects at the receptor site

B. Adverse reactions: sedation, drowsiness, dry mouth, blurred vision, urinary retention, constipation; can also stimulate the nervous system, especially in children, causing insomnia, irritability, and nervousness

C. Agents

Examples	Clinical indications
Brompheniramine maleate (Dimetane)	Colds, allergies
Carbinoxamine maleate (Clistin)	Colds, allergies
Chlorpheniramine maleate (Chlor-Trimeton, Teldrin, Chlortab)	Colds, allergies
Cyproheptadine hydrochloride (Periactin)	Pruritus
Dexchlorpheniramine maleate (Polaramine)	Colds, allergies
Dimethindene maleate (Forhistal)	Colds, allergies
Diphenhydramine hydrochloride (Benadryl)	Allergic reactions, motion sickness, mild parkinsonism
Meclizine hydrochloride (Bonine)	Motion sickness
Methdilazine (Tacaryl) hydrochloride	Pruritus
Promethazine hydrochloride (Phenergan, Promine, Remsed, Zipan)	Sedation, pruritus, motion sickness, nausea, vomiting
Trimeprazine tartrate (Temaril)	Pruritus
Tripelennamine hydrochloride (Pyribenzamine)	Colds, allergies

D. Nursing assessment: obtain vital signs; assess respiratory and cardiovascular status; ascertain if resident has history of allergy and extent and type of rash if present; instruct resident on dangers of operating machinery and to wear medical identification tag in presence of allergies

E. Nursing management: monitor respiratory response, vital signs, urinary and bowel function

F. Nursing evaluation: observe for therapeutic effects and adverse reaction

NASAL DECONGESTANTS

A. Action: sympathomimetic agents (see pp. 156-157) when applied to nasal mucosa or taken orally constrict the smooth muscle of arterioles in the nasal mucosa and thus reduce blood flow and edema

B. Adverse reactions: rebound nasal congestion if used too often; nervousness, irritability

C. Agents: the following are a few examples of the numerous preparations available
1. Allerest
2. Afrin
3. Contac
4. Coricidin
5. Dristan
6. Neo-Synephrine
7. Privine
8. Sine-Off
9. Sinutab
10. Sudafed

D. Nursing assessment: obtain history of irritants or environmental conditions contributing to symptoms and such objective data as respiratory rate and vital signs

E. Nursing management: instruct resident regarding medication use

F. Nursing evaluation: monitor for therapeutic effects and adverse reactions

EXPECTORANTS, ANTITUSSIVES, MUCOLYTIC DRUGS

A. Definitions
1. Expectorant: increases output of respiratory tract fluid that coats the bronchi and trachea
2. Antitussive: suppresses cough
3. Mucolytic: breaks up viscous mucus to allow for ease in expectoration of drainage

B. Adverse reactions
1. Expectorants: nausea, drowsiness; iodide base drugs: skin rash, metallic taste, fever, skin eruptions, mucous membrane ulcerations, salivary gland swelling
2. Antitussives: nausea, dizziness, constipation
3. Mucolytics: gastrointestinal upset

C. Agents: the following are examples
1. Expectorants: Robitussin, iodinated glycerol (Organidin), potassium iodide, SSKI

2. Antitussives: codeine, hydrocodone bitartrate, dextromethorphan hydrobromide (Romilar), Benylin, benzonatate (Tessalon)
3. Mucolytics: acetylcysteine (Mucomyst), Alevaire

D. Nursing assessment: obtain history relevant to cough, vital signs, and such objective data as character and quantity of secretions

E. Nursing management: monitor symptoms, vital signs, and amount of secretions with mucolytics

F. Education: instruct resident regarding drugs, how/when to take them and when they should be discontinued; encourage residents with persistent coughs to seek follow-up treatment

BRONCHODILATORS

A. Action: act on bronchial cells to dilate the bronchioles

B. Adverse reactions: CNS stimulation, increased heart rate, muscle tremors, headache, nausea, epigastric pain, bronchospasms

C. Agents: the following are examples
1. Aminophylline
2. Dyphylline (Dilin, Protophylline) Ephedrine sulfate (Slo-Fedrin)
3. Epinephrine (Sus-Phrine)
4. Epinephrine bitartrate (AsthmaHaler, Medihaler-Epi, Primatene Mist)
5. Epinephrine hydrochloride (Adrenalin Chloride)
6. Isoetharine hydrochloride (Bronkosol)
7. Isoetharine mesylate (Bronkometer)
8. Isoproterenol hydrochloride (Iprenol, Isuprel Hydrochloride)
9. Metaproterenol sulfate (Alupent, Metaprel)
10. Oxtriphylline (Choledyl)
11. Terbutaline sulfate (Brethine, Bricanyl)
12. Theophylline (many preparations)

D. Nursing assessment: obtain relevant history and vital signs; note amount and characteristics of secretions

E. Nursing management: monitor vital signs and closely monitor intravenous drugs; instruct resident regarding drug knowledge and usage

F. Nursing evaluation: observe for therapeutic effects

Cardiovascular System
DRUGS TO IMPROVE CIRCULATION

A. Action: vasoconstriction (direct- and indirect-acting sympathomimetic amines cause release of norepinephrine, which stimulates alpha receptors and thus produces vasoconstriction)
B. Adverse reactions: headache, anxiety, palpitation, nausea, vomiting, insomnia, tremors
C. Agents: the following are examples
   1. Dobutamine hydrochloride (Dubutrex)
   2. Dopamine hydrochloride (Intropin)
   3. Epinephrine hydrochloride (Adrenalin Chloride)
   4. Isoproterenol hydrochloride (Isuprel Hydrochloride)
   5. Mephentermine sulfate (Wyamine)
   6. Metaraminol bitartrate (Aramine)
   7. Methoxamine hydrochloride (Vasoxyl)
   8. Norepinephrine bitartrate (Levarterenol bitartrate; Levophed)
   9. Phenylephrine hydrochloride (Neo-Synephrine Hydrochloride, Isophrin)
D. Principal clinical use: treatment of cardiogenic and anaphylactic shock; to maintain blood pressure in life-threatening situations and during anesthesia
E. Nursing assessment: obtain pulse, respirations, and blood pressure; note level of consciousness
F. Nursing management: use infusion-control device to monitor IV administration; monitor vital signs frequently
G. Nursing evaluation: observe for therapeutic effects

VASODILATOR DRUGS (ANTIANGINAL DRUGS)

A. Action: dilate arterioles and veins to lower blood pressure, which reduces workload on the heart and decreases the heart's oxygen demand; increases circulation to cardiac muscle
B. Adverse reactions: flushing, headache, dizziness
C. Agents: the following are examples
   1. Amyl nitrite (Vaporole)
   2. Erythrityl tetranitrate (Cardilate)
   3. Isosorbide dinitrate (Iso-Bid, Isordil, Sorbide, Sorbitrate)
   4. Mannitol hexanitrate (Nitranitol)
   5. Nitroglycerin (Nitro-Bid)
   6. Nitroglycerine lingual aerosol (Nitrolingual Spray)
   7. Nitroglycerin ointment, 2% (Nitrol)
   8. Pentaerythritol tetranitrate (Peritrate)
   9. Trolnitrate phosphate (Metamine)
D. Nursing assessment: obtain vital signs and history relevant to onset and duration of pain
E. Nursing management: observe and monitor for additional angina attacks; instruct resident about prescribed drugs
F. Nursing evaluation: observe for therapeutic effects

VASODILATOR DRUGS FOR PERIPHERAL VASCULAR DISEASE

A. Action: work directly on vascular smooth muscle to cause relaxation or stimulate beta receptors in blood vessels to produce vasodilation
B. Adverse reactions: gastrointestinal upset, flushing, hypotension, dizziness, increased heart rate, headache
C. Agents: the following are examples
   1. Cyclandelate (Cyclospasmol)
   2. Ergoloid mesylates (dihydrogenated ergot alkaloids; Hydergine)
   3. Isoxsuprine hydrochloride (Vasodilan)
   4. Nylidrin hydrochloride (Arlidin, Rolidrin)
   5. Papaverine hydrochloride (many trade names)
   6. Tolazoline hydrochloride (Priscoline)
D. Nursing assessment: obtain history of onset and course of vascular disease; assess blood pressure, pulses, including peripheral pulses, mental status, and color of affected extremities
E. Nursing evaluation: observe for therapeutic and adverse effects
F. Nursing management: monitor presenting signs and symptoms; instruct resident regarding medications

ANTIHYPERTENSIVES

There are several subgroups of drugs that can lower blood pressure
A. Action
   1. Adrenergic drugs
      a. Beta-1 adrenergic receptor antagonists (beta-blockers): reduce cardiac output; reduce renin release from kidney (blocks response to sympathetic impulses)
      b. Alpha-1 adrenergic receptor antagonists: prevent norepinephrine from constricting blood vessels to increase resistance to blood flow

2. Centrally acting antihypertensive drugs that inhibit the activity of the sympathetic nervous system: decrease sympathetic tone and activate alpha receptors in the medulla that decrease heart rate and cardiac output
3. Vasodilators: relax arteriolar smooth muscle
4. Vasodilators in hypertensive emergencies: rapidly relax smooth muscle

B. Adverse reactions: bradycardia, hypotension, nasal congestion, reflex tachycardia, dry mouth, fluid retention, arthralgia, depression, drowsiness

C. Agents: the following are examples
1. Beta adrenergic receptor antagonists
   a. Metoprolol tartrate (Lopressor)
   b. Nadolol (Corgard)
   c. Propranolol hydrochloride (Inderal)
2. Alpha adrenergic receptor antagonists
   a. Phenoxybenzamine hydrochloride (Dibenzyline)
   b. Phentolamine mesylate (Regitine)
   c. Prazosin hydrochloride (Minipress)
3. Drugs interfering with norepinephrine
   a. Deserpidine (Harmonyl)
   b. Guanethidine monosulfate (Ismelin)
   c. Rauwolfia serpentina (Raudixin)
   d. Reserpine (Serpasil, Sandril)
4. Centrally acting antihypertensive drugs
   a. Clonidine hydrochloride (Catapres)
   b. Methyldopa (Aldomet)
5. Vasodilators
   a. Hydralazine hydrochloride (Apresoline)
   b. Minoxidil (Loniten)
6. Vasodilators: hypertensive emergencies
   a. Diazoxide (Hyperstat)
   b. Sodium nitroprusside (Nipride)
   c. Trimethaphan camsylate (Arfonad)

D. Nursing assessment: obtain vital signs and additional baseline data, such as weight, diet, and blood studies

E. Nursing management: monitor vital signs, intake and output, weight, blood studies; instruct resident regarding drugs

F. Nursing evaluation: observe for therapeutic effects and adverse reactions

G. Education: stress the importance of knowing acceptable ranges of blood pressure and pulse; taking medication as ordered; preventing orthostatic hypotension; and reporting asthmalike signs and symptoms

DIURETICS

A. Action: increase the excretion of sodium ion and thus increase urine flow

B. Agents

Examples	Clinical indications
Ethacrynic acid (Edecrin)	Dehydration, thrombosis, emboli, electrolyte imbalance
Furosemide (Lasix)	Acute dehydration, sodium and potassium depletion, calcium loss, dermatitis, blood dyscrasias
1. Thiazide diuretics Bendroflumethiazide (Naturetin) Benzthiazide (Aquatag, Urazide) Chlorothiazide (Diuril) Chlorthalidone (Hygroton) Cyclothiazide (Anhydron) Hydrochlorothiazide (Esidrix, HydroDiuril) Hydroflumethiazide (Saluron) Methyclothiazide (Enduron) Metolazone (Zaroxolyn) Polythiazide (Renese) Trichlormethiazide (Diurese, Naqua)	Fluid and electrolyte imbalance, increased calcium serum levels, gastrointestinal irritation, dizziness, headache, paresthesias, blood dyscrasias, allergy, hypotension
2. Carbonic anhydrase inhibitors Acetazolamide (Diamox) Ethoxzolamide (Cardrase, Ethamide)	
3. Organomercurials Mercaptormerin sodium (Thiomerin) Merethoxylline (Dicurin) procaine	Electrolyte imbalance, skin irritation, bone marrow toxicity, kidney toxicity

Agents—cont'd

Examples	Clinical indications
4. Potassium-sparing diuretics Spironolactone (Aldactone) Triamterene (Dyrenium)	Hyperkalemia, fatal cardiac dysrhythmias, endocrine alterations, blood dyscrasias

C. Nursing assessment: perform total resident assessment with emphasis on presenting signs and symptoms, vital signs, and laboratory blood studies
D. Nursing management: foster drug therapy such as by restrictions of fluid and diet; monitor weight, intake and output, and vital signs; instruct resident regarding drugs and diet
E. Nursing evaluation: observe for therapeutic effects and adverse reactions

CARDIOTONIC DRUGS (CARDIAC GLYCOSIDES)

A. Action: act directly on myocardial cells to increase contractility and thus cardiac output; slows heart rate
B. Adverse reactions: anorexia, nausea, vomiting, bradycardia, weakness, fatigue, visual dimming, double vision, altered color vision, mood alterations, hallucinations, dysrhythmias
C. Agents: the following are examples
   1. Digitoxin (Crystodigin)
   2. Digoxin (Lanoxin)
D. Nursing assessment: obtain baseline data, weight, vital signs, electrocardiogram (ECG) results
E. Nursing management: monitor vital signs, weight, fluid intake and output, serum electrolyte level, especially potassium; instruct resident regarding drugs
F. Nursing evaluation: observation for therapeutic effects and adverse reactions

DRUGS TO CONTROL DYSRHYTHMIAS

A. Action: slow conduction through atrioventricular (AV) node; block effects of vagal nerve stimulation; block beta adrenergic stimulation; suppress automaticity; increase electrical threshold for stimulation

B. Agents

Examples	Adverse reactions
Atropine	Dry mouth, cycloplegia, mydriasis, fever, urinary retention
Bretylium tosylate (Bretylol)	Anginal attacks, bradycardia, hypotension
Deslanoside (Cedilanid-D)	Bradycardia, premature ventricular beats, atrioventricular tachycardia, anorexia, nausea, vomiting
Digitoxin (Crystodigin, Purodigin)	
Digoxin (Lanoxin)	
Disopyramide phosphate (Norpace)	Dry mouth, constipation, urinary retention, blurred vision
Lidocaine (Xylocaine without epinephrine)	Muscle twitching, respiratory depression, convulsions, coma
Phenytoin (Dilantin)	Bradycardia, cardiac arrest, nausea, dizziness, drowsiness
Procainamide hydrochloride (Pronestyl)	Hypotension, decreased cardiac output, gastrointestinal distress
Propranolol hydrochloride (Inderal)	Bradycardia, lowered cardiac output, bronchospasm
Quinidine sulfate (Cin-Quin, Quinora) Quinidine gluconate (Duraquin) Quinidine polygalacturonate (Cardioquin)	Peripheral vasodilation, hypotension, gastrointestinal distress

C. Nursing assessment: obtain baseline data, history of subjective and objective symptoms, vital signs
D. Nursing management: monitor vital signs; instruct resident regarding drugs
E. Nursing evaluation: observe for therapeutic effects and adverse reactions

ANTICOAGULANTS

A. Action: inhibit the aggregation of platelets; interfere with any of the steps leading to the formation of fibrin
B. Adverse reactions: hemorrhage, hematuria, melena, rashes, depression of bone marrow

C. Agents: the following are examples
1. Antiplatelet drugs
   a. Aspirin
   b. Dipyridamole (Persantine)
   c. Sulfinpyrazone (Anturane)
2. Heparin sodium (Liquaemin Sodium, Panheprin, Lipo-Hepin)
3. Coumarins
   a. Dicumarol
   b. Phenprocoumon (Liquamar)
   c. Warfarin sodium (Coumadin, Panwarfin)
4. Indanediones
   a. Anisindione (Miradon)
   b. Phenindione (Hedulin)
D. Nursing assessment: obtain baseline data relevant to general condition of the resident, history of problems with clots, and blood coagulation studies: prothrombin time (PT), partial thromboplastin time (PTT), platelet count, and clotting times
E. Nursing management: monitor blood coagulation studies carefully; use infusion monitoring device for constant infusions of heparin; have drug antidotes readily available
F. Nursing evaluation: observe for therapeutic effects and adverse reactions
G. Education: stress home safety factors to prevent tissue trauma and bleeding; advise to avoid foods high in vitamin K; instruct resident to observe excreta for signs of bleeding
H. Drug interactions
1. Drugs potentiating response: clofibrate (Atromid-S), disulfiram (Antabuse), neomycin sulfate, phenylbutazone (Butazolidin), salicylates, sulfisoxazole (Gantrisin)
2. Drugs diminishing response: barbiturates, cholestyramine (Questran), ethchlorvynol (Placidyl), glutethimide (Doriden), griseofulvin (Grifulvin-V)
I. Antidotes
1. Heparin: protamine sulfate
2. Coumarins: vitamin K

THROMBOLYTIC DRUGS

A. Action: promote the digestion of fibrin to dissolve the clot
B. Agents: enzymes urokinase and streptokinase
C. Adverse reaction: hemorrhage

D. Special considerations: reserved for use in acute pulmonary embolism, deep vein thrombosis, or peripheral arterial occlusion; posttreatment: treated with heparin
E. Nursing assessment: obtain baseline data relevant to size, location, and symptoms of clot
F. Nursing management: used only in acute care setting; monitor laboratory blood studies and for signs of clot dissolution
G. Nursing evaluation: observe for therapeutic effects and adverse reactions

HEMOSTATIC AGENTS

A. Action: inhibit the dissolution of blood clots
B. Adverse reactions: nausea, cramps, dizziness, tinnitus, thrombophlebitis, flushing, vascular collapse
C. Agents

Examples	Clinical indications
1. Systemic agents Aminocaproic acid (Amicar)	Used in special surgical situations
Menadiol sodium diphosphate (Synkayvite) Menadione sodium bisulfite (Hykinone)	Correction of secondary hypoprothrombinemia, correction of severe vitamin K deficiency
Phytonadione; vitamin K (Aqua MEPHYTON, Konakion, Mephyton)	Oral anticoagulant overdose emergency
2. Local hemostatic agents Absorbable gelatin sponge (Gelfoam)	Control bleeding in wound or at operative site
Microfibrillar collagen hemostat (Avitene)	Control bleeding in wound or at operative site
Oxidized cellulose (Oxycel)	Control hemorrhage and absorb blood
Thrombin	Control bleeding in wound or at operative site

D. Nursing assessment: obtain baseline data relevant to type, location, and amount of bleeding, appropriate laboratory blood studies, and general condition of resident

E. Nursing management: monitor appropriate laboratory blood studies

F. Nursing evaluation: observe for therapeutic effects and adverse reactions

DRUGS THAT LOWER BLOOD LIPID LEVELS

A. Action: in general these drugs lower blood lipid concentrations

NOTE: no present proof that lowering blood lipid concentrations will reverse or halt atherosclerosis

B. Adverse reactions: bloating, nausea, constipation, muscle cramps, impotence, flushing, weight loss, insomnia, water retention

C. Agents: the following are examples
1. Aluminum nicotinate (Nicalex)
2. Beta sitosterol (Cytellin)
3. Cholestyramine resin (Questran)
4. Clofibrate (Atromid-S)
5. Colestipol hydrochloride (Colestid)
6. Dextrothyroxine (Choloxin)
7. Niacin; nicotinic acid (Nicobid, Niac, Nicolar)
8. Probucol (Lorelco)

D. Nursing assessment: obtain baseline data relevant to weight, serum cholesterol and triglyceride levels, blood pressure, and dietary history

E. Nursing management: observe for any new symptoms; instruct resident regarding drugs

F. Nursing evaluation: observe for adverse effects; monitor blood levels for therapeutic effects

DRUGS THAT TREAT NUTRITIONAL ANEMIAS

A. Action: supplement or replace essential vitamins and minerals

B. Agents

Examples	Clinical indications
1. Iron salts	Acute toxicity: acute nausea and vomiting, metabolic acidosis, extensive liver and kidney damage
Ferrous sulfate (Feosol, Fer-In-Sol, Fero-Gradumet, Mol-Iron)	
Ferrous gluconate (Fergon, Ferralet Plus, Entron)	Chronic toxicity: bronze coloration of skin, development of diabetes mellitus, heart failure
Ferrocholinate (Chel-Iron, Kelex)	

B. Agents—cont'd

Examples	Clinical indications
Ferrous fumarate (Ferranol, Feostat)	
Iron dextran injection (Imferon)	
2. Antidote for iron toxicity	
Deferoxamine mesylate (Desferal)	
3. Vitamin B$_{12}$	Virtually free of adverse reactions
Cyanocobalamin (Betalin 12 Crystalline, Redisol, Rubramin PC, Sytobex)	
Hydroxocobalamin (alphaRedisol)	
4. Folic acid for anemia	Nontoxic
Folic acid (Folvite)	
Leucovorin calcium	

C. Nursing assessment: obtain baseline data for vital signs, weight, dietary history, blood studies, and presence of neurologic symptoms

D. Nursing management: monitor blood studies, vital signs

E. Nursing evaluation: observe for therapeutic effects and adverse reactions; instruct resident regarding medications

F. Education: expect dark or black stools and the possibility of gastrointestinal distress

Gastrointestinal System
DRUGS THAT INCREASE TONE AND MOTILITY

A. Action: cholinomimetic action to stimulate or restore intestinal tone or urinary bladder tone

B. Adverse reactions: salivation, skin flushing, sweating, diarrhea, abdominal cramps

C. Agents: bethanechol chloride (Urecholine); neostigmine methylsulfate (Prostigmin)

D. Nursing assessment: obtain baseline data regarding vital signs, bowel sounds, fluid intake and output, bowel activity

E. Nursing management: stay with resident at least 15 minutes after administration to observe for adverse reactions; monitor vital signs, fluid intake and output, bowel activity

F. Nursing evaluation: observe for therapeutic effects and adverse reactions

DRUGS THAT DECREASE TONE AND MOTILITY (ANTICHOLINERGICS)

A. Action: inhibit gastric secretion and depress gastrointestinal motility
B. Adverse reactions: dry mouth, mydriasis, blurred vision, tachycardia, constipation, and acute urinary retention
C. Agents: the following are examples
    1. Anisotropine methylbromide (Valpin 50)
    2. Atropine sulfate
    3. Belladonna extract
    4. Belladonna tincture
    5. Dicyclomine hydrochloride (Bentyl, Di-Spaz)
    6. Diphemanil methylsulfate (Prantal)
    7. Glycopyrrolate (Robinul)
    8. Homatropine methylbromide (Homapin)
    9. Hyoscyamine hydrobromide
    10. Hyoscyamine sulfate (Anaspaz, Levsin)
    11. Mepenzolate bromide (Cantil)
    12. Methantheline bromide (Banthine)
    13. Methixene hydrochloride (Trest)
    14. Methscopolamine bromide (Pamine)
    15. Oxyphencyclimine hydrochloride (Daricon)
    16. Propantheline bromide (Pro-Banthine)
    17. Thiphenamil hydrochloride (Trocinate)
    18. Tridihexethyl chloride (Pathilon)
D. Nursing assessment: obtain baseline data for vital signs, frequency and character of stools, and presence of occult blood in stools
E. Nursing management: monitor vital signs; instruct resident regarding medication
F. Nursing evaluation: observe for therapeutic effects and adverse reactions

DRUGS TO TREAT ULCERS

A. Action:
    1. Antacids: neutralize gastric hydrochloric acid
    2. Anticholinergic drugs: see above and drugs under the Autonomic Nervous System, p. 156
    3. Antihistamines: block the histamines' receptors and decrease gastric acid production
B. Adverse reactions: constipation, diarrhea; can interfere with absorption of some drugs: tetracycline, digoxin, quinidine

C. Agents (antacids): the following are examples

Aluminum hydroxide (Amphojel) / Calcium carbonate (Dicarbosil, Tums) — Aluminum hydroxide / Magnesium hydroxide (Maalox)

Dihydroxyaluminum aminoacetate (Robalate) / Dihydroxyaluminum sodium carbonate (Rolaids) — Aluminum hydroxide / Magnesium trisilicate (Trisogel)

Magnesium hydroxide (Milk of Magnesia) / Aluminum hydroxide — Aluminum hydroxide gel / Magnesium hydroxide / Simethicone (Maalox Plus, Mylanta, Gelusil)

Calcium carbonate / Magnesium hydroxide (Camalox) — Aluminum phosphate gel (Phosphaljel) / Magaldrate (Riopan)

D. Agents (Histamine H_2-receptor antagonists): the following are examples
    1. Cimetidine (Tagamet)
    2. Famotodine (Pepcid)
    3. Ranitidine hydrochloride (Zantac)
E. Eradicating *Helicobacter pylori* bacteria
    1. Combination drugs
        a. Dual therapy
            (1) Omeprazole
            (2) Amoxicillin or clarithromycin
            (3) Two-week regimen
        b. Triple therapy
            (1) Bismuth subsalicylate
            (2) Metronidazole
            (3) Tetracycline or amoxicillin
            (4) 1- to 4-week regimen
        c. Quadruple therapy
            (1) Bismuth subsalicylate
            (2) Metronidazole
            (3) Tetracycline or amoxicillin
            (4) Omeprazole or ranitidine
            (5) 1-to 4-week regimen
    2. Administration caution
        a. Separate bismuth subsalicylate and tetracycline by 2 hours
        b. Administer tetracycline between meals (on an empty stomach) to avoid incompatibility with other agents
F. Nursing assessment: obtain baseline data relevant to vital signs, level of consciousness, character and quality of emesis and stool, appropriate laboratory blood studies

G. Nursing management: monitor vital signs, fluid intake and output, level of consciousness, and character of stools and vomitus

H. Nursing evaluation: observe for therapeutic effects and adverse reactions

ANTIEMETICS

A. Action: control nausea and vomiting by reducing stimulation of labyrinthine receptors; dopamine antagonists, which act on the chemoreceptor trigger zone in the medulla

B. Adverse reactions: drowsiness, blurred vision, dilated pupils, dry mouth, extrapyramidal symptoms

C. Agents: the following are examples
   1. Anticholinergics
      Scopolamine hydrobromide
   2. Antihistamines
      a. Dimenhydrinate (Dramamine)
      b. Diphenhydramine hydrochloride (Benadryl)
      c. Hydroxyzine pamoate (Vistaril)
      d. Meclizine hydrochloride (Antivert, Bonine)
      e. Promethazine hydrochloride (Phenergan)
   3. Miscellaneous drugs
      a. Benzquinamide hydrochloride (Emete-Con)
      b. Diphenidol hydrochloride (Vontrol)
      c. Trimethobenzamide hydrochloride (Tigan)
   4. Dopamine antagonists
      a. Chlorpromazine hydrochloride (Thorazine)
      b. Fluphenazine hydrochloride (Prolixin)
      c. Haloperidol (Haldol)
      d. Perphenazine (Trilafon)
      e. Prochlorperazine (Compazine)
      f. Promazine hydrochloride (Sparine)
      g. Triflupromazine hydrochloride (Vesprin)

D. Nursing assessment: obtain baseline data regarding vital signs, character and quantity of any emesis, presence of bowel sounds, fluid intake and output

E. Nursing management: monitor vital signs and fluid intake and output

F. Nursing evaluation: observe for therapeutic effects and adverse reactions

ANTIDIARRHETIC AGENTS

A. Action: decrease tone of small and large bowel; depress smooth muscle contraction; decrease release of acetylcholine; absorb toxins

B. Adverse reactions: respiratory depression, constipation, impaction

C. Agents: the following are examples
   1. Bismuth subsalicylate (Pepto-Bismol)
   2. Codeine phosphate
   3. Codeine sulfate
   4. Diphenoxylate hydrochloride with atropine sulfate (Diphenatol, Lomotil, Lofene)
   5. Loperamide hydrochloride (Imodium)

D. Nursing assessment: obtain baseline data relevant to vital signs, fluid and solid intake and output, nature and character of stools

E. Nursing management: monitor vital signs, intake and output, frequency and character of stools

F. Nursing evaluation: observe for therapeutic effects and adverse reactions

LAXATIVES

A. Action: retain water to keep stools large and soft; stimulate motility in large intestine; inhibit reabsorption of water; attract water by osmosis; soften feces

B. Adverse reactions: loss of bowel tone, dehydration, hypokalemia, hyponatremia, malabsorption of fat-soluble vitamins

C. Agents: the following are examples
   1. Bulk-forming agents
      a. Gum karaya
      b. Plantago seed (psyllium)
      c. Psyllium hydrocolloid (Effer-Syllium)
      d. Psyllium hydrophilic mucilloid (Metamucil)
   2. Stimulant cathartics (irritants)
      a. Bisacodyl (Bisco-Lax, Dulcolax)
      b. Cascara sagrada
      c. Castor oil
      d. Glycerin suppositories
      e. Phenolphthalein (Ex-Lax, Feen-A-Mint, Phenolax)
      f. Senna concentrate (Senokot)
      g. Senna pod
   3. Saline cathartics
      a. Magnesium hydroxide (Milk of Magnesia)

b. Magnesium sulfate (Epsom salt)
c. Monosodium phosphate (Sal Hepatica)
d. Sodium phosphate with sodium biphosphate (Phospho-Soda)

4. Lubricants
a. Mineral oil (Agoral Plain, Petrogalar Plain)

5. Fecal softeners
a. Docusate calcium (dioctyl calcium sulfosuccinate; Surfak)
b. Docusate sodium (dioctyl sodium sulfosuccinate; Colace, Comfolax, D-S-S)

D. Nursing assessment: obtain baseline data relevant to vital signs, intake and output, presence of bowel sounds, bowel habits, dietary history, medications

E. Nursing management: monitor diet and fluid intake; instruct resident regarding drugs

F. Nursing evaluation: observe for therapeutic effects and adverse reactions

Endocrine System
DRUGS AFFECTING PITUITARY GLAND

A. Action
1. Antidiuretic hormone (ADH): increases renal tubule's permeability and thus its ability to reabsorb water
2. Oxytocin: promotes uterine contractions during last stages of labor when cervix is fully dilated
3. Growth hormone: anabolic agent that increases cell size and cell numbers
4. Gonadotropic hormone (GTH): regulates maturation and function of male and female sexual organs
5. Adrenocorticotropic hormone (ACTH): stimulates adrenal cortex to release its hormone

B. Adverse reactions: hyponatremia, water retention, glycosuria, vasoconstriction, nausea

C. Agents

Examples	**Clinical indications**
Desmopressin acetate (DDAVP)	Diabetes insipidus
Lypressin (Diapid)	Diabetes insipidus
Posterior pituitary extract (Pituitrin)	Smooth muscle contraction
Vasopressin (Pitressin)	Short-term maintenance of unconscious resident

D. Nursing assessment: obtain baseline data relative to excesses or deficiencies of specific hormone

E. Nursing management: monitor fluid intake and output, laboratory values; instruct resident regarding medications

F. Nursing evaluation: observe for therapeutic effects and adverse reactions

DRUGS AFFECTING ADRENAL GLANDS

A. Action: replace the body's normal amount of hormones; block inflammatory responses; antineoplastic; antagonize autoimmune responses

B. Adverse reactions: impaired glucose tolerance or hyperglycemia; fat deposition; muscle weakness or wasting; peptic ulcer; growth inhibition; mood changes or psychosis; osteoporosis; sodium retention; potassium loss

C. Agents: dosage is individualized to resident and diagnosis; the following are examples
1. Betamethasone valerate (Valisone)
2. Cortisone (Cortone)
3. Desoxycorticosterone acetate (Doca, Percorten)
4. Dexamethasone (Decadron, Hexadrol)
5. Fludrocortisone acetate (Florinef)
6. Hydrocortisone (cortisol; Cortef, Cortril, Hydrocortone)
7. Hydrocortisone (Cortef) acetate
8. Methylprednisolone (Medrol, Wyacort)
9. Methylprednisolone acetate (Depo-Medrol)
10. Methylprednisolone sodium succinate (Solu-Medrol)
11. Prednisolone (Delta-Cortef, Paracortol)
12. Prednisolone sodium phosphate (Hydeltrasol)
13. Prednisone (Meticorten, Delta-Dome)
14. Triamcinolone (Aristocort, Kenacort)
15. Triamcinolone acetonide (Kenalog)
16. Triamcinolone hexacetonide (Aristospan)

D. Nursing assessment: obtain baseline data relevant to vital signs, weight, glycosuria

E. Nursing management: monitor vital signs, weight, serum electrolyte levels, sugar concentrations in blood and urine, signs of masked infection; instruct resident regarding medications

F. Nursing evaluations: observe for therapeutic effects and adverse reactions

DRUGS AFFECTING THYROID GLAND

A. Action
  1. Hypothyroidism: replace the body's normal amount of hormone
  2. Hyperthyroidism
      a. Control the symptoms of hyperthyroidisim
      b. Inhibit the synthesis of thyroid hormones
      c. Inhibit iodine uptake by thyroid gland
      d. Inhibit thyroid hormone release and symptoms
      e. Suppress continued uptake of iodine
      f. Destroy surrounding tissue by emission of low-energy radiation
B. Adverse reactions to drugs for hyperthyroidism: agranulocytosis, skin rash, nausea, vomiting, twitching muscles, bronchospasm, iodism, symptoms of hyperthyroidism
C. Adverse reactions to drugs for hypothyroidism: dysrhythmias, hypertension, headache, insomnia, irritability, vomiting, weight loss
D. Agents: the following are examples
  1. Hypothyroidism
      a. Natural thyroid hormones
          (1) Thyroglobulin (Proloid)
          (2) Thyroid (Delcoid, Thyrar, Thyrocrine)
      b. Synthetic thyroid hormones
          (1) Levothyroxine sodium (Eltroxin, Levoid, Synthroid)
          (2) Liothyronine sodium (Cytomel)
          (3) Liotrix (Euthroid, Thyrolar)
      c. Adenohypophyseal hormone
          (1) Thyroid-stimulating hormone (TSH) (thyrotropin; Thytropar)
          (2) Protirelin (Thypinone)
  2. Hyperthyroidism
      a. Thioamides
          (1) Methimazole (Tapazole)
          (2) Propylthiouracil
      b. Beta adrenergic blocker
          (1) Propranolol hydrochloride (Inderal)
      c. Iodine
          (1) Potassium or sodium iodide (Lugol's solution)
      d. Radioactive iodine (13I)
E. Nursing assessment: obtain baseline data relevant to vital signs, weight, level of energy, and symptoms of hypofunctioning or hyperfunctioning of gland
F. Nursing management: monitor vital signs, weight; instruct resident regarding medications
G. Nursing evaluation: observe for therapeutic effects and adverse reactions

DRUGS AFFECTING PARATHYROID GLAND

A. Action: maintain blood calcium levels in the blood
B. Adverse reactions: nausea, local irritation at injection sites, drowsiness; gastrointestinal complaints, hypertension
C. Agents: the following are examples
  1. Calcitonin (Calcimar)
  2. Calcitriol (Rocaltrol)
  3. Parathyroid hormone
D. Nursing assessment: obtain baseline data relevant to vital signs and blood calcium levels
E. Nursing management: monitor vital signs, blood calcium levels instruct resident regarding medications
F. Nursing evaluation: observe for therapeutic effects (e.g., decreased muscle cramping) and adverse reactions;

Female Hormones
ESTROGENS

A. Action: replace or supplement natural body hormones; alter cell environment in neoplastic processes
B. Adverse reactions: breast tenderness, increased risk of endometrial cancer, nausea, vomiting, anorexia, malaise, depression, salt and water retention
C. Agents: the following are examples
  1. Chlorotrianisene (TACE)
  2. Diethylstilbestrol (DES) (Stilbestrol)
  3. Estradiol (Estrace)
  4. Estrogen, conjugated (Premarin)
  5. Estrone (Theelin, Femogen)
  6. Ethinyl estradiol (Estinyl)

PROGESTINS

A. Action: suppress endometrial bleeding; withdrawal of drug induces tissue sloughing
B. Adverse reactions: edema, breast tenderness, depression, midcycle bleeding
C. Agents: the following are examples
  1. Dydrogesterone (Gynorest)
  2. Hydroxyprogesterone caproate (Delalutin, Gesterol LA)

3. Medroxyprogesterone acetate (Depo-Provera, Provera)
4. Megestrol acetate (Megace)
5. Norethindrone (Norlutin)
6. Progesterone (Gesterol-50, Lipo-Lutin)

The Eye
ANTICHOLINERGIC DRUGS

A. Action: cause mydriasis (dilated pupils) and cycloplegia (blurred vision)
B. Adverse reaction: dry mouth and skin, fever, thirst, confusion, hyperactivity
C. Agents: the following are examples
  1. Atropine sulfate (Atropisol, Isopto Atropine)
  2. Cyclopentolate hydrochloride (Cyclogyl)
  3. Homatropine hydrobromide (Isopto Homatropine, Homatrocel)
  4. Scopolamine hydrobromide (hyoscine hydrobromide; Isopto Hyoscine)
  5. Tropicamide (Mydriacyl)

ADRENERGIC DRUGS

A. Action: cause mydriasis
B. Adverse reactions: rare
C. Agents: the following are examples
  1. Hydroxyamphetamine hydrobromide (Paredrine)
  2. Phenylephrine hydrochloride (Alconefrin, Mydfrin, Neo-Synephrine Hydrochloride)

DRUGS USED TO TREAT GLAUCOMA

A. Action: cause miosis (pupil constriction); reduce resistance to outflow of aqueous humor; decrease production of aqueous humor
B. Adverse reactions: blood vessel congestion causing increased intraocular pressure, ocular pain, headache, tachycardia or bradycardia, hypertension, diaphoresis, anorexia, gastrointestinal upset, lethargy, depression, diuresis, dehydration
C. Agents: the following are examples
  1. Acetazolamide (Diamox)
  2. Carbachol (Isopto Carbachol)
  3. Demecarium bromide (Humorsol)
  4. Dichlorphenamide (Daranide, Oratrol)
  5. Echothiophate iodide (Phospholine Iodide)
  6. Epinephrine bitartrate (Epitrate, Primatene Mist Suspension)
  7. Epinephryl borate (Epinal, Eppy/N)
  8. Epinephrine hydrochloride (Epifrin, Glaucon)
  9. Ethoxzolamide (Cardrase, Ethamide)
  10. Glycerin (Dlyrol, Osmoglyn)
  11. Isoflurophate (Floropryl)
  12. Isosorbide (Ismotic)
  13. Mannitol (Osmitrol)
  14. Methazolamide (Neptazane)
  15. Physostigmine sulfate (Eserine)
  16. Pilocarpine hydrochloride (Isopto Carpine, Pilocar)
  17. Timolol maleate (Timoptic)
  18. Urea (Ureaphil, Urevert)
D. Nursing assessment: obtain history of eye-related symptoms, such as difficulty in driving or ambulating; examine eyes for signs of infection, exudate, tearing, or drying
E. Nursing management: advise resident about effects of drugs such as blurred vision and photophobia; instruct resident regarding drugs (i.e., do not skip doses)
F. Nursing evaluation: observe for therapeutic effects and adverse reactions

Drugs Used to Control Muscle Tone
ACETYLCHOLINESTERASE INHIBITORS (ANTICHOLINERGIC AGENTS)

A. Action: allow the accumulation of acetylcholine at neuromuscular junctions and thus ensure muscle contractility; drugs are not used during pregnancy or with residents that have hyperexcitability of muscular symptoms
B. Adverse reactions: muscle cramps, fasciculations (rapid, small contractions), weakness; excessive salivation, perspiration, nausea, vomiting
C. Agents: the following are examples
  1. Ambenonium chloride (Mytelase)
  2. Edrophonium chloride (Tensilon)
  3. Neostigmine bromide (Prostigmin)
  4. Pyridostigmine bromide (Mestinon, Regonol)
D. Nursing assessment: obtain baseline data relevant to vital signs, ability to swallow, muscle strength, and eyelid ptosis
E. Nursing management: monitor disease symptoms and vital signs; have suction and intubation equipment at bedside
F. Nursing evaluation: observe for therapeutic effects and adverse reactions

NEUROMUSCULAR BLOCKING AGENTS

A. Action: produce muscle paralysis
B. Adverse reactions: hypotension, bronchospasm, tachycardia, bradycardia, cardiac dysrhythmias, respiratory distress
C. Agents: the following are examples
   1. Decamethonium bromide (Syncurine)
   2. Gallamine triethiodide (Flaxedil)
   3. Pancuronium bromide (Pavulon)
   4. Succinylcholine chloride (Anectine Quelicin, Sucostrin)
   5. Tubocurarine chloride (Tubarine)
D. Nursing assessment: obtain baseline data relevant to pulse, respiration, and blood pressure
E. Nursing management: monitor vital signs; observe rate, quality, and depth of respiration
F. Nursing evaluation: observe for therapeutic effects: sufficient muscle relaxation to allow procedure to be done; observe for adverse reactions: cough and inability to breathe unassisted and to handle secretions

Diabetes Mellitus
INSULIN

A. Action: restores the cell's ability to use glucose and to correct the metabolic changes that occur with diabetes mellitus
B. Adverse reactions: allergic reactions, insulin resistance, injection-site lipoatrophy
C. Agents

	Onset of action	Peak action	Duration of action
Rapid acting			
Insulin injection (Regular Insulin)	Within 1 hr	2-4 hr	6-8 hr
Prompt insulin zinc suspension (Semilente Iletin, Semilente Insulin)	1.5-2 hr	4-7 hr	12-16 hr
Intermediate acting			
Globin zinc insulin injection	2-4 hr	10-14 hr	14-22 hr
Isophane insulin suspension (NPH Iletin, NPH Insulin)	1-2 hr	10-16 hr	18-30 hr
Insulin zinc suspension (Lente Iletin, Lente Insulin)	1-2 hr	10-16 hr	18-30 hr

C. Agents—cont'd

	Onset of action	Peak action	Duration of action
Long acting			
Protamine zinc insulin suspension (Protamine Zinc Iletin, Protamine Zinc Insulin, PZI)	6-8 hr	14-24 hr	24-36 hr or longer
Extended insulin zinc suspension (Ultralente Iletin, Ultralente Insulin)	5-8 hr	16-18 hr	24-36 hr or longer

ORAL HYPOGLYCEMIC AGENTS

A. Action: stimulate release of insulin from pancreas
B. Adverse reactions: gastrointestinal distress, muscle weakness, paresthesias, skin reactions, hypoglycemia
C. Agents

Examples	Duration of action
Tolbutamide (Orinase)	6 to 12 hours
Acetohexamide (Dymelor)	12 to 24 hours
Tolazamide (Tolinase)	12 to 24 hours
Glyburide (Micronase)	up to 24 hours
Chlorpropamide (Diabinese)	up to 72 hours

D. Nursing assessment: obtain baseline data relevant to vital signs, weight, blood and urine glucose levels, and other signs and symptoms of the disease
E. Nursing management: monitor vital signs, blood and urine glucose levels, and other appropriate laboratory results; instruct resident regarding medications and administration
F. Nursing evaluation: observe for therapeutic effects and adverse reactions

Prevention and Treatment of Infections (Antimicrobials/Antiinfectives)
PENICILLINS AND CEPHALOSPORINS

A. Action: bacteriocidal by interfering with the synthesis of the bacterial cell wall
B. Adverse reactions: allergies—rash, anaphylaxis; convulsions with high parenteral doses; gastrointestinal distress—nausea, vomiting, and diarrhea

C. Agents: the following are examples
   1. Penicillins
      a. Amoxicillin (Amoxil, Larotid, Polymox, Trimox)
      b. Ampicillin (Amcill, Omnipen, Polycillin, Principen)
      c. Carbenicillin disodium (Geopen)
      d. Cloxacillin sodium (Cloxapen, Tegopen)
      e. Dicloxacillin sodium (Dycill, Dynapen)
      f. Methicillin sodium (Celbenin, Staphcillin)
      g. Nafcillin sodium (Nafcil, Unipen)
      h. Oxacillin sodium (Bactocill, Prostaphlin)
      i. Penicillin G potassium (Pentids, Pfizerpen)
      j. Penicillin G benzathine (Bicillin)
      k. Penicillin G procaine (Crysticillin, Duracillin, Wycillin)
      l. Penicillin V (Pen-Vee K, V-Cillin, Veetids)
   2. Cephalosporins
      a. Cefaclor (Ceclor)
      b. Cefamandole nafate (Mandol)
      c. Cefazolin sodium (Ancef, Kefzol)
      d. Cefoxitin (Mefoxin)
      e. Cephalexin (Keflex)
      f. Cephaloridine (Loridine)
      g. Cephalothin sodium (Keflin)
      h. Cephapirin sodium (Cefadyl)
      i. Cephradrine (Anspor, Velosef)
D. Clinical indications
   1. Wound and skin infections
   2. Respiratory infections
   3. Prophylaxis for residents with rheumatic fever or congenital heart disease
   4. Gram-positive infections caused by streptococci and some staphylococci
   5. Gram-negative infections caused by *Haemophilus influenza, Escherichia coli,* and *Neisseria gonorrhoeae*

ERYTHROMYCIN, CLINDAMYCIN (PENICILLIN SUBSTITUTES)

A. Action: bacteriostatic or bacteriocidal (dosage related) by inhibiting protein synthesis
B. Adverse reactions: abdominal discomfort, cramping, nausea, vomiting, diarrhea, urticaria, anaphylaxis, colitis, liver dysfunction, deafness (vancomycin), permanent kidney damage (systemic bacitracin)

C. Agents: the following are examples
   1. Erythromycins
      a. Erthromycin (E-Mycin, Ilotycin, Robimycin, RP-Mycin)
      b. Erythromycin estolate (Ilosone)
      c. Erythromycin ethylsuccinate (EES)
      d. Erythromycin stearate (Erythrocin)
   2. Clindamycins/Lincomycins
      a. Clindamycin (Cleocin)
      b. Lincomycin hydrochloride (Lincocin)
   3. Penicillin substitutes
      a. Bacitracin
      b. Novobiocin sodium (Albamycin)
      c. Spectinomycin hydrochloride (Trobicin)
      d. Vancomycin hydrochloride (Vancocin)
D. Clinical indications
   1. See clinical indications, below left, for penicillins
   2. Used for residents allergic to penicillin

TETRACYCLINES AND CHLORAMPHENICOL

A. Action: bacteriostatic by preventing the start of protein synthesis (tetracyclines) or inhibiting protein synthesis (chloramphenicol)
B. Adverse reactions
   1. Tetracyclines: nausea, vomiting, stomach pain, diarrhea, superimposed infections, impaired kidney functions, jaundice, delayed blood coagulation, brown discoloration of teeth in children under 8 years of age
   2. Chloramphenicol: bone marrow toxicity, aplastic anemia, allergies, gastrointestinal irritation, headache, mental confusion, depression
C. Agents: the following are examples
   1. Chloramphenicol (Chloromycetin)
   2. Chlortetracycline hydrochloride (Aureomycin)
   3. Demeclocycline hydrochloride (Declomycin)
   4. Doxycycline hyclate (Vibramycin, Doxychel)
   5. Methacycline hydrochloride (Rondomycin)
   6. Minocycline hydrochloride (Minocin, Vectrin)
   7. Oxytetracycline hydrochloride (Terramycin, Oxlopar)
   8. Tetracycline hydrochloride (Achromycin, Panmycin Hydrochloride, Sumycin, Tetracyn)

D. Clinical indications
   1. Gram-negative and gram-positive infections
   2. Severe acne vulgaris
   3. Used for residents allergic to penicillin

AMINOGLYCOSIDES AND POLYMYXINS

A. Action
   1. Aminoglycosides: inhibit early stages of protein synthesis
   2. Polymyxins: alter bacterial cell membrane permeability
B. Adverse reactions: eighth cranial nerve damage, renal damage, respiratory paralysis
C. Agents: the following are examples
   1. Aminoglycosides
      a. Amikacin sulfate (Amikin)
      b. Gentamicin sulfate (Garamycin)
      c. Kanamycin sulfate (Kantrex)
      d. Neomycin sulfate (Mycifradin, Neobiotic)
      e. Streptomycin
      f. Tobramycin sulfate (Nebcin)
   2. Polymyxins
      a. Colistimethate sodium (Coly-Mycin M)
      b. Colistin sulfate (Coly-Mycin S)
      c. Polymyxin B sulfate (Aerosporin)
D. Clinical indications: drugs are potentially dangerous and are used only in cases of severe infections, such as gram-negative bone and joint infections and septicemia

SULFONAMIDES, TRIMETHOPRIM, NITROFURANTOINS, NALIDIXIC ACID

A. Action: block bacterial synthesis of folic acid; inhibit bacterial enzymes required for proper metabolism of sugar; interfere directly with DNA synthesis
B. Adverse reactions
   1. Sulfonamides, trimethoprim, nitrofurantoins: allergies, nausea, vomiting, diarrhea, stomatitis, blood dyscrasias, renal calculi, and hematuria
   2. Nalidixic acid: convulsions, mental instability, headache, dizziness, visual disturbances, photosensitivity
C. Agents: the following are examples
   1. Sulfonamides
      a. Sulfadiazine

b. Sulfameter (Sulla)
c. Sulfamethizole (Microsul, Thiosulfil, Forte)
d. Sulfamethoxazole (Gantanol)
e. Sulfamethoxazole-phenazopyridine (Azo Gantanol)
f. Sulfamethoxazole-trimethoprim (Bactrim, Septra)
g. Sulfamethoxypyridazine (Midicel) acetyl
h. Sulfasalazine (Azulfidine, Salazopyrin)
i. Sulfisoxazole (Gantrisin, Rosoxol, Sulfalar)
j. Sulfisoxazole—phenazopyridine hydrochloride (Azo Gantrisin, SK-Soxazole, Azosul)
   2. Sulfonamides: topical agents
      a. Mafenide (Sulfamylon)
      b. Nitrofurantoin (Furadantin, Furalan, Nephronex)
      c. Nitrofurantoin macrocrystals (Macrodantin)
      d. Nalidixic acid (NegGram)
      e. Silver sulfadiazine (Silvadene)
      f. Sulfacetamide (Sulamyd) sodium
      g. Sulfisoxazole diolamine (Gantrisin Ophthalmic)
      h. Trimethoprim (Proloprim, Trimpex)
D. Clinical indications
   1. Used to treat acute and chronic urinary tract infections
   2. Other uses include trachoma, chancroid, toxoplasmosis, acute otitis media, and prophylactic therapy in cases of recurrent rheumatic fever
   3. Treatment of ulcerative colitis
   4. Prophylaxis for residents scheduled for bowel surgery

DRUGS USED TO TREAT TUBERCULOSIS AND LEPROSY

A. Action: alter several metabolic processes in mycobacteria
B. Adverse reactions: peripheral neuropathies, visual disturbances, gastrointestinal distress, ototoxicity, headache
C. Agents: the following are examples
   1. First-line antitubercular drugs
      a. Ethambutol hydrochloride (Myambutol)

    b. Isoniazid (Isotamine, Niconyl, Nydrazid)

    c. Para-aminosalicylic acid (PAS) (aminosalicylic acid, Teebacin acid)

    d. Rifampin (Rifadin, Rimactane)

    e. Streptomycin

  2. Second-line antitubercular drugs

    a. Capreomycin (Capastat)

    b. Cycloserine (Seromycin)

    c. Ethionamide (Trecator-SC)

    d. Pyrazinamide

  3. Antileprosy agents

    a. Clofazimine (Lamprene)

    b. Dapsone (Avlosulfon)

    c. Rifampin (Rifadin, Rimactane)

    d. Sulfoxone (Diasone) sodium

D. Education: stress importance of long-term compliance and follow-up visits with the physician; report any adverse reactions promptly; refrain from using alcohol; refrain from taking other medications without the knowledge and permission of the physician; wear a medical identification tag indicating medication being taken

ANTIFUNGAL DRUGS

A. Action: selectively damages the membranes of fungi

B. Adverse reactions: renal damage, anemia, nausea, diarrhea

C. Agents: the following are examples

  1. Systemic agents

    a. Amphotericin B (Fungizone)

    b. Flucytosine (Ancobon)

    c. Hydroxystilbamidine isethionate

    d. Miconazole (Monistat IV)

  2. Topical agents

    a. Acrisorcin (Akrinol)

    b. Amphotericin B (Fungizone)

    c. Candicidin (Vanobid)

    d. Clioquinol (Vioform)

    e. Clotrimazole (Gyne-Lotrimin, Lotrimin)

    f. Griseofulvin (Fulvicin-P/G, Grifulvin V, Grisactin)

    g. Haloprogin (Halotex)

    h. Miconazole nitrate (Micatin, Monistat)

    i. Nystatin (Mycostatin, Nilstat)

    j. Tolnaftate (Aftate, Tinactin)

    k. Undecylenic acid—zinc undecylenate (Desenex, Ting, Cruex)

DRUGS USED TO TREAT VIRAL DISEASES

A. Action: selective toxicity in various processes of virus reproduction

B. Adverse reactions: ataxia, slurred speech, lethargy, local irritation, anorexia, nausea, vomiting, diarrhea

C. Agents: the following are examples

  1. Acyclovir (Zovirax)

  2. Amantadine (Symmetrel)

  3. Idoxuridine (Dendrid, Herplex Liquifilm, Stoxil)

  4. Methisazone

  5. Vidarabine (Vira-A)

  6. Zidovudine* (AZT, Retrovir)

ANTIPROTOZOAL AND ANTHELMINTIC AGENTS

A. Action: destroy the protozoa and helminths at various stages of development

B. Adverse reactions: gastrointestinal distress, flatulence, vision changes, irritability, hemolysis, skin eruptions, blood dyscrasias

C. Agents: the following are examples

  1. Amebic infestations

    a. Chloroquine (Aralen) phosphate

    b. Diloxanide (Furamide)

    c. Emetine hydrochloride

    d. Iodoquinol (Yodoxin)

    e. Metronidazole (Flagyl)

  2. Malaria

    a. Amodiaquine hydrochloride (Camoquin)

    b. Chloroquine hydrochloride (Aralen)

    c. Primaquine phosphate

    d. Quinine

  3. Others

    a. Povidone-iodine (Betadine, Proviodine)

    b. Quinacrine hydrochloride

  4. Anthelmintics

    a. Mebendazole (Vermox)

    b. Niclosamide (Yomesan)

    c. Piperazine citrate (Antepar)

    d. Pyrantel pamoate (Antiminth)

    e. Pyrvinium pamoate (Povan)

---

*Used in treatment of acquired immunodeficiency syndrome (AIDS); prevents replication of human immunodeficiency virus (HIV), thus delaying disease progression.

D. Nursing assessment: obtain history of allergies; evaluate baseline data relevant to signs and symptoms of infection, vital signs, pertinent laboratory tests, appearance of wounds, incisions or lesions, amount and description of drainage, swelling, erythema, subjective symptoms of pain or pressure

E. Nursing management: obtain culture for specimens before starting antibiotics; maintain supportive measures such as rest, comfort, nutrition, fluids and electrolyte balance; maintain proper administration regarding route, time, and dosage; monitor vital signs and laboratory results; instruct resident regarding medications to ensure compliance

F. Nursing evaluation: observe for therapeutic effects and adverse reactions

Neoplastic Diseases
SPECIFIC ANTINEOPLASTIC AGENTS

A. Action: selective toxicity during various stages of the cell cycle

B. Agents

Examples	Adverse reactions
Asparaginase (Elspar)	Central nervous system depression
Bleomycin sulfate (Blenoxane)	Pulmonary toxicity, skin reactions
Busulfan (Myleran)	Bone marrow and kidney toxicity
Calusterone (Methosarb)	Mild virilism, edema, hypercalcemia, nausea, vomiting
Carmustine (BiCNU)	Bone marrow suppression, nausea
Chlorambucil (Leukeran)	Bone marrow suppression
Cisplatin (Platinol)	Renal damage, nausea and vomiting, ototoxicity, neurotoxicity, and anaphylactic reactions
Cyclophosphamide (Cytoxan)	Hemorrhagic cystitis, bladder fibrosis
Cytarabine (Cytosar-U)	Bone marrow suppression
Dacarbazine (DTIC-Dome)	Bone marrow suppression
Dactinomycin (Cosmegen)	Bone marrow suppression, gastrointestinal irritation, skin reactions

B. Agents—cont'd

Examples	Adverse reactions
Diethylstilbestrol diphosphate (Stilphostrol)	Risk of thromboembolic disease, edema, mood changes
Doxorubicin hydrochloride (Adriamycin)	Bone marrow suppression, gastrointestinal distress, alopecia
Dromostanolone propionate (Drolban)	Mild virilism, edema, hypercalcemia
Estradiol (Progynon)	Risk of thromboembolic disease, edema, mood changes
Etoposide	Bone marrow suppression
Floxuridine (FUDR)	Gastrointestinal and hematologic toxicity
Fluorouracil (5-FU, Adrucil)	Gastrointestinal and hematologic toxicity
Hydroxyurea (Hydrea)	Bone marrow suppression
Lomustine (CeeNU)	Myelosuppression, nausea
Mechlorethamine hydrochloride or nitrogen mustard (Mustargen)	Bone marrow suppression
Medroxyprogesterone (Depo-Provera)	Menstrual irregularities, rashes, and thrombolic diseases
Megestrol acetate (Megace)	Thromboembolic disease
Melphalan (Alkeran)	Leukopenia, anemia, menstrual irregularities
Mercaptopurine (Purinethol)	Hematologic toxicity, immunosuppression
Methotrexate	Gastrointestinal toxicity, bone marrow suppression, immunosuppression
Mitomycin (Mutamycin)	Bone marrow suppression, gastrointestinal irritation, alopecia, renal toxicity
Mitotane (Lysodren)	Gastrointestinal disturbances, skin reactions
Plicamycin (mithramycin; Mithracin)	Gastrointestinal, skin, liver, and kidney toxicity

B. Agents—cont'd

Examples	Adverse reactions
Polyestradiol phosphate (Estradurin)	Risk of thromboembolic disease, edema, mood changes
Prednisone (Deltasone, Panasol, Meticorten)	Cushing's syndrome
Procarbazine hydrochloride (Matulane)	Bone marrow suppression, gastrointestinal disturbances
Tamoxifen citrate (Nolvadex)	Hot flashes, nausea, vomiting
Teniposide	Bone marrow suppression
Testolactone (Teslac)	Pain and irritation at injection site, hypercalemia
Thioguanine	Hematologic toxicity
Thiotepa	Bone marrow toxicity
Vinblastine sulfate (Velban)	Peripheral neuropathy and bone marrow suppression
Vincristine sulfate (Oncovin)	Alopecia, abdominal pain, peripheral neuropathy

C. Nursing assessment: obtain baseline data regarding possible adverse reactions of drugs; evaluate condition of hair, skin, nails, weight, vital signs, and necessary blood laboratory studies (especially WBC and RBC count)

D. Nursing management: monitor weight, vital signs, and laboratory studies; institute regular inspection of mouth; maintain good medical asepsis; use infusion monitoring device for IV administration; provide resident/family teaching and psychologic support

E. Nursing evaluation: observe for therapeutic effects and adverse reactions

VITAMINS

A. General information
1. Group of substances that act as coenzymes to help in the conversion of carbohydrate and fat into energy and to form bones and tissues; necessary for metabolism of fat, carbohydrate, and protein; normally obtained from foods
2. Subclassified as the following:
   a. Fat-soluble: A, D, E, K
   b. Water-soluble: B complex, C

B. Agents
1. Fat-soluble vitamins: the following are examples
   a. Vitamin A (Alphalin, Aquasol A)
   b. Vitamin E (Tocopherol, Aquasol E)
   c. Vitamin K
      (1) Menadiol sodium diphosphate (Synkayvite)
      (2) Phytonadione (Mephyton, AquaMEPHYTON)
2. Water-soluble vitamins: the following are examples
   a. B-complex
      (1) Calcium pantothenate
         (a) B_5
         (b) Pantholin
      (2) Cyanocobalamin
         (a) B_{12}
         (b) Rubramin PC, Betalin 12
      (3) Folic acid (Folvite)
      (4) Niacin
      (5) Pyridoxine hydrochloride
         (a) B_6
         (b) Hexa-Betalin
      (6) Riboflavin (Riobin-50, B_2)
      (7) Thiamine hydrochloride B_1 (Betalin S)
   b. Vitamin C: ascorbic acid

MINERALS AND ELECTROLYTES

A. General information: (1) basic constituents of living tissues and components of many enzymes; (2) function to maintain fluid, electrolyte, and acid-base balance; maintain muscle and nerve function; (3) assist in transfer of materials across cell membranes; and (4) contribute to the growth process

B. Agents: the following are examples
1. Ammonium chloride
2. Deferoxamine mesylate (Desferal)
3. Ferrous gluconate (Fergon)
4. Ferrous sulfate (Feosol)
5. Iron dextran injection (Imferon)
6. Magnesium sulfate
7. Potassium bicarbonate—potassium citrate (K-Lyte)
8. Potassium chloride (Kay Ciel, K-Lor)
9. Potassium gluconate (Kaon)
10. Sodium bicarbonate

11. Sodium polystyrene sulfonate (Kayexalate)
12. Tromethamine (THAM)
13. Multiple mineral-electrolyte preparations
    a. Normosol-R
    b. Pedialyte (oral)
    c. Plasma-Lyte 56
    d. Plasma-Lyte 148
    e. Polysal M
    f. Ringer's lactate

IMMUNIZATIONS

A. Influenza:
   1. Places frail older adults at major risk because of reduced respiratory activity, decreased ability to remove secretions, decreased resistance and presence of other conditions that reduce activity
   2. Candidates for influenza vaccination
      a. Those with chronic cardiovascular or pulmonary disorders
      b. Residents of long term care facilities
      c. Persons age 65 and older with chronic metabolic disorders, anemia, renal failure, or immunosuppression
      d. Older persons who are otherwise healthy
      e. Health-care professionals with extensive contacts with high-risk individuals
   3. New influenza vaccine developed every year, based on information about strains of viruses most likely to affect population
   4. Vaccine made from inactivated viruses; should have minimal side effects
   5. There is 2- to 3-week delay in development of antibody response; vaccines do not provide immediate protection
   6. Because of albumin in the vaccine, it should not be given to individuals allergic to eggs or egg products
   7. Should be administered annually during months between September and November

B. Pneumococcal vaccine
   1. Recommended as prevention against most common causative organism for pneumococcal pneumonia and bacteremia in older adults
   2. Candidates for receiving pneumococcal vaccine include individuals with:
      a. Chronic cardiopulmonary disease
      b. Alcoholism
      c. Multiple myeloma, lymphoma

d. Splenic dysfunction, immunosuppression, renal failure, and chronic liver disease
      e. Healthy persons over age 65
   3. May be administered at some time as influenza vaccine—at different sites
   4. Pneumococcal vaccine usually required only once in an adult
   5. Side effect may include local redness and pain, fever, myalgia, and, rarely, anaphylaxis

C. Hepatitis B vaccine (HBV)
   1. Recommended as preventive against spread of Hepatitis B
   2. Candidates for receiving HBV
      a. Adolescents and high risk individuals
      b. Health care workers
      c. Household and sexual contacts of HBV carriers
      d. Infants
      e. Residents in contact with known HBV carriers
   3. Vaccine is inactivated viral surface antigen derived by means of recombinant DNA technology
   4. Schedule of injections
      a. Primary (mother not infected): at 0-2 days, then at 1-2 months, and 6-18 months; alternative: 1-2 months; 2-4 months and 6-18 months.
      b. Primary (mother infected): on day of birth, then at 1-6 months
      c. All other residents—receive three injections scheduled at periodic intervals
   5. Contraindications
      a. Anaphylactic reaction to previous HBV
      b. Moderate-to-severe illness with or without fever
      c. Pregnant women should receive vaccine only if clearly needed
   6. Side effects
      a. Local soreness and redness
      b. Headache
      c. Fever, malaise
      d. Upper respiratory infection
      e. Gastrointestinal distress
      f. Rarely, joint pain and neurological reactions such as vertigo and paresthesia

Review Questions

1. A resident receiving high-dosage chlorpromazine hydrochloride (Thorazine) has developed tremors of the hands. The nurse should:
   ① Report the symptoms to the physician
   ② Withhold the medication
   ③ Tell the resident it is transitory
   ④ Give the resident finger exercises to perform

2. A resident is to receive 2000 ml of IV fluid in 12 hours. The drop factor is 10 gtt/ml. The nurse should regulate the flow so the number of drops per minute is approximately:
   ① 27 to 29
   ② 30 to 32
   ③ 40 to 42
   ④ 48 to 50

3. A resident with emphysema is receiving aminophylline. The nurse knows this medication will act to:
   ① Relax the diaphragm and intercostals to increase chest expansion
   ② Decrease contraction of the smooth muscles of the bronchi
   ③ Increase the contraction of the bronchi and alveoli
   ④ Decrease the amount of mucous secretion from the bronchi

4. After the first two doses of haloperidol (Haldol), a resident begins to pace, feeling "antsy," and cannot sit still. The neck becomes stiff and twists to one side, then the eyes roll upward. These symptoms are consistent with:
   ① A severe allergic reaction
   ② An extrapyramidal reaction
   ③ A worsening of the resident's psychosis
   ④ A rare side effect

5. Whenever a medication is ordered for its diuretic effect, the nurse should understand the importance of:
   ① Forcing fluids
   ② Placing the resident on bed rest
   ③ Measuring all fluid output
   ④ Daily urinalysis

6. While distributing medications, the nurse observes that a resident who has been taking digoxin has not touched any breakfast and that a partially filled emesis basin is on the bedside table. Acting on knowledge of this drug, the nurse would be correct to:
   ① Give the drug if the radial pulse is above 60 and reports to the head nurse
   ② Omit the drug, checks the apical pulse, and reports to the head nurse

③ Postpone the administration of the drug until after lunch
④ Await the results of the daily ECG and then administers half the dose

7. Some adrenergic drugs can be used in stopping bleeding and relieving nasal and ocular congestion by causing:
   ① Constriction of blood vessels
   ② Vasodilation of blood vessels
   ③ Astringent action on mucous membranes
   ④ A rise in arterial blood pressure

8. The major adverse reaction associated with the use of sedative-hypnotics is:
   ① Hypertension
   ② Hypotension
   ③ Respiratory depression
   ④ Hypothermia

9. Common adverse reactions to corticosteroid therapy include:
   ① Tachycardia, insomnia
   ② Bradycardia, mental dullness
   ③ "Moon face," obese trunk
   ④ Anorexia, polyuria

10. Daily assessment of the integrity of the oral mucous membranes is important when the resident is receiving:
    ① Antibiotics
    ② Cancer drugs
    ③ Antiparkinsonian drugs
    ④ Vitamins

11. A nursing observation that would support evidence of the therapeutic effects of antianxiety drug therapy is:
    ① Crying, facial grimaces, and rigid posture
    ② Anger, aggressive behavior
    ③ Decrease in blood pressure, pulse, and respirations
    ④ Verbal statements such as "more worried" or "resting poorly"

12. Frequently used medications for myocardial infarctions are:
    ① Salicylates, antiinflammatory agents, and gold salts
    ② Antidysrhythmics, analgesics, and anticoagulants
    ③ Cardial glycosides, diuretics, and nitrates
    ④ Anticoagulants, vasodilators, and fibronolytics

13. The nurse knows that oral care is essential when a resident is receiving long-term Dilantin therapy because of:
    ① Formation of dental caries
    ② Gingival hypertrophy

③ Eroding of the tooth enamel

④ The possibility of xerostomia

14. Toxicity to digitalis occurs more rapidly when the body stores of what ion are depleted?
    ① Sodium
    ② Potassium
    ③ Calcium
    ④ Chloride

15. Side effects of the antidepressant group MAO inhibitors that the nurse must observe are:
    ① Lowered blood pressure, increased ocular pressure, and tachycardia
    ② Flushing, diaphoresis, and dry mouth
    ③ Drowsiness
    ④ Confusion

16. Lorazepam (Ativan) is ordered for a resident by the physician. A common CNS side effect to Ativan is:
    ① Drowsiness
    ② Dry mouth
    ③ Dizziness
    ④ Urine retention

17. Drugs such as trihexyphenidyl (Artane), biperiden (Akineton), and benztropine (Cogentin) are often prescribed in conjunction with:
    ① Major tranquilizers
    ② Minor tranquilizers
    ③ Barbiturates
    ④ Antidepressants

18. The nurse should teach a male resident with angina pectoris that he will know the prescribed nitroglycerin sublingual tablet is effective when his:
    ① Pain subsides because his arterioles and venules dilate
    ② Pulse rate increases because the cardiac output is stimulated
    ③ Sublingual area tingles because sensory nerves are being triggered
    ④ Capacity for activity escalates because of increased collateral circulation

19. The major adverse reactions with the use of meperidine hydrochloride (Demerol) are:
    ① Increased perspiration, euphoria, nausea
    ② Increased blood pressure and decreased respirations
    ③ Diarrhea and decreased blood pressure
    ④ Dysphagia and urinary retention

20. The therapeutic effectiveness of the bronchodilating drugs can be assessed by observing for:
    ① Cardiac dysrhythmias
    ② Nausea and vomiting

③ Insomnia, restlessness

④ Decreased dyspnea and wheezing

21. A major adverse reaction commonly seen with the use of antineoplastic drugs is:
    ① Bone marrow depression
    ② Oliguria
    ③ Lethargy
    ④ Photosensitivity

22. A potassium-sparing (retaining) diuretic used to reduce hypertension and/or edema is:
    ① Furosemide (Lasix)
    ② Spironolactone (Aldactone)
    ③ Sulfisoxazole (Gantrisin)
    ④ Methenamine (Mandelamine)

23. The main pharmacologic treatment for tuberculosis (TB) includes isoniazid (INH) and para-aminosalicylate sodium (PAS). In planning care for a resident receiving these medications, the nurse is aware that they are used:
    ① To prevent TB organisms from multiplying
    ② For 6 to 8 weeks
    ③ To destroy the TB organisms
    ④ For the rest of the resident's life

24. A resident with essential hypertension is to receive 1 g of methyldopa (Aldomet) daily. Because each dose is 250 mg, the nurse will administer:
    ① 1 tablet daily
    ② 3 tablets daily
    ③ 4 tablets daily
    ④ 8 tablets daily

25. A resident is receiving a major tranquilizer bid. Two thirds of the daily dose is given in the evening, one third in the morning. This is done to:
    ① Help the resident sleep at night
    ② Reduce sedation during the daytime
    ③ Maintain diurnal rhythms
    ④ Reduce increased assaultiveness in the evening

26. A resident who is actively hallucinating approaches the nurse and states, "I am hearing voices that are saying bad things about me." The nurse should:
    ① Simply state, "I do not hear the voices."
    ② Encourage the resident not to listen to what the voices are saying.
    ③ Suggest the resident join other residents playing cards.
    ④ State, "The staff understands that you are frightened and will stay with you while the voices are speaking."

ANSWERS AND RATIONALES FOR REVIEW QUESTIONS

1. **1** The physician is responsible for medication orders but depends on the nurse's observations in making decisions.
   2 This would not be a severe enough symptom to warrant withholding the drug.
   3 It is a reaction to the Thorazine and must be treated.
   4 This would have no effect on the tremors.

2. **1** $\dfrac{\text{Amount to be infused} \times \text{Drop factor}}{\text{Amount of time (in minutes)}}$

   $$\dfrac{2000 \times 10}{12 \times 60} = \dfrac{20,000}{720} = 27.77 \text{ drops/min}$$

   2 Incorrect calculation; would result in excessive fluid administration.
   3 Incorrect calculation; would result in excessive fluid administration.
   4 Incorrect calculation; would result in excessive fluid administration.

3. **3** Aminophylline is a bronchodilator and relaxes the smooth muscles of the bronchi.
   1 Lung expansion is limited (decreased) by the disease process; the drug will not affect lung expansion.
   2. The action of the drug relaxes the smooth muscles allowing for increased air flow (see rationale to answer 3)
   4 There is usually an *increase* in mucous secretion from increased air flow

4. **2** Extrapyramidal reactions are common side effects of major tranquilizers. Although they are not life-threatening, they are acutely uncomfortable for the resident. They require rapid intervention with medications such as diphenhydramine (Benadryl), benztropine (Cogentin), or trihexyphenidyl (Artane).
   1 Many residents believe this experience represents an allergic reaction. This is not the case.
   3 Sometimes the resident's pacing and odd movements are mistaken for a worsening of the psychosis. This can be an unfortunate error and can lead to the resident's being improperly treated.

4 Rare side effects include agranulocytosis, cholestatic jaundice, and the occasionally fatal neuroleptic malignant syndrome.

5. **3** Action assists in determining drug effectiveness
   1 Forcing fluids may or may not be indicated and does not assist in evaluating drug action.
   2 Residents receiving diuretics are not required to be on bedrest as a direct result of diuretic therapy.
   4 Daily urinalysis is not required unless such is warranted for other medical reasons.

6. **2** Early signs of digitalis toxicity.
   1 This action would increase the already toxic effects of the drug.
   3 Not reporting resident status could lead to a life-threatening situation for the resident.
   4 This action could also result in a life-threatening situation; determining dosage is not a nursing responsibility.

7. **1** Action of the drug.
   2 This action would be opposite to that which is desired.
   3 Action is directed to the blood vessels, not the mucous membranes.
   4 This action is a direct result of the primary action (see answer 1) of the drug.

8. **3** Depresses the medulla oblongata.
   1 No significant effect.
   2 No significant effect.
   4 No significant effect.

9. **3** Caused by abnormal fat deposits.
   1 Tachycardia can occur with rapid IV administration of high doses; insomnia is a common side effect, not an adverse reaction
   2 Bradycardia is not an adverse reaction; mental changes such as depression are rare.
   4 *Increase* in appetite is a side effect, whereas increased urination (polyuria) can be an adverse reaction (less frequent)

10. **2** Altered integrity of oral mucosa (ulcerations) due to stomatitis is an indicator of drug toxicity.
    1 Diarrhea, nausea, and vomiting are commonly noted side effects of antibiotics.
    3 Blurred vision, dry skin, nausea, and vomiting are commonly noted side effects of anticholinergic drugs.
    4 Side effects/adverse reactions to vitamins are not commonly seen unless very large doses are given over a period of time; integrity of the oral mucosa is not usually affected.

Chapter Fourteen Answers

11. **3** Antianxiety drugs decrease physiological manifestations of anxiety such as elevated levels of blood pressure, pulse, and respiration.
    1 These are signs of anxiety.
    2 These are paradoxical reactions that would not support evidence of positive effects of drug therapy.
    4 These are signs of anxiety.

12. **2** Anticoagulants such as heparin or warfarin (Coumadin) are given to reduce chances of clotting; analgesic drugs such as morphine are given to control pain; and antidysrhythmics such as lidocaine (Xylocaine) IV is used to treat ventricular dysrhythmias.
    1 These are frequently used medications for rheumatoid arthritis.
    3 These are medication therapy for congestive heart failure.
    4 These are medications for pheripheral artery disease.

13. **2** Common side effect in long-term therapy.
    1 Is not a characteristic side effect.
    3 Is not a characteristic side effect.
    4 Is not a characteristic side effect.

14. **2** Hypokalemia can increase risk of toxicity; potassium supplements are usually recommended for cardiac residents also on diuretics.
    1 Sodium diuresis is a desired action of diuretic therapy.
    3 Excess calcium in the presence of digitalis may cause sinus bradycardia, atrioventricular conduction block, and ectopic dysrhythmia.
    4 Various diuretics, one of which could be ammonium chloride, is used to induce diuresis.

15. **1** These antidepressants mainly affect the CNS.
    2 These are side effects of the tricyclic antidepressant drugs.
    3 This is a side effect of trazadone hydrochloride antidepressant drugs.
    4 This is a side effect of the tricyclic antidepressant drugs.

16. **1** Drowsiness is the only CNS side effect listed.
    2 Dry mouth is a gastrointestinal side effect.
    3 Dizziness is a cardiovascular side effect.
    4 Urine retention is a genitourinary side effect.

17. **1** These drugs are used to control the extrapyramidal (parkinsonism-like) symptoms that often develop as a side effect of major tranquilizer therapy.
    2 There is no documented use with minor tranquilizers, because they do not have extrapyramidal side effects.
    3 Barbiturates do not have extrapyramidal side effects, which would respond to these drugs.
    4 Antiparkinson drugs (e.g., Cogentin) are not usually prescribed in conjunction with antidepressants; gastrointestinal tract depression can result in paralytic ileus.

18. **1** Nitroglycerin causes vasodilation, increasing the flow of blood and oxygen to the myocardium and reducing anginal pain.
    2 An increased pulse rate does not indicate effectiveness; it is a side effect of nitroglycerin.
    3 The tingling indicates that the medication is fresh; relief of pain is the only indicator of effectiveness.
    4 Nitroglycerin does not promote the formation of new blood vessels.

19. **1** Common side effects.
    2 Among the most serious adverse reactions to the drug are respiratory and circulatory depression and constipation.
    3 Among the most serious adverse reactions to the drug are respiratory and circulatory depression and constipation.
    4 Difficulty swallowing (dysphagia) and urinary retention are not adverse reactions associated with this drug.

20. **4** Expected outcome.
    1 Adverse reaction.
    2 Adverse reaction.
    3 Adverse reaction.

21. **1** Major adverse reaction.
    2 Oliguria and photosensitivity are not adverse reactions commonly noted with antineoplastic drugs.
    3 Lethargy may be seen with high dose or long-term antineoplastic drug therapy.
    4 Oliguria and photosensitivity are not adverse reactions commonly noted with antineoplastic drugs.

22. **2** Spironolactone (Aldactone) is a potassium-sparing diuretic.

    1 Furosemide (Lasix) is a potassium-eliminating diuretic.

    3 Sulfisoxazole (Gantrisin) is classified as an antiinfective.

    4 Methenamine (Mandelamine) is classified as a urinary antiseptic.

23. **1** These medications inhibit the enzyme needed for growth of the bacilli.

    2 The treatment regimen is usually 9 months or longer.

    3 These drugs nearly, but never completely, eliminate the TB organism.

    4 The treatment regimen is usually 9 months or longer.

24. **3** Using the method, desired over available, the nurse would calculate the following: 1 g = 1000 mg; 1000 mg divided by 250 mg = 4 tablets.

    1 This dose is only 250 mg.

    2 This dose is only 750 mg.

    4 This amount exceeds the required dose.

25. **2** Major tranquilizers tend to make the resident listless or drowsy and can interfere with the ability to participate in the therapeutic regimen.

    1 Major tranquilizers do not really induce sleep; just listlessness.

    3 Major tranquilizers do not appreciably affect diurnal rhythms.

    4 Assaultiveness is associated with increased anxiety; unrelated to time.

26. **4** When the resident's perceptions are especially frightening, the nurse must let the resident know that the fears are recognized as real and frightening even if the nurse does not share these perceptions. Staying with the resident will convey concern as well as reduce the fears.

    1 Nontherapeutic; the voices are real to the resident.

    2 Nontherapeutic; the resident is unable to separate the voices from reality.

    3 The resident will be unable to play cards because the resident cannot concentrate when the voices are speaking.

chapter fifteen

Physiologic Changes of Aging

The percentage of the population over age 65 has topped 13% and continues to constitute our fastest-growing age group. As the life expectancy of Americans continues to lengthen, we should be increasingly aware that by the year 2020 one of every five individuals in our society will be an older adult.

It is nursing's challenge to meet the care needs of our older adults, who are so vulnerable to the biases of our fast-paced, youth-oriented society. As nurses we have an opportunity to play a significant role in determining whether these will be years of continued growth and development, years of happiness and accomplishment, or years of forced shame, illness, and neglect.

Normal aging changes are gradual and begin in early middle age. This chapter focuses on aging as a normal process and strives to increase the practitioner's knowledge of and understanding for a stage of life we will all pass through.

Most Commonly Occurring Health Problems of Older Adults

A. Arthritis
B. Hypertension
C. Heart disease
D. Hearing impairment
E. Orthopedic impairments
F. Cataracts
G. Sinusitis
H. Diabetes
I. Tinnitus

Important Primary Components of the Health History for the Older Adult

A. Focused data collection
B. Subjective view of current health
C. Current use of health care system
D. Chief concern or complaint
E. Other symptomatology
F. Past illnesses, accidents, and use of health care system
G. Medication review
H. Nutritional status screen
I. Functional deficits and strengths
J. Social support network
K. Health maintenance activities
L. Compliance with prescribed medication regimen
M. Reasons for medication noncompliance
   1. Does not understand the purpose/benefit of the medication
   2. Does not understand the exact instructions for taking the medicine (e.g., 3 times a day, before meals, every 4 hours)
   3. Does not have enough money to buy the medicine (many prescriptions are never filled because residents spend their limited financial resources on food instead of medicine)
   4. Tries to save on the amount of money spent on medications by cutting a pill in two or four, skipping a dose, or taking a regularly scheduled medication only when feeling ill
   5. Cannot remove the cap on a bottle of medicine (the pharmacist should be instructed not to use a childproof cap)
   6. Cannot read the instructions on the label of a medication bottle (the pharmacist should be requested to use a large-print label)
   7. Fears that asking the physician or nurse questions about the medication regimen will result in being labeled "senile"

8. Does not remember whether a medication has been taken because of confusion or drowsiness that may be caused by the medication; may omit or double a dose
9. Does not believe the medicine is needed
10. Does not trust the physician, nurse, or care giver
11. Takes more than the prescribed dose when feeling ill or takes none at all when feeling well
12. Takes over-the-counter medications advertised on television instead of medications prescribed by the physician

N. Impact of discomfort and pain
   1. Diminished enjoyment of activities (recreational activities and social events)
   2. Impaired ambulation (e.g., walking, transfers)
   3. Impaired posture
   4. Sleep disturbance
   5. Depression
   6. Anxiety
   7. Impaired bowel function (constipation)
   8. Impaired appetite
   9. Impaired memory
   10. Impaired bladder function (incontinence)
   11. Impaired dressing or grooming

O. Misconceptions about pain in older adults
   1. Myth: Pain is expected with aging
      Fact: Pain is not normal with aging; the presence of pain in older persons necessitates aggressive assessment, diagnosis, and management similar to that for younger persons
   2. Myth: Pain sensitivity and perception decrease with aging
      Fact: This assumption is dangerous, because data conflict regarding age-associated changes in pain perception, sensitivity, and tolerance; consequences of this assumption are needless suffering and undertreatment of both pain and the underlying cause
   3. Myth: If a resident does not complain of pain, he must not have much pain
      Fact: This is erroneous for all ages but particularly for older adults; older residents may not report pain for a variety of reasons, including fear of the meaning of the pain, fear of diagnostic workups, fear of pain treatments, and a belief that pain is normal

4. Myth: A person who has no functional impairment, appears occupied, or is otherwise distracted from pain must not have significant pain
   Fact: People have a variety of reactions to pain: many older adults are stoic and refuse to "give in" to their pain; over extended periods of time, they may mask any outward signs of pain
5. Myth: Narcotic medications are inappropriate for residents with chronic nonmalignant pain
   Fact: Opioid analgesics are often indicated in nonmalignant pain
6. Myth: Potential side effects of narcotic medications make them too dangerous to use for older adults
   Fact: Narcotics may be used safely; although older residents may be more sensitive to narcotics, this does not justify withholding narcotics and failing to relieve pain

P. Barriers to effective management of cancer pain
   1. Residents and family members
      a. Lack of awareness that cancer pain can be managed, with the result that residents may suffer in silence
      b. Fear that use of narcotic analgesics will lead to addiction
      c. Fear that use of narcotic analgesics will lead to mental confusion, disorientation, and personality change
      d. Failure to report pain because of the desire to be "good" and not distract the physician from the primary task of treating the disease
      e. Underreporting of pain because of fear that increasing pain suggests the disease is progressing
   2. Health care professionals
      a. Lack of understanding of the pathophysiology of cancer pain
      b. Lack of knowledge of the clinical pharmacology of narcotic analgesics
      c. Lack of knowledge of new methods of pain relief, including the use of adjuvant drugs and neurosurgical procedures
      d. Insufficient professional education in cancer pain therapy

e. Lack of knowledge of the difference between physical dependence and addiction
f. Excessive concern about development of tolerance to narcotic analgesics
g. Excessive concern about addicting residents to narcotic analgesics
h. Excessive concern about the side effects of narcotic analgesics
i. The belief that cancer pain should be moderate to severe before residents receive medication
j. The belief that residents are not good judges of the severity of their pain
k. Assignment of low priority to pain management
l. Lack of thorough and frequent reevaluation of residents' pain status
m. The difficult and frustrating nature of certain pain management problems

Q. Nursing responsibilities in administering medications to older adults
1. Take a complete medication history
   a. Past medications
   b. Present medications (prescription and over-the-counter)
   c. Allergies of all kinds
   d. Resident's understanding of medications being taken (name, purpose, dosage, method, times)
2. Space oral medications so that not more than one or two are taken at one time
3. Have the resident drink a little fluid before taking oral medications (to ease swallowing)
4. Encourage the resident to drink at least 5 to 6 ounces of fluid after taking the medication (to ensure that the medications have left the esophagus and are in the stomach and to speed absorption of the medications)
5. Do not routinely give analgesics for pain q4h; because of delayed absorption and distribution and the half-life of the medicine, there may be an adverse cumulative effect
6. If the resident has difficulty swallowing a large capsule or tablet, ask the physician to substitute a liquid medication if at all possible (cutting the tablet in half or crushing it and placing it in applesauce or fruit juice may distort the action of some medications, reduce the dose, or cause choking or aspiration of particles of medication or applesauce)
7. Teach alternatives to medications
   a. Proper diet instead of vitamins
   b. Exercise instead of laxatives
   c. Bedtime snacks instead of hypnotics
   d. Decrease in weight, salt, fat, stress, and smoking, and increased exercise, instead of hypertensive agents (if approved by physician)

Integumentary System

A. Decreased vascularity of dermis (loss of capillaries) results in pallor
B. Decreased melanin (melanocytes) results in skin sallowness and changes in hair color (to gray or white)
C. Decreased sebaceous and sweat gland function results in decreased perspiration, dry skin, and less efficient body cooling
D. Decreased subcutaneous fat results in increased wrinkling, deepening of hollows, and more prominent contours
E. Decreased thickness of epidermis results in increased susceptibility to trauma and tissue fragility
F. Decreased density of hair and changes in texture results in thinning or balding on head and loss of body hair
G. Decreased hormone production results in loss of moisture of vaginal mucosa
H. Decreased peripheral circulation results in thick, brittle, split nails, increased thickening and yellowing of nails, longitudinal ridges of nails, and increased sensation of coolness
I. Decreased rate of nail growth results in increased brittleness of nails
J. Increased localized pigmentation results in keratoses, senile lentigines
K. Increased androgen to estrogen ratio results in appearance of facial hair in women and decreased facial hair in men

Musculoskeletal System

A. Alterations
1. Loss of lean muscle mass and muscle cells: decreased muscle strength, size, and tone

2. Loss of elastic fibers in muscle tissue: increased stiffness and decreased flexibility
3. Thinning of long bones: brittle, porous bones
4. Thinning of intervertebral disks: height loss and changes in posture

B. Selected disorders
1. Decreased bone calcium—osteoporosis, kyphosis
2. Decreased fluid in intervertebral disks—decreased height
3. Decreased blood supply to muscles—decreased strength
4. Decreased tissue elasticity—decreased mobility and flexibility
5. Decreased muscle mass—decreased strength, increased risk of falls

C. Contributing factors
1. Nutritional patterns
2. Endocrine system changes: decreased estrogen and testosterone
3. Gastrointestinal system changes: decreased absorption of vitamins and minerals
4. Cardiovascular system changes: poor circulation
5. Neurologic deficits causing safety hazards
6. Decreased level of activity and periods of prolonged bed rest
7. Side effects of medications (e.g., steroids)

D. Resulting problems
1. Increased susceptibility to fractures
2. Altered body image
3. Pain and discomfort
4. Decreased mobility
5. Impaired ability to perform activities of daily living (ADLs)
6. Increasing feelings of dependency
7. Calcium deposits in blood vessels and renal structures
8. Weakened muscles affecting other systems
   a. Diaphragm
   b. Bladder
   c. Myocardium
   d. Abdominal wall

E. Nursing management
1. Handle resident gently
2. Reduce environmental safety hazards
3. Encourage mobility and exercise
4. Allow extra time for performing activities
5. Assist with ADLs and exercises as needed
6. Provide encouragement and support for accomplishments
7. Prevent deformities
   a. Proper positioning
   b. Exercises such as range of motion (ROM)
8. Alleviate pain
   a. Rest periods
   b. Positioning
9. Encourage liberal fluid intake

Pulmonary System

A. Alterations
1. Structural alterations (scoliosis, kyphosis, osteoporosis): decrease in lung expansion and capacity
2. Alveoli enlarge and thin out: decreased oxygen and carbon dioxide diffusion
3. Loss of bronchiole elasticity: decreased breathing capacity, increased residual air
4. Diaphragm becomes fibrotic and weakened; diminished efficiency
5. Respiratory muscle structure and function decreases: diminished strength for breathing and coughing, increased pooling of secretions in lower lobes
6. Changes in larynx: weaker, higher-pitched voice
7. Decrease in ciliary function: increased susceptibility to upper respiratory tract infection
8. Increased rigidity of rib cage and calcification of cartilage
9. Decreased body fluids with decreased ability to humidify air

B. Selected disorders
1. Contributing factors
   a. Decreased resistance to infection
   b. Musculoskeletal system changes: weakened muscles and postural changes
   c. Longer history of smoking and exposure to pollutants
   d. Periods of prolonged bed rest
   e. Cardiovascular system changes
   f. Side effects of medications (e.g., sedatives and hypnotics)
2. Resulting problems
   a. Dyspnea
   b. Chronic cough

c. Fatigue and debilitation
d. Cerebral hypoxia
   (1) Confusion
   (2) Restlessness
   (3) Behavioral changes
e. Decreased activity tolerance
f. Cardiovascular problems (e.g., congestive heart failure)
g. Anorexia
3. Nursing management
   a. Assist with ADLs as necessary
   b. Encourage breathing exercises
   c. Administer oxygen and respiratory therapy treatments
   d. Change position frequently
   e. Encourage liberal fluid intake
   f. Discourage smoking
   g. Position for maximum comfort and efficiency of respiration (e.g., extra pillows, Fowler's position); use of postural drainage
   h. Allow rest periods
   i. Assess pulmonary status when assessing behavioral changes

Cardiovascular System

A. Alterations
1. Decrease in enzymatic stimulation: longer and less forceful contractions of heart
2. Increase in fat and collagen amounts: decline in cardiac output
3. Increase in oxygen demands of coronary arteries and brain: decreased peripheral circulation
4. Loss of elasticity of vessel walls; decrease in contraction and recoiling responses
5. Reduced or unaltered heart rate at rest
6. Mild tachycardia on activity
7. Decreased heart size with result of decreased oxygenation
8. Decreased cardiac output with result of increased chance of heart failure and decreased peripheral circulation
9. Decreased elasticity of heart muscle and blood vessels resulting in a decreased venous return, increased dependent edema, increased incidence of orthostatic hypotension, and increased varicosities and hemorrhoids
10. Increased atherosclerosis resulting in increased blood pressure

B. Selected disorders
1. Contributing factors
   a. Poor nutritional patterns
   b. Anxiety and stress
   c. Decreased activity level
   d. Arteriosclerosis and hypertension
   e. Pulmonary system changes
   f. Side effects of medications
2. Resulting problems
   a. Fatigue and decreased activity tolerance
   b. Increased anxiety
   c. Edema
   d. Hypertension: increased risk of cerebrovascular accident (CVA)
   e. Behavioral changes
   f. Poor circulation to other systems and extremities: delayed healing
3. Nursing management
   a. Assist with ADLs prn
   b. Encourage moderate activity and exercise
   c. Resident teaching considerations
      (1) Confusion
      (2) Forgetfulness
      (3) Resistance to change
   d. Avoid excess pressure on the skin
      (1) Change position frequently
      (2) Sheepskin; water mattress
      (3) Bed cradle
   e. Assess cardiovascular status when assessing behavioral changes
   f. Avoid tight, constrictive clothing and shoes
   g. Special foot care
      (1) Prevent trauma
      (2) Prevent infection

Gastrointestinal System

A. Alterations
1. Muscle atrophy in the tongue, cheeks, mouth
2. Esophageal wall thinning
3. Decrease in ptyalin and amylase secretion by salivary gland: alkaline saliva
4. Decrease in saliva secretion: thicker mucus and dryness
5. Oral sensitivity loss
6. Increased dental caries and tooth loss, with decreased ability to chew normally and decreased nutritional status

7. Ill-fitting dentures, periodontal disease, and nutritional deficiencies
8. Shrinkage of bony structure of mouth
9. Decreased gag reflex, resulting in increased incidence of choking and aspiration
10. Gastric mucosa shrinks: decline in digestive enzyme secretion leads to delayed digestion
11. Decrease in lipase secretion: fat intolerance
12. Decrease in gastric acid: diminished ability to use calcium
13. Decrease in intrinsic factor: pernicious anemia
14. Decrease in iron absorption: iron deficiency anemia
15. Sphincter muscle tone loss: alterations in bowel evacuation, esophageal reflux
16. Decreased gastric secretions, causing decreased digestion
17. Decreased peristalsis, resulting in increased constipation and bowel impaction

B. Selected disorders
  1. Contributing factors
    a. Decreased level of activity
    b. Dental problems
    c. Poor nutritional patterns
    d. Weakened muscles
    e. Nervous system changes
    f. Overuse of laxative and enemas
    g. Anorexia
    h. Side effects of medications (e.g., opiates and steroids)
  2. Resulting problems
    a. Discomfort
    b. Constipation and impaction
    c. Fecal incontinence
    d. Anorexia
    e. Increased risk of aspiration
  3. Nursing management
    a. Promote nutritional intake
      (1) Alter consistency of food
      (2) Ability to manage utensils
      (3) Allow extra time for feeding (oral and tube)
    b. Provide good oral hygiene
    c. Encourage mobility and exercise
    d. Provide adequate fluid intake
    e. Educate resident regarding constipation and laxative abuse

f. Check bowel habits regularly
g. Give prompt assistance to bathroom or with bedpan
h. Prevent skin and mucosal breakdown
  (1) Prompt, thorough cleansing of anal area
  (2) Extra gentleness when inserting rectal and feeding tubes

Renal System

A. Alterations
  1. Decrease in kidney size
  2. Decline in renal blood flow and supply with decreased removal of body wastes and increased concentration of urine
  3. Decreased number of functional nephrons with decreased filtration rate
  4. Reduced ability of nephron to filter urine: decreased clearance
  5. Reduced ability of tubule cells to selectively secrete and reabsorb: fluid and electrolyte alterations
  6. Decreased muscle tone and tissue elasticity resulting in increased amount of residual urine, as well as decreased bladder capacity leading to frequency and urgency
  7. Loss of muscle tone of bladder and uterus
  8. Loss of pelvic muscle tone
  9. Decreased urine concentration ability
  10. Prostate gland enlargement: increased risk of infection, decreased stream of urine, increased hesitancy and frequency

B. Selected disorders
  1. Contributing factors
    a. Periods of prolonged bed rest
      (1) Increased urinary stasis
      (2) Renal calculi formation
    b. Cardiovascular system changes (e.g., decreased renal perfusion)
    c. Nervous system changes
    d. Decreased fluid intake
    e. Muscle weakness
    f. Social withdrawal and apathy (e.g., sensory deprivation)
    g. Side effects of medication (e.g., diuretics, antiparkinsonian drugs)
  2. Resulting problems
    a. Hyperglycemia
    b. Behavioral changes (e.g., confusion, elevated BUN, electrolyte imbalance)
    c. Interference with sleep and recreational patterns

      (1) Urinary frequency
      (2) Urinary urgency
      (3) Nocturia
  d. Increased chance of skin breakdown (e.g., incontinence)
  e. Feelings of embarrassment, rejection, and withdrawal

C. Nursing management
1. Prevent urinary stasis
  a. Encourage liberal fluid intake
  b. Encourage frequent change of position
  c. Encourage ambulation
2. Prevent skin breakdown: prompt and thorough cleansing
3. Bladder retraining
4. Promptly respond to call for bathroom or bedpan
5. Leave nightlight on if resident is experiencing nocturia
6. Assess renal status when assessing behavior changes
7. Early recognition of urinary tract infection
8. Risk factors for urinary tract infections
  a. Inadequate or improper hygiene related to difficulty cleansing self after toileting
  b. Urinary stasis and incomplete emptying of bladder due to physiologic changes and decreased mobility
  c. Coexisting diseases, such as diabetes, hypertension, stroke, and dementia
  d. Medical interventions, including catheterization and repeated use of antibiotics (which can lead to resistant strains of bacteria)
  e. Increased exposure to microorganisms in hospitals or long-term care facilities

Neurologic System

A. Alterations
1. Decrease in weight and size of brain
2. Decline in number of neurons with decreased reflexes and coordination
3. Decreased amounts of neuroreceptors with decreased perception of stimuli and motor responses
4. Diminished nerve conduction speed
  a. Voluntary movement slower
  b. Increased reaction time
  c. Delayed decisions
5. Alterations in sleep-wake cycle
  a. Less rapid eye movement (REM) sleep
  b. Less deep sleep: tendency to catnap
  c. Easily awakened
  d. Difficulty falling asleep
  e. Average 5 to 7 hours
6. Brain tissue atrophy and meningeal thickening: short-term memory loss

B. Selected disorders
1. Contributing factors
  a. Poor nutrition patterns
  b. Cardiovascular system changes (e.g., decreased circulation)
  c. Pulmonary system changes (e.g., cerebral hypoxia)
  d. Sensory deprivation
  e. Side effects of medications (e.g., sedatives)
2. Resulting problems
  a. Safety hazards
      (1) Impaired senses (e.g., vision, hearing, pain, and temperature)
      (2) Forgetfulness and confusion
  b. Anorexia (e.g., decreased taste buds)
  c. Social isolation and rejection
  d. Impaired ability to perform ADLs
      (1) Decreased coordination
      (2) Safety hazards
  e. Increased sense of dependency
  f. Incontinence
  g. Altered self-image and declining confidence
  h. Behavioral changes (e.g., forgetfulness, confusion)
3. Nursing management
  a. Provide for safety
  b. Establish means of communication if resident has hearing impairment
  c. Assess all systems when assessing behavioral changes
  d. Maintain sense of independence when possible
  e. Assist with ADLs only when necessary; allow extra time
  f. Encourage socialization
  g. Provide sensory stimulation
  h. Consider forgetfulness and confusion when teaching
      (1) Be consistent
      (2) Provide repetition when necessary
      (3) Be patient

(4)   Provide positive reinforcement and encouragement

i.   Assess other symptoms carefully when assessing for infection and trauma: decreased temperature control and pain perception mask these symptoms

j.   Carefully check temperature of bath water and forms of heat therapy to avoid burns: discrepancy in sensation of heat and cold

k.   Maximize use of environmental aids

Endocrine System

A.   Alterations
1.   Decline in growth hormone secretion
2.   Estrogen secretion diminishes
3.   Uterus becomes smaller
4.   Fallopian tubes decrease in size and motility
5.   Vagina loses elasticity
6.   Vulva and external genitalia shrink with loss of subcutaneous fat
7.   Vaginal secretions diminish
8.   Response to sexual stimulation takes longer
9.   Elasticity of breast tissue is reduced
10.   Testosterone secretion decreases
11.   Testes become smaller and less firm
12.   Sperm production is slowed
13.   Erection takes longer to achieve and subsides more rapidly
14.   Ejaculation is shorter and less forceful
15.   Time between erection and orgasm lengthens
16.   Basal metabolism rate is decreased
17.   Woman loses ability to procreate
18.   Glucose metabolism diminishes
19.   Pancreatic secretions decrease
20.   Decreased pituitary secretions with decreased muscle mass
21.   Decreased production of thyroid-stimulating hormone resulting in decreased basal metabolic rate
22.   Decreased production of parathyroid hormone (seen with osteoporosis) as well as increased blood calcium levels

B.   Selected disorders
1.   Contributing factors: glandular changes as result of aging process
2.   Resulting problems
     a.   Adult-onset diabetes mellitus
     b.   Musculoskeletal system changes
     c.   Hypothyroidism

C.   Nursing management of diabetes mellitus: special considerations
1.   Poor vision
2.   Lack of coordination
3.   Poor nutritional patterns
4.   Forgetfulness and confusion
5.   Resistance to change
6.   Masking of symptoms by physiologic changes of aging and disease
7.   Decreased activity level
8.   Stress and anxiety
9.   Increased susceptibility to complications

Hematopoietic and Lymph System

A.   Alterations
1.   Diminished immunoglobulin production
2.   Weakened antibody response
3.   Atypical signs and symptoms frequently a response to infection (e.g., subnormal temperature, behavior changes, decreased pain sensation)
4.   Increased plasma viscosity causing increased risk of vascular occlusion
5.   Decreased red blood cell production with increased incidence of anemia
6.   Increase in immature T cells resulting in decreased immune response

B.   Selected disorders
1.   Contributing factors
     a.   Weakened antibody response
     b.   Reduced immunoglobulin production
          (1)   Thymus gland wasting
          (2)   Reticuloendothelial system alterations
2.   Resulting problems
     a.   Self-destructive autoaggressive phenomenon
     b.   Increased susceptibility to infection
     c.   Increased susceptibility to disease
     d.   Misdiagnosis
          (1)   Older adults with pneumonia may not have a fever or chills
          (2)   Dysuria is often absent in the older person with a urinary tract infection

(3) Pain may be absent with peritonitis or appendicitis, even though the individual is obviously ill

(4) Physiologic response of the older adult to tuberculosis skin testing may be less intense than that of younger individuals

C. Nursing management
1. Be careful in observation and assessment
2. Be aware that atypical symptoms of infection are common among older adults; for example, with otitis media, difficulty in hearing is too often dismissed as a typical aging problem
3. Use early nursing intervention

Sense Organs

A. Vision
1. Alterations
   a. Pupil size diminishes: loss of responsiveness to light
   b. Decline in peripheral vision
   c. Accommodation ability decreases, causing presbyopia (farsightedness)
   d. Decrease in tear production with increased risk of eye irritation
   e. Decrease in lens transparency and elasticity
   f. Decline in ability to focus quickly
   g. Decline in color discrimination
   h. Difficulty in adjusting to light changes
   i. Decreased number of eyelashes, leading to increased risk of eye injury
   j. Increased discoloration of lens, causing decreased color perception
   k. Decreased tissue elasticity, resulting in increased blurring
   l. Decreased muscle tone, causing a decreased diameter of pupil, increased refractive errors, decreased night vision, and increased sensitivity to glare
2. Selected disorders
   a. Cataracts
   b. Glaucoma
   c. Senile macular degeneration
   d. Presbyopia
   e. Floaters and flashes
   f. Ectropion
   g. Entropion
3. Low-vision optical aids
   a. Magnifying devices
      (1) Hand held
      (2) Glasses
      (3) Flat bars
   b. Telescopic lenses for distance vision
   c. Microscopic lenses for close vision
   d. High-intensity reading lamps
   e. Closed-circuit television
   f. Computers
   g. Large-print books, newspapers, magazines, checks (ask at a bank), telephone dials, clocks, watches, oven timers, playing cards, bingo cards
   h. Signature guide
   i. Self-threading sewing needles
   j. Talking clocks and wristwatches
4. Care and management considerations
   a. Bright, diffused light is best
   b. Place items on better-vision side
   c. Avoid glare
   d. Strips on stairs improve depth perception
   e. Glasses should be kept clean (older residents frequently forget or ignore this)
   f. Use colors that increase visual acuity (e.g., red, orange, and yellow)
   g. Avoid night driving
   h. Use resources and aids for visually impaired
   i. Preserve independence
   j. Visual losses increase susceptibility to illusions, disorientation, confusion, and isolation
   k. Place objects directly in front of individual with decreased peripheral vision
   l. Stimulate other senses

B. Hearing
1. Auditory alterations
   a. Progressive loss of hearing, starting with high-frequency tones due to decreased tissue elasticity
      (1) Presbycusis (loss of sound perception)
      (2) Otosclerosis (bone cell overgrowth)
      (3) Cerumen accumulation

b. Eardrum thickens and becomes more opaque

c. Decreased joint mobility causing decreased hearing ability

d. Decreased number of hair cells in inner ear with increased problems with balance—Ménière's disease

2. Hearing devices

a. Hearing aids (multiple types are available)

b. Telephone, television, radio amplifiers

c. Captioned television

d. Teletypewriters

e. Doorbell and telephone that light as well as ring

f. Flashing smoke detectors and alarm clocks

g. Burglar alarms that light up as well as sound

3. Care and management considerations

a. Older persons usually do poorly on hearing tests because of their cautious responsiveness

b. Reduce distractions

c. Do not fatigue with unnecessary noise and talk

d. Speak in a normal tone of voice; shouting is misinterpreted by those who have normal hearing

e. Observe for signs of developing hearing loss

(1) Leaning forward

(2) Inappropriate responses

(3) Cupping ear when listening

(4) Loud speaking voice

(5) Requests to repeat what has been said

f. Reduce background noise before speaking (e.g., television and radio)

g. Hearing deficits increase social isolation, suspiciousness, and fear

h. Speak toward the better ear

i. Be sure to have the person's attention before speaking

j. Use resources and aids for the hearing impaired (e.g., television and telephone amplifiers, sound lamps, and alarm clocks that shake the bed)

C. Other sense organs

1. Taste bud alterations

a. Number of taste buds declines

b. Taste sensation is dulled

c. Taste detection declines with bitter, sour, salty, flavors

d. Sweet flavor awareness remains intact

2. Olfactory alterations

a. Olfactory nerve fibers decrease

b. Sense of smell diminishes

3. Tactile alterations

a. Sense of touch dulled

b. Pain threshold higher

c. Sense of vibration diminished

4. Vestibular/kinesthetic alterations

a. Diminished proprioception

b. Decrease in coordination

c. Decline in equilibrium

Special Considerations
NUTRITION

A. Diet

1. Nutrition needs same as those of other adults (vitamins and minerals)

2. Adequate protein to prevent muscle wasting and weakness

3. Adequate fats for tissue, insulation, and energy

4. Adequate carbohydrates from unprocessed foods for energy: older adults have a tendency to buy high-carbohydrate, empty-calorie foods because they are:

a. Less costly

b. Filling

c. Easy to chew

d. Easy to prepare

B. Physiologic changes affect nutrition of older adults

1. Aging slows the basal metabolic rate (BMR); combined with decreased activity, the result is decreased energy requirements and decreased number of calories needed

2. Taste may be adversely affected by gradual diminishment of the senses of smell, sight, and taste

3. Loss of teeth may affect food intake or its enjoyment

4. Decreased body secretions make swallowing more difficult and digestion less efficient

5. Decreased movement of wastes through intestines contributes to constipation

C. Economic and social considerations
   1. Decrease in income among older adults, combined with an increase in the amount spent for medical care, leaves less for adequate nutrition; tendency is to eat less protein (which is expensive) and more carbohydrates (which are cheaper and easier to prepare)
   2. Loss of spouse, friends, or mobility results in isolation, depression, and often decreased will to obtain adequate nutrition
   3. Financial assistance and planning
   4. Transportation to and from grocery store
   5. Assistance with packages because of weakness and physical disabilities
   6. Assistance for the confused, forgetful, and ill
   7. Encourage regular meals—older adults have a tendency to skip meals
   8. Education classes on purchasing healthful foods on limited income
D. Planning diets
   1. Diet should be well balanced in protein, vitamins, and minerals (especially calcium and iron) to allow for diminished absorption
   2. Calories sufficient to maintain energy and activity (reduced from those previously required)
   3. Soft bulk in diet to prevent constipation (cooked fruits and vegetables) as well as fiber and roughage
   4. Increased fluid intake required to eliminate metabolic wastes—2500 to 3000 ml per day
   5. Meals should be light and easily digested; that is, contain a small amount of fats
   6. Individual preferences should be respected and the diet built around them; make changes slowly
   7. Meals eaten with others are often more appetizing than those eaten alone
   8. Ethnic, cultural, and lifestyle preferences should be encouraged for identity reinforcement and appetite stimulation
   9. Tendency to reduce intake because of urinary frequency, urgency, and incontinence
   10. Vitamin supplements to prevent deficiencies
   11. Lactose intolerance common: calcium can be obtained from other sources (e.g., spinach, asparagus, broccoli, and sardines)
   12. Consistency and preparation in accordance with chewing, swallowing, and digestive abilities
   13. Small, frequent meals are easier to digest and conserve energy
   14. Unhurried atmosphere to increase appetite and incentive to eat
   15. Caution against food fads and megavitamin therapy
   16. Assess facilities for appropriateness
       a. Storage
       b. Cooking
       c. Refrigeration
   17. Monitor weight and adjust food intake as required

FLUID VOLUME

A. Older adults likely to experience fluid volume deficit:
   1. Have altered swallow reflex (stroke victims)
   2. Are nauseated and unwilling to eat or drink
   3. Are under acute emotional distress and have decreased interest in personal needs
   4. Are unable to obtain adequate fluids without assistance (bedridden residents)
   5. Have altered cognition (Alzheimer's disease or dementia) and are not aware of the need for fluids
   6. Have draining wounds, open sores, or ulcers
   7. Are receiving diuretic medications
   8. Have kidney disease
   9. Are receiving tube feedings of preparations with low sodium content
B. Older adults likely to experience fluid volume excess:
   1. Have increased fluid intake secondary to excess sodium intake, hyperglycemia, or medications
   2. Drink water compulsively
   3. Have decreased urine output secondary to kidney dysfunction
   4. Have heart failure
   5. Have insufficient protein intake or excessive protein loss

6. Are on steroid therapy
7. Have a history of alcoholism or liver disease
8. Have kidney disease
9. Are experiencing diaphoresis
10. Are experiencing intermittent or persistent vomiting
11. Have intermittent or persistent diarrhea

C. Nursing interventions
1. Assess
2. Monitor vital signs
3. Monitor intake and output
4. Monitor laboratory values
5. Weigh resident daily
6. Measure leg and abdominal girth for changes
7. Maintain required fluid intake

ACTIVITIES OF DAILY LIVING AND SELF-CARE

A. Older adults may ignore appearance because of fatigue, unawareness, or lack of incentive
B. Clean clothing is essential for maintaining pride and dignity
C. Choosing what to wear provides a source of control over one's life, fosters independence, and increases self-confidence and self-esteem
D. Lifelong sleeping attire (or lack of attire) should be encouraged
1. Reinforces individuality
2. Reduces sleep interference
E. Standard clothing sizes no longer fit; loose-fitting, comfortable clothing should be encouraged
F. Front closures are more easily managed
G. Cotton socks absorb perspiration
H. Zippers, velcro, and large buttons make dressing easier
I. Layering provides warmth in cold weather
J. Daily exercise should be encouraged and paced
K. Older adults likely to experience self-care deficits
1. Have decreased strength or endurance because of respiratory or cardiovascular changes
2. Have altered neuromuscular or musculoskeletal function related to disease or aging
3. Are experiencing pain
4. Have cognitive or perceptual problems (Alzheimer's disease or dementia)

5. Are experiencing severe anxiety or depression
6. Have impaired mobility

HYGIENE

A. Skin
1. Water temperature 100° to 105° F (37.7° to 40.5° C)
2. Daily baths not necessary
3. Oil-base or emollient lotion
4. Alcohol and dusting powder not appropriate because they dry out the skin
5. Avoid friction
6. Avoid pressure
7. Neutral-reaction or oil-base soap
8. Susceptible to bruising and skin tears
B. Nose: blunt-end scissors to trim nasal hairs that extend beyond nares
C. Oral hygiene
1. Dentures
2. Soft nylon toothbrush, electric toothbrush, or adaptive toothbrush
3. Half-strength hydrogen peroxide rinses
4. Lanolin to lips
5. Encourage semiannual dental visits
6. Frequent mouth inspection for food accumulation, injury, disease, and infection
B. Ears
1. Clean with warm, soapy water and dry with towel
2. Do not use cotton swabs because they force cerumen back against the tympanum
3. Trim ear hair growth in men
4. Hearing aids
   a. Wash mold and receiver with mild soap and warm water
   b. Check cannula for patency, and clean and dry with pipe cleaner
   c. Remove batteries when aid is not in use
   d. Store batteries in refrigerator to retain freshness
   e. Turn aid to off position when inserting in resident's ear
   f. Turn aid on to adjust volume
   g. Store aid in its original box away from cold, heat, and sunlight
C. Eyes
1. More frequent cleaning of eyeglasses required
2. Use cool water to clean eyeglasses

3. Store only in eyeglass case
D. Nails
1. Daily care
2. Use moisturizer on nails and cuticles
3. Encourage circulation with buffing of nails
4. File with emery board (cutting makes them more brittle and risks injury)
E. Hair
1. Use mild shampoo that is not irritating to the eyes
2. Remove facial hair from women with tweezers or waxing
3. Use of a shaving brush is recommended for men
4. Moisturizers are beneficial for men's facial skin
F. Feet
1. Give daily care
2. Inspect between and under toes for abrasions, cracking, lacerations, and scaling
3. Clip toenails straight across
4. Pumice stone should be used to remove dry, hard skin
5. Discourage use of irritants
6. Avoid elastic-top socks or knee-high stockings
7. Emphasize the danger of roll garters
8. Recommend properly fitting shoes with low, broad, rubber heels for safety, comfort, and fatigue reduction

SLEEP

A. Stages of sleep
1. Stage 1: non-REM
   a. Lightest level of sleep
   b. Lasts a few minutes
   c. Decreased physiologic activity beginning with a gradual fall in vital signs and metabolism
   d. Person easily aroused by sensory stimuli such as noise
   e. If person awakes, feels as though daydreaming
2. Stage 2: non-REM
   a. Period of sound sleep
   b. Relaxation progresses
   c. Arousal still easy
   d. Lasts 10 to 20 minutes
   e. Body functions still slowing
3. Stage 3: non-REM
   a. Initial stages of deep sleep
   b. Sleeper difficult to arouse and rarely moves
   c. Muscles completely relaxed
   d. Vital signs declining but remaining regular
   e. Lasts 15 to 30 minutes
4. Stage 4: non-REM
   a. Deepest stage of sleep
   b. Very difficult to arouse sleeper
   c. If sleep loss has occurred, sleeper will spend considerable portion of night in this stage
   d. Restores and rests the body
   e. Vital signs significantly lower than during waking hours
   f. Lasts approximately 15 to 30 minutes
   g. Possible sleepwalking and enuresis
5. REM sleep
   a. Stage of vivid, full-color dreaming (less vivid dreaming may occur in other stages)
   b. Usually begins every 50 to 90 minutes after sleep has begun
   c. Typified by autonomic response of rapidly moving eyes, fluctuating heart and respiratory rates, and blood pressure
   d. Loss of skeletal muscle tone
   e. Responsible for mental restoration
   f. Sleeper most difficult to arouse
   g. Duration increasing with each cycle and averaging 20 minutes
B. Older adults likely to experience problems related to sleep or rest:
1. Are experiencing pain
2. Are under increased physical or psychologic stress
3. Have recently experienced environmental changes such as a change of residence or hospitalization
4. Are physically inactive
C. Nursing interventions
1. Identify specific factors that make sleep difficult
2. Ask if resident can identify any changes that would aid sleep
3. Consider room change if possible
4. Close door to reduce extraneous noise
5. Discourage daytime napping

6. Encourage daytime physical activities
7. Recommend avoidance of caffeine after dinner
8. Teach relaxation techniques
9. Provide comfort measures at bedtime
10. Assess need for further sleeping aids

ACTIVITY AND EXERCISE

A. Older adults likely to have problems related to activity intolerance:
   1. Have a sedentary lifestyle
   2. Have a decreased sense of self-worth, self-esteem, or independence
   3. Have generalized weakness, are immobile, or are restricted to bed rest
   4. Have problems related to oxygenation
   5. Have cognitive impairment (Alzheimer's disease or dementia)
   6. Are malnourished
B. Older adults likely to have problems related to diversional activities:
   1. Are restricted in mobility
   2. Are confined to an environment with limited activities
   3. Are suffering from anxiety, depression, or grief
   4. Have limited financial or transportation resources
   5. Have cognitive or perceptual problems
C. Older adults likely to have problems related to impaired physical mobility:
   1. Cannot tolerate physical activity because of medical conditions that decrease endurance or strength
   2. Are experiencing pain
   3. Have neuromuscular or musculoskeletal conditions
   4. Have cognitive impairment (Alzheimer's disease or dementia)
   5. Have severe anxiety or depression
   6. Are on prescribed bed rest
   7. Use restrictive devices (restraints, casts, splints, immobilizers)
D. Interventions
   1. Cognitive training
      a. Consists of memory exercises, problem-solving situations, and memory training
      b. Leader must be familiar with resident's past leisure time utilization, hobbies, and occupations
      c. Individual, small, or large groups
      d. Purpose is to maintain mental activity
   2. Relaxation therapy
      a. Promotes sense of physical well-being, reduces stress, releases tension
      b. Small groups
      c. Involves rhythmic breathing, tension-relaxation exercises, and altered state of consciousness
   3. Reminiscence
      a. Small group sessions
      b. Based on life review process
      c. Older adults with cognitive dysfunction retain long-term memory and through reminiscence can adapt to the aging process
      d. Purposes
         (1) Conflict resolution
         (2) Sharing of memories
         (3) Sense of identity and self-importance achieved
         (4) Focus is on a life that has meaning as opposed to a life viewed as a waste of time
         (5) Natural for older persons to reminisce
            (a) Feels comfortable
            (b) They're good at it
            (c) Reinforces sense of belonging (everyone talks about life's trials and tribulations)
         (6) Therapeutic relationship with leader more likely to develop as residents realize their memories are important and valued
         (7) Depressed residents find a caring listener and an opportunity to externalize their anger
         (8) Psychologically disturbed residents receive acceptance, group validation, and a forum for expression: encourage active exploration of past strengths
         (9) Strive to change outlook on the past rather than establishing new future directions
         (10) Psychologic assessment tool (e.g., insight into past coping mechanisms)
         (11) Reduces isolation, insecurity, and negative self-esteem

(12) Confused residents can be assisted to explore a memory that will stimulate latent thoughts, become more oriented, and improve ability to focus

(13) Current circumstances are often reflected through memories

e. If residents have difficulty focusing their thoughts, assist by selecting a specific memory

f. Stimulation of dormant thoughts to the surface decreases disorientation

g. Residents who are reluctant to talk can usually be stimulated with topics of food, movies, or music

h. Program implementation is not limited to a particular setting

4. Reality orientation
   a. Emphasizes orientation to time, place, and person
   b. Orientation boards are used to provide contact with reality (e.g., time, date, locations, weather, last meal, and next meal)
   c. Program success depends on total staff commitment and 24-hour implementation
   d. Program implementation not limited to a particular setting
   e. Components
      (1) Formal classroom sessions
      (2) Morning sessions recommended (older adults are more alert in the morning)
      (3) Positive verbal feedback emphasized
      (4) Confusion never reinforced
   f. All personnel who come in contact with residents participating in the program are expected to use reality orientation
      (1) Address resident by name and title
      (2) Orient resident to time, place, and person
      (3) Give positive verbal feedback
      (4) Do not reinforce confusion
   g. Structured
   h. Refreshments or food may be served for identification
   i. Appreciation of the work of the world;

constantly reminded of who they are, where they are, why they are there, and what is expected of them

j. Class range from 3 to 5 residents, depending on degree/level of confusion or disorientation from any cause

k. Meeting $1/2$ hour daily at same time in same place

l. Planned procedures: reality-centered objects

m. Consistence of approach and response of resident responsibility of teacher

n. Periodic reality orientation test pertaining to resident's level of confusion or disorientation

o. Use of portion of mind function still intact

p. Residents thanked for coming, and extended handshake and/or physical contact according to attitude approach in group

q. Conducted by trained staff

5. Remotivation
   a. Similar to reality orientation
   b. Normal behavior reinforced through structured group program
   c. Stimulating participation and interest in the environment are key components
   d. Sessions average 20 minutes
   e. Visual aids (items that stimulate sensory responses) are used
   f. Resident behavior recorded
   g. Staff support and involvement essential
   h. Orientation to reality for community living; present oriented
   i. Definite structure
   j. Refreshments not served
   k. Appreciation of the work of the group stimulates the desire to return to function in society
   l. Group size: 5 to 12 residents
   m. Preselected and reality-centered objects
   n. No exploration of feelings
   o. Topic: no discussion of religion, politics, or death
   p. No physical contact permitted; acceptance and acknowledgment of everyone's contribution
   q. Conducted by trained staff

Review Questions

1. Nursing actions for older residents should include health education and promotion of self-care. When dealing with older residents the nurse should:
   ① Encourage exercise and naps
   ② Strengthen the concept of ageism
   ③ Reinforce residents' strengths and promote reminiscing
   ④ Teach about a high-carbohydrate diet and focus on the present

2. The nutritional status of the older resident requires regular monitoring. It's important for the nurse to know that:
   ① Caloric requirements are greater than for younger residents
   ② Caloric requirements are less than for younger residents
   ③ Caloric requirements are the same as for younger residents
   ④ Nutritional requirements are greater for older residents than for younger residents

3. A deprivation particular to older adults is:
   ① Nutritional diet
   ② Touch
   ③ Intellectual stimulation
   ④ Olfaction

4. When removing an older resident's meal tray the nurse notices that the resident did not eat any of the chicken. When asked why the chicken was not eaten, the resident stated, "I only eat meat once a week because old people don't need protein every day." Based on this statement the nurse knows that the resident should be taught about the:
   ① Need for home-delivered meals
   ② Effect of aging on the need for some foods
   ③ Foods included in the Food Guide Pyramid
   ④ Need for meat at least once per day throughout life

5. The older adult may perform certain cognitive tasks more slowly because of:
   ① Increased motor response to sensory stimulation
   ② Increase of visual and auditory acuity
   ③ Loss of the family unit
   ④ Recent memory loss

6. A resident is scheduled for cataract surgery. The resident tells the nurse that he is too old to go through a surgical procedure and hesitates to learn about postoperative care. The nurse's response should be:
   ① "Oh, you're not too old! There's not that much to learn."
   ② "You'll be surprised how well you will do."
   ③ "The physician and nursing staff will assist you."
   ④ "You seem concerned about your surgery and your postoperative care. Do you want to talk about it?"

7. A resident has bladder and bowel incontinence. At a nursing care planning conference the staff decides to proceed with a bowel-retraining program. Bowel retraining is initiated before bladder retraining because:
   ① Bowel retraining is easier than bladder retraining
   ② Bowel incontinence is more demoralizing to the resident
   ③ Bowel retraining may solve the resident's urinary incontinence
   ④ The resident is usually more cooperative

8. The nurse teaches a resident how to use a nebulizer. The nurse would recognize that the nebulizer is not being used correctly and that additional instruction is needed when the resident:
   ① Holds the inspired breath for at least 3 seconds
   ② Positions the tip of the nebulizer beyond the lips
   ③ Inhales with the lips tightly sealed around the mouthpiece
   ④ Exhales slowly through the mouth with lips pursed slightly

9. You find an elderly man with heat exhaustion. Which of the following are signs and symptoms the nurse might expect the victim to manifest related to his diagnosis?
   ① Marked diaphoresis; cool, pale, damp skin; possible temperature elevation
   ② Cessation of sweating; flushed, hot, dry skin; elevated temperature
   ③ Red, blistering skin with wet appearance and edema
   ④ Hyperemic skin with blister formation and edema

10. An older resident receiving antihypertensive drugs should be cautioned to avoid sudden changes in position, especially from a supine to an upright position, because:
    1. A thrombus may become dislodged
    2. Severe nausea may result
    3. Postural hypotension may occur
    4. Increased diuresis occurs

11. While taking amitriptyline hydrochloride (Elavil), a resident in a nursing home reports a dry mouth. An appropriate nursing intervention would be to:
    1. Tell the resident that this is just his imagination and to ignore it
    2. Tell the resident to suck on hard candies
    3. Recommend chewing sugarless gum or drinking plenty of fluids
    4. Instruct the resident to rinse the mouth with saltwater

12. An older adult has recently become a resident of a nursing home. While visiting with the resident, a nurse learns he is very depressed and feels worthless and unloved by his family. The resident is receiving amitriptyline hydrochloride (Elavil) prescribed by the physician. When would this drug be most likely to achieve the goal of lifting depression?
    1. After a 6- to 7-week period
    2. In 2 to 4 weeks
    3. Within a few days
    4. Almost immediately

13. An older adult has recently moved into a nursing home and is feeling depressed. The physician has prescribed amitriptyline hydrochloride (Elavil). An adverse effect of this antidepressant may be:
    1. Diarrhea
    2. Insomnia
    3. Hypertension
    4. Urinary retention

ANSWERS AND RATIONALES FOR REVIEW QUESTIONS

1. **3** Reinforcing strengths promotes self-esteem; reminiscing is a therapeutic tool that provides a life review, which assists adaptation and helps achieve the task of integrity associated with older adults.
   1 Exercise should be encouraged, but naps tend to interfere with adequate sleep at night.
   2 Reinforcing ageism would enhance devaluation of the older adult.
   4 A well-balanced diet that also includes protein and fiber should be encouraged; older adults need to put the past in perspective, and a positive self-assessment should be supported.

2. **2** Older adults have a decreased need for calories
   1 Caloric needs are decreased
   3 Caloric needs are decreased
   4 Nutritional needs are the same.

3. **2** Touch, because of relational losses.
   1 May be deprived, but not the most correct answer.
   3 May or may not be true.
   4 May or may not be true.

4. **3** The need for the six basic food groups in the Food Guide Pyramid continues throughout life.
   1 The priority is to educate the resident, although home-delivered meals may be one way to provide adequate nutrition.
   2 Aging does not necessarily have an effect on the specific nutrients needed; however, it may influence digestion and/or absorption of food.
   4 Protein is needed every day, but it need not be in the form of meat.

5. **4** Unless there are physical or neurologic changes such as a recent memory loss, the functions of habit, judgment, creativity, and problem-solving are maintained.
   1 Motor response decreases with age.
   2 Visual and auditory acuity decrease with age.
   3 This is not pertinent to cognitive tasks.

6. **4** This response allows the resident to talk about feelings and raises questions that need to be addressed.
   1 This response cuts the resident off and does not allow him to state what is really bothering him.
   2 This gives false reassurance.
   3 This response does not address the resident's concerns.

7. **1** Bowel retraining is easier, and success is usually met in a much shorter period of time.
   2 Both are demoralizing.
   3 Bowel retraining does not solve urinary incontinence.
   4 Cooperation does not usually vary.

8. **3** This technique promotes nasal breathing, which negates the effects of aerosol medication; a loose seal around the mouthpiece allows for inhalation through the mouth.
   1 This is a correct technique; it promotes contact of medication with the bronchial mucosa.
   2 This is a correct technique; the nebulizer tip must be past the lips to deliver medication.
   4 This is a correct technique; it prolongs and improves delivery of the medication to the respiratory mucosa.

9. **1** These are signs and symptoms of heat exhaustion.
   2 These are signs and symptoms of heat stroke.
   3 These are signs and symptoms of second-degree burns.
   4 These are signs and symptoms of second-degree burns.

10. **3** Adverse reaction commonly noted
    1 Sudden change in position is not a known cause for a thrombus to become an embolism.
    2 Not usually noted due to a sudden change in position.
    4 This will not occur simply due to a change in position; diuretics in combination with an antihypertensive medication accounts for the increase in diuresis.

11. **3** This is the best answer because these measures are helpful in overcoming thirst and a dry mouth.
    1 Untrue; this is a common side effect.
    2 Sucking on hard candies will increase thirst and predispose the resident to dental caries.
    4 Rinsing the mouth with plain water may be beneficial. This should not include saltwater because many older adults also have conditions such as congestive heart failure or kidney disease that would cause fluid retention.

12. **2** Elavil is an antidepressant with sedative effects. It usually takes 2 to 4 weeks to achieve favorable results.
    1 This is incorrect. Although the sedative effect may be apparent before the antidepressant effect is noted, an adequate therapeutic effect may take as long as 30 days to develop.
    3 This is incorrect. Although the sedative effect may be apparent before the antidepressant effect is noted, an adequate therapeutic effect may take as long as 30 days to develop.
    4 This is incorrect. Although the sedative effect may be apparent before the antidepressant effect is noted, an adequate therapeutic effect may take as long as 30 days to develop.

13. **4** An adverse effect of the medication is urine retention; this is a serious problem and should be reported promptly.
    1 This is not associated with amitriptyline therapy.
    2 This is not associated with amitriptyline therapy.
    3 This is not associated with amitriptyline therapy.

chapter sixteen

Pediatric Overview

Assessment of Child and Family

A. Functions and structure of family
1. The functions and structure of the family are vital to the normal growth and development of the child
2. Three primary functions of the family are:
   a. Providing physical care such as food, clothing, shelter, safety, prevention of illness, and care during illness
   b. Education and training: language, values, morals, and formal education
   c. Protecting psychologic and emotional health
B. Physical assessment of child
1. Performing a health history, including the child's past history as well as current complaints or problems, is done by the nurse, physician, or nurse practitioner
2. Assessment of child's physical growth and development level is done by the physician or nurse practitioner
C. Concepts of child development
1. Freud's theory of development is based on the child's psychosexual development
2. Erikson's theory of development is based on psychosocial development as a series of developmental tasks
3. Piaget's theory of development is based on intellectual (cognitive) development: how the child learns and develops intelligence

With advances in early diagnosis and treatment of many chronic illnesses and with improved technology there is an increased demand of the nurse to know and manage the care of the child with special needs.

Impact of Chronic Illness on the Child and Family
CHRONIC ILLNESSES

Scope of care for the chronically ill child includes early detection of problem, assessment and identification, diagnostic studies, and supportive pertinent interventions.

NEUROLOGIC MALFORMATIONS
Spina Bifida

A. Malformation of the spine in which the posterior portion of the laminae of the vertebrae fails to close; most common site is the lumbosacral area
B. Associated defects include weakness or paralysis below the defect, bowel and bladder dysfunction, clubfeet, dislocated hip, and hydrocephalus
C. Classifications
1. Spina bifida occulta: spinal cord and meninges are intact
2. Meningocele
3. Meningomyelocele
D. Clinical findings
1. Degree of neurologic dysfunction directly related to level of defect
2. Defective nerve supply to bladder affects sphincter and muscle tone
3. Frequently poor anal sphincter control
E. Therapeutic management
1. Multidisciplinary approach including rehabilitation
2. Surgical repair of the sac to maintain neurologic function and prevent infection

Nursing Care of Infants and Children with Spina Bifida

A. Assessment
1. Condition of the myelomeningocele sac
2. Level of neurologic involvement
3. Elimination
   a. Urine: dribble or stream
   b. Anal reflexes
4. Monitor head circumference and fontanels at least daily
B. Analysis/nursing diagnoses
1. Risk for infection related to exposed myelomeningocele sac
2. Risk for trauma related to spinal cord lesion
3. Risk for impaired skin integrity related to paralysis, incontinence
4. Alterated family relationships due to having a critically ill child
C. Planning/implementation
1. Protect against infection because breakdown of the sac leaves the spinal cord open to the environment
   a. Area must be kept clean, especially from urine and feces
   b. Diaper is not used, but sterile gauze with antibiotic solution may be placed over the sac
   c. Avoid pressure on sac
2. Maintain function through proper position: place in prone position, hips slightly flexed and abducted, feet hanging free of mattress, and a slight Trendelenburg slope to reduce spinal fluid pressure

Hydrocephalus

A. Definition: disorder caused by an obstruction of cerebrospinal fluid drainage; characterized by an excess of cerebrospinal fluid (CSF) within the cranial cavity, which causes an enlarged head and potential brain damage or retardation
B. Symptoms
1. Bulging of the anterior fontanel
2. Enlargement of the head
3. Irritability
4. Opisthotonos, "setting sun" sign (sclera can be seen above the iris because of increased intracranial pressure)

C. Diagnosis—based on:
1. Symptoms
2. Frequent measurement of head circumference
3. CAT scans
D. Treatment/nursing interventions
1. Surgical repair is necessary to relieve the obstruction or to shunt the CSF from the ventricles of the brain into the heart (ventriculoarterial shunt) or the abdomen (ventriculoperitoneal shunt)
2. Postoperative care includes frequent position changes to prevent pressure on the head, care of the shunt, and general postoperative care

Cerebral Palsy

A. Definition: a group of nonprogressive disorders caused by a malfunction of the motor centers of the brain; oxygen deprivation (anoxia) damages the brain's motor centers prenatally, during, or immediately after delivery or during childhood after an accident or disease
B. Symptoms: difficulty in controlling voluntary muscle movements, delays in development, hearing and vision impairment, seizures, and in some cases mental retardation
C. Diagnosis: based on the mother's prenatal history, birth history, history of an accident or disease, presence of delays in growth and development, and abnormal neurologic examination
D. Types of cerebral palsy
1. Spastic: hyperactive muscle and tendon reflexes, accompanied by continuous spasms and muscle contractures
2. Dyskinetic (athetoid): the body muscles are in a constant state of motion and slow muscle contractions
3. Ataxia: a lack of coordination and balance when walking
E. Treatment/nursing interventions
1. Treatment and care are supportive to ensure optimal level of development for the child
2. Physical and occupational therapy to help the child learn some control over muscle movements
3. Braces as needed to hold extremities in correct positions of function

Developmental aspects of chronic illness or disability on children

Age/Developmental Tasks	Potential Effects of Chronic Illness or Disability	Supportive Interventions
Infancy		
Develop a sense of trust	Multiple care givers and frequent separations, especially if hospitalized Deprived of consistent nurturing	Encourage consistent care givers in hospital or other care settings Encourage parents to visit frequently or "room in" during hospitalization and to participate in care
Bond/attach to parent	Delayed because of separation, parental grief for loss of "dream" child, parental inability to accept the condition, especially a visible defect	Emphasize healthy, perfect qualities of infant Help parents learn special care needs of infant for them to feel competent
Learn through sensorimotor experiences	Increased exposure to painful experiences over pleasurable ones Limited contact with environment from restricted movement or confinement	Expose infant to pleasurable experiences through all senses (touch, hearing, sight, taste, movement) Encourage age-appropriate developmental skills (e.g., holding bottle, finger feeding, crawling)
Begin to develop a sense of separateness from parent	Increased dependency on parent to care Overinvolvement of parent in care	Encourage all family members to participate in care to prevent overinvolvement of one member Encourage periodic respite from demands of care responsibilities
Toddlerhood		
Develop autonomy	Increased dependency on parent	Encourage independence in as many areas as possible (e.g., toileting, dressing, feeding)
Master locomotor and language skills	Limited opportunity to test own abilities and limits	Provide gross motor skill activity and modification of toys or equipment, such as modified swing or rocking horse Give choices to allow simple feeling of control (e.g., choice of what book to look at or what kind of sandwich to eat)
Learn through sensorimotor experience, beginning preoperational thought	Increased exposure to painful experiences	Institute age-appropriate discipline and limit setting Recognize that negative and ritualistic behavior are normal Provide sensory experiences (e.g., water play, sandbox, finger paint)
Preschool		
Develop initiative and purpose Master self-care skills	Limited opportunities for success in accomplishing simple tasks or mastering self-care skills	Encourage mastery of self-help skills Provide devices that make task easier (e.g., self-dressing)
Begin to develop peer relationships	Limited opportunities for socialization with peers; may appear "like a baby" to age-mates Protection within tolerant and secure family may cause child to fear criticism and to withdraw	Encourage socialization, such as inviting friends to play, daycare experience, trips to park Provide age-appropriate play, especially associative play opportunities
Develop sense of body image and sexual identification	Awareness of body may center on pain, anxiety, and failure Sex role identification focused primarily on mothering skills	Emphasize child's abilities; dress appropriately to enhance desirable appearance Encourage relationships with same-sex and opposite-sex peers and adults Help child deal with criticisms; realize that too much protection prevents child from realities of world

Learn through preoperational thought (magical thinking)	Guilt (child thinks he caused the illness/disability or is being punished for wrongdoing)	Clarify that cause of child's illness or disability is not his fault or a punishment
School age		
Develop a sense of accomplishment	Limited opportunities to achieve and compete (e.g., many school absences or inability to join regular athletic activities)	Encourage school attendance; schedule medical visits at times other than school; encourage to make up missed work Educate teachers and classmates about child's condition, abilities, and special needs Encourage sports activities (e.g., Special Olympics)
Form peer relationships	Limited opportunities for socialization	Encourage socialization (e.g., Girl Scouts, Campfire, Boy Scouts, 4-H Clubs, having a best friend or a club)
Learn through concrete operations	Incomplete comprehension of the imposed physical limitations or treatment of the disorder	Provide child with knowledge about condition Encourage creative activities (e.g., Very Special Arts)
Adolescence		
Develop personal and sexual identity	Increased sense of feeling different from peers and less able to compete with peers in appearance, abilities, special skills	Realize that many of the difficulties the teenager is experiencing are part of normal adolescence (rebelliousness, risk taking, lack of cooperation, hostility toward authority) Provide instruction on interpersonal and coping skills Encourage socialization with peers, including peers with special needs and those without special needs Provide instruction on decision making, assertiveness, and other skills necessary to manage personal plans
Achieve independence from family	Increased dependency on family; limited job/career opportunities	Encourage increased responsibility for care and management of the disease or condition, such as assuming responsibility for making and keeping appointments (ideally alone), sharing assessment and planning stages of health care delivery, and contacting resources Encourage activities appropriate for age, such as attending mixed-sex parties, sports activities, and driving a car
Form heterosexual relationships	Limited opportunities for heterosexual friendships; less opportunity to discuss sexual concerns with peers	Be alert to cues that signal readiness for information regarding implications of condition on sexuality and reproduction Emphasize good appearance: wearing stylish clothes, use of makeup Understand that adolescent has same sexual needs and concerns as any other teenager Discuss planning for future and how condition can affect choices
Learn through abstract thinking	Increased concern with issues such as why he has the disorder and whether he can marry and have a family Decreased opportunity for earlier stages of cognition may impede achieving level of abstract thinking	

4. Use of wheelchairs, walkers, and crutches as needed for ambulation/locomotion
5. Speech therapy as needed
6. Emotional support for the family and child; most often, cerebral palsy children are of normal intelligence and have only physical limitations
7. Encourage the child to live as normal a life as possible; refer the family to supportive groups such as the Easter Seal Society

Down's Syndrome

A. Definition: an abnormality caused by an extra chromosome 21 (trisomy 21). It is associated most commonly with advanced maternal age; however, in a small percent of cases the abnormality has been noted in younger women
B. Symptoms (defects)
   1. Hypotonia
   2. Small, low-set ears
   3. Slanted eyes
   4. Protruding tongue
   5. Small, flattened nose
   6. Short, broad neck
   7. Single transverse palmar crease
   8. Dry, cracked skin
   9. Congenital heart defects
   10. Mental retardation

ACQUIRED IMMUNODEFICIENCY SYNDROME (AIDS)

A. Infection with human immunodeficiency virus (HIV)
B. Generalized dysfunction of the immune system, including helper T cells
C. Abnormal B-cell function in pediatric AIDS
D. Three populations of pediatric patients
   1. Children exposed in the perinatal period
   2. Children who have received blood products before 1987, especially children with hemophilia
   3. Adolescents who are infected after engaging in high-risk behavior
E. Clinical findings
   1. Failure to thrive
   2. Interstitial pneumonitis
   3. Hepatosplenomegaly
   4. Diffuse lymphadenopathy

Nursing Care of Infants and Children With AIDS

A. Assessment
   1. Family support; who is able to care for child
   2. History to determine source of infection
   3. Health status
B. Analysis/nursing diagnoses
   1. Risk for infection related to
      a. Risk factors for AIDS
      b. Impaired immune response
   2. Body image disturbance related to having a serious illness
   3. Altered family processes related to having a child with life-threatening disease
   4. Anticipatory grieving related to having a child with a potentially fatal illness
C. Planning/implementation
   1. Prevent transmission of virus
      a. Blood and body secretion precautions
      b. Education of child and parent about modes of transmission
   2. Support child and family
   3. Monitor child for signs and symptoms of sepsis and other complications
D. Evaluation/outcomes
   1. Child does not transmit the HIV infection
   2. Child remains free of opportunistic infection
   3. Child has positive interpersonal relationships
   4. Family can demonstrate appropriate care for child
   5. Family demonstrates positive bereavement behavior

DEVELOPMENTAL ASPECTS OF CHRONIC ILLNESS OR DISABILITY ON CHILDREN
(See pp. 202-203)

STRESSES OF FAMILIES WITH A CHILD WITH SPECIAL NEEDS

A. Day-to-day stresses
   1. Constant attention
   2. Reactions of other children and the larger community
   3. Social relations
   4. Effect on siblings
   5. Marital relations
B. Life maintenance stresses
   1. Financial stress, insurance

2. Housing
3. Transportation
4. Clothing and appliances
5. Need for support
C. Worries about the future
1. Future children
2. Schooling and vocational training
3. Residential care
D. Anticipated parental stress points
1. Diagnosis of the condition—requires considerable learning, as well as dealing with emotional response
2. Developmental milestones—times children normally achieve walking, talking, self-care are delayed or impossible for the child
3. Start of schooling—particularly stressful are situations in which appropriate schooling will not be in a regular class placement
4. Reaching the ultimate attainment—situations must be handled (e.g., realizing that ambulation will be impossible or that the child will not learn to read)
5. Adolescence—issues such as sexuality and independence become prominent
6. Future placement—decisions about placement must be made when the child becomes an adult or when the parents can no longer care for the child
7. Death of the child
E. Anticipated sibling stress points
1. Birth of another child—may be the affected sibling or the subsequent birth of an unaffected child
2. Diagnosis of condition—in certain illnesses, times of remission and exacerbations are difficult
3. Start of schooling—particularly stressful if friends reject the child with special needs
4. Adolescence—when dating begins, may be embarrassed to bring dates home
5. Future placement—may worry about responsibility for the affected sibling, especially if the parents are ill or die
6. Death of the child

Review Questions

1. Nursing interventions for a child with an upper respiratory tract infection may include:
   ① Administering antibiotics, instilling ear drops, encouraging fluids, and eliminating environmental allergies
   ② Providing emotional support for the parents, decreasing fluids, positioning on the side, and decreasing stimuli
   ③ Antipyretics, bed rest, oral decongestants, cool air humidifier, proper nutrition, and fluids
   ④ Breathing exercises, liquid diet, steroid medications, bronchodilator medications, and intermittent positive-pressure breathing treatments

2. The nurse should recognize that the most common serious anomaly associated with Down's syndrome is:
   ① Renal disease
   ② Hepatic defects
   ③ Congenital heart disease
   ④ Endocrine gland malfunction

3. An initial nursing assessment of an infant with severe dehydration will most likely reveal:
   ① Stools that are frothy
   ② A weak, decreased pulse
   ③ Bulging of the occipital fontanel
   ④ An elevated urine specific gravity

4. To best ascertain the magnitude of fluid loss in an infant with gastroenteritis and diarrhea, the nurse should:
   ① Evaluate the infant's skin turgor carefully
   ② Note the elevation of the infant's hematocrit
   ③ Assess the moistness of the infant's mucous membranes
   ④ Compare the infant's pre-illness weight with current weight

5. After performing range of motion on a 13-year-old paraplegic, the nurse notices that his right foot is in a plantar flexion most of the time. The nurse should initiate which of the following interventions?
   ① Position him in proper alignment while he is asleep; increase his exercise while he is awake
   ② Inform the charge nurse of the need for intervention; increase exercise
   ③ Offer the range of motion more frequently; change the type of exercise

④ Place a foot board at the end of the bed; position the feet in a dorsal flexion position

6. The nurse has an order for acetaminophen (Tylenol) chewable tablets, two PO q4h for T >101° F (38.3° C) for a pediatric resident. The nurse assistant reports a rectal temperature of 39.2° C. The nurse would proceed with which of the following?
   ① Give two Tylenol tablets
   ② Give one Tylenol tablet
   ③ Do not give any Tylenol tablets
   ④ Check the temperature orally first

7. An antibiotic ordered for a pediatric resident comes in liquid form. The label reads 125 mg/5 ml. The physician orders 150 mg q6h. How many ml would the nurse give for each dose?
   ① 0.5 ml
   ② 5 ml
   ③ 6 ml
   ④ 10 ml

8. A school-age child is receiving a low-sodium diet. The child has requested an evening snack. In planning the diet, which of the following foods would the nurse consider?
   ① Banana
   ② Candy bar
   ③ Ham sandwich
   ④ Tuna salad

9. The nurse would assess a 4-year-old child's pain by:
   ① Asking the child to point to where the pain is
   ② Auscultating the abdomen for bowel sounds
   ③ Asking the parents about the child's bowel movements
   ④ Observing the position and behavior while the child is moving

10. During a tonic-clonic seizure a child becomes cyanotic. The nurse should:
    ① Insert an oral airway
    ② Administer oxygen by mask
    ③ Continue to observe the seizure
    ④ Notify the physician immediately

11. A nurse suspects that a child with diabetes mellitus might be hypoglycemic when the child manifests:
    ① Redness of the face and deep, rapid breathing
    ② A change in behavior, hunger, and diaphoresis
    ③ Increased thirst, sleepiness, and some vomiting
    ④ A decreased level of consciousness and dry mouth

12. Immediately after being placed flat a child experiences shortness of breath and must sit up to breathe. The nurse knows that the term that best describes this phenomenon is:
    ① Apnea
    ② Dyspnea
    ③ Orthopnea
    ④ Hyperpnea

13. In caring for a 5-year-old, the nurse knows that the normal pulse rate for a child of this age is:
    ① 76 to 90 beats/min
    ② 90 to 100 beats/min
    ③ 110 to 140 beats/min
    ④ 120 to 150 beats/min

14. A 15-year-old insulin-dependent diabetic has a history of noncompliance with therapy. The nurse is aware that the noncompliance is developmentally related to:
    ① The need for attention
    ② A denial of the diabetes
    ③ The struggle for identity
    ④ A regression associated with illness

15. Which of the following is the most important factor for the nurse to remember when planning how best to work with adolescent residents?
    ① Their general dislike of adults
    ② Their need to experiment with substances
    ③ Their level of cognitive ability to consider consequences
    ④ Their natural mistrust of health care providers

16. A resident has been having low-grade fever, weight loss, and pain in his arms and legs. He recently had a sore throat and was diagnosed as having rheumatic fever. In planning care for this resident, the nurse knows that the organism most likely responsible for the sore throat is:
    ① A virus
    ② *Pneumococcus*
    ③ *Staphylococcus*
    ④ *Streptococcus*

17. The nurse is aware that the most reliable indicator of pain in a 4-year-old child is:
    1. Crying and sobbing
    2. Changes in behavior
    3. Decreased heart rate
    4. Verbal reports of pain

18. A 4-year-old with AIDS is placed on appropriate isolation precautions. These precautions include:
    1. Gloves should be worn whenever approaching the bedside
    2. Gloves should be worn when in contact with blood and body fluids
    3. Limited physical contact should be made when care is administered
    4. Gowns, masks, and gloves should be worn when providing direct care

19. When planning long-term care for a child with cerebral palsy, it is important for the nurse to recognize that the:
    1. Effects of cerebral palsy are unstable and unpredictable
    2. Child should have genetic counseling before planning a family
    3. Illness is not progressively degenerative
    4. Child probably has some degree of mental retardation

ANSWERS AND RATIONALES FOR REVIEW QUESTIONS

1. **3** Increased fluids are needed because there is a potential fluid volume deficit related to decreased oral intake and because it is necessary to liquify secretions and aid in their expectoration. A cool-air humidifier helps to moisten mucous membranes and prevent further irritation. Adequate rest and nutrition are primary measures to encourage healing.
   1 This intervention is for otitis media.
   2 This intervention is for meningitis.
   4 This intervention is for asthma.

2. **3** Forty percent of children with Down's syndrome have cardiac anomalies.
   1 This is not a characteristic finding in children with Down's syndrome.
   2 This is not a characteristic finding in children with Down's syndrome.
   4 This is not a characteristic finding in children with Down's syndrome.

3. **4** This is a normal adaptation to a state of dehydration; the urine will be concentrated.
   1 There is no indication of celiac disease.
   2 The initial response to decreased circulating fluids would be an increased pulse rate.
   3 One of the signs of dehydration in an infant is a sunken, not a bulging, fontanel.

4. **4** Loss of weight is the best way to evaluate the magnitude of fluid loss in the infant; 1 liter of fluid weighs 2.2 pounds.
   1 This is a subjective assessment; measurement of weight is an objective assessment.
   2 Although this would indicate dehydration, it is not an effective monitoring method for assessing fluid loss.
   3 This is a subjective and inaccurate assessment.

5. **4** Further footdrop can be prevented by proper positioning of the feet. A foot board is helpful in maintaining this proper alignment.
   1 This should be done regardless of footdrop, but it will not guarantee that the footdrop will not worsen.
   2 This may help and is an appropriate choice, but it should not limit the nurse in independent measures as explained in the correct response.
   3 This option may help, but the footdrop will worsen if the foot is not properly positioned between exercises.

6. **1** The temperature would be 102.6° F (39.2° C), and the Tylenol should be given as ordered.
   2 The nurse could be held liable for any consequences that may occur if the orders were clear and not followed.
   3 The nurse could have made an error in calculation, but she would be held accountable for the error.
   4 A rectal or axillary temperature is usually preferred in children unless the child is old enough to safely follow instructions for an oral temperature.

7. **3** $150 \text{ mg} \times \dfrac{5 \text{ ml}}{125 \text{ mg}} = 6 \text{ ml}$

   1 Incorrect calculation; dose is too low.
   2 Incorrect calculation; dose is too low.
   4 Incorrect calculation; dose is too high.

8. **1** A banana would be considered more nutritious, and it does not contain sodium.
   2 A candy bar would not be considered nutritious; it may contain some sodium.
   3 A ham sandwich would be omitted because ham contains sodium.
   4 Tuna salad would be omitted because tuna is found in salt water.

9. **4** The child with abdominal pain may assume the side-lying position with the knees flexed to the abdomen and/or may self-splint when moving.
   1 A 4-year-old may be unable to define the exact location of the pain; in addition, the pain may be generalized rather than localized.
   2 This might be included in the physical assessment, but it is not specific to the assessment of pain.
   3 This might be included in the health history, but it is not specific to the assessment of pain.

10. **3** The child's status and the progression of the seizure should be monitored; the child will not breathe until the seizure is over and cyanosis should subside at that time.
    1 Attempting to open clenched jaws could result in injury to the child.
    2 Oxygen will be useless until the child breathes when the seizure is over.
    4 The physician can be notified later; provision of safety and observation are the priorities.

11. **2** These are the most common signs of hypoglycemia in children.
    1 These are signs of hyperglycemia.
    3 These are signs of hyperglycemia.
    4 These are signs of hyperglycemia.

12. **3** Orthopnea is shortness of breath in any position except the erect sitting or standing position.
   1 This is a temporary cessation of breathing.
   2 This is labored or difficult breathing regardless of the position.
   4 This is an increased respiratory rate, not shortness of breath.

13. **2** 90 to 100 beats/min for age 2 to 6.
   1 76 to 90 beats/min for children over age 10.
   3 110 to 140 beats/min for an infant (1 month to 1 year of age).
   4 120 to 150 beats/min for a neonate (birth to 1 month of age).

14. **3** Striving to attain identity and independence is a task of the adolescent, and rebellion against established norms may be exhibited.
   1 This behavior is not a bid for attention; it is instead an attempt to establish an identity, which is a normal developmental task of the adolescent.
   2 Although the adolescent may be using denial, denial is not developmentally related to adolescence.
   4 This behavior is not regression; it is an attempt to attain identity by rebellion against established norms.

15. **3** Many developmentalists have suggested that adolescents have not reached a cognitive level at which they can fully understand what will happen as a result of their actions.
   1 This is not necessarily true.
   2 Not all adolescents need to do this.
   4 Adolescents as a group are more likely to be trusting of health care providers than of other adults.

16. **4** The pathology of rheumatic fever is not clearly understood, but the disease tends to follow a recent infection with the beta-hemolytic *Streptococcus*.
   1 Virus is not a cause.
   2 Pneumococcus organism is one of the many causes of pneumonia.
   3 Staphylococcus organism is one of a genus of nonmotile, nonsporeforming gram-positive bacteria.

17. **2** Although none of the choices is always indicative of pain, a change in behavior is the indicator that occurs most often in children.
   1 Many things can cause crying, including pain, fear, separation, and unhappiness; crying does not always indicate pain.
   3 Vital signs are often normal in children, even in the presence of pain.
   4 Children often hide their pain; they may perceive it as punishment, or they may fear the injection that would be given to relieve the pain.

18. **2** The Centers for Disease Control and Prevention have determined that health care professionals should use gloves when coming into direct contact with body fluids and blood of HIV-infected individuals because these fluids contain the virus.
   1 Approaching the bedside does not expose the health care worker to the virus.
   3 Contact should not be limited; this does not allow for optimal care of the child.
   4 A mask and an impervious gown are needed in addition to gloves only when there is a potential for the health care worker to be splashed with body fluids or blood.

19. **3** The damage is fixed. It does not become progressively greater.
   1 Cerebral palsy is a nonprogressive chronic condition.
   2 The etiology of cerebral palsy is related to anoxia in the prenatal, perinatal, or postnatal periods.
   4 Although mental retardation may be present in some children with cerebral palsy, it cannot be assumed that all children with this disorder are mentally retarded.

Psychosocial Integrity

chapter *seventeen*

Psychosocial Aspects and the Developmental Continuum in Long-Term Care

The nurse working in long-term care requires knowledge of mental health, personality development, self-perception, tasks, psychosocial alterations, and sexuality. The nurse must also examine personal attitudes and beliefs about the life-span continuum and aging.

Holism

A. Definition: a concept of health—holds that illness results from a complex interaction between the mind and body and the internal and external alterations that disturb the natural balance
B. Approaches to treatment: multifaceted approaches are used to treat disturbances, rather than simply relying on treatments aimed at specific symptoms; these approaches include the following dimensions:
    1. Physical
    2. Psychologic
    3. Cultural
    4. Socioeconomic

Mental Health Continuum

A. Mental health and mental illness are seen as opposite poles on a continuum
B. The precise point at which an individual is deemed mentally ill is determined not only by the specific behavior exhibited but also by the context in which the behavior is seen
C. Some behaviors considered deviant in one setting are considered normal in another setting
D. Variations are based on the culture, the time or era, the specific personal characteristics of the individual, and many other variables

E. Behaviors of the ill individual are exaggerations of normal human behaviors

Mental Health

A. Definition: an individual's ability to manage life's problems and to derive satisfaction from living throughout various life stages
B. Persons may experience times of greater or lesser satisfaction with life; at times of lesser satisfaction, may seek the assistance of a therapist
C. No clear set of characteristics specific to mental health can be identified
    1. All behavior is considered meaningful and may be interpreted as the individual's effort to adapt or cope with the environment
    2. At times some adaptations fail; others are continued long after the need for them has passed; still others may be directed to an undesired end

Criteria of Mental Health

A. Positive attitudes toward self
B. Growth, development, and self-actualization
C. Integration
D. Autonomy
E. Reality perception
F. Environmental mastery

Ageism

A. Ageism is a term used to denote discrimination against the elderly. Although fascination with youth in the United States has waned, this country still does not have a culture that values

213

everyone regardless of age or ethnic background

B. It is important that you examine your attitude about aging; how you see older residents wittingly or unwittingly influences how you react and treat them

C. Personal independence is highly valued in this country; when people can no longer live independently and require some assistance, they are viewed as inferior

D. Older persons remind us of our own mortality

E. The person who has contact with older persons who are well has the most positive regard for all older persons

Personality Development

A. Definition: a consistent set of behaviors peculiar to a specific individual; the sum of thoughts, feelings, physical characteristics, and sociocultural biases on which all behavior is built

B. Heredity
  1. Personality is influenced by inherited characteristics, both physical and psychologic
  2. Controversy exists over the extent of genetic influence on specific human behaviors

C. Environment
  1. The environment is a strong determining factor in the individual's development
  2. Environment includes the intrauterine environment as well as all the external factors that influence the individual after birth

D. Physical basis: personality develops normally if the necessary physical basis is present
  1. The brain is the major organ of thought and is necessary to the development of personality
  2. Other influential factors include a normally functioning endocrine system, which strongly influences behavior

E. Elements of personality
  1. Levels of consciousness
    a. The unconscious: always outside the awareness of the individual; influences actions in ways the individual may not understand; thought to include dreams
    b. The preconscious: usually outside awareness; available to conscious mind in special circumstances such as under hypnosis or during therapy

    c. The conscious: ordinary awareness
  2. Structures: some theorists refer to personality structures
    a. Freud: id, ego, superego
    b. Berne: child, adult, parent
  3. Functions: each structure is thought to perform specific functions
    a. Id/child: basic, innate psychic energy; emotional
    b. Ego/adult: mediates between person's perception and objective reality; always rational
    c. Superego/parent: incorporates societal values; judgmental and critical

G. Developmental levels: various theorists describe levels of development
  1. Freud: oral, anal, phallic, latency, genital
  2. Erikson: basic trust vs. mistrust; autonomy vs. shame and doubt; initiative vs. guilt; industry vs. inferiority; identity vs. role diffusion; intimacy vs. isolation; generativity vs. stagnation; ego integrity vs. despair

H. Development of the self-concept
  1. A family provides the basis of self-concept by offering:
    a. Feelings of adequacy or inadequacy
    b. Feelings of acceptance or rejection
    c. Opportunities for identification
    d. Expectations of values, goals, and behaviors
  2. Self-concept consists of
    a. Body image: one's perception of one's body
    b. Self-ideal: one's idea of what is "good" behavior
    c. Self-esteem: personal judgment of one's own worth
    d. Role: one's perception of how one fits into the society
    e. Identity: the combination of all of the above into a unified whole

I. The self-actualized individual (Maslow)
  1. Has accurate perception of reality
  2. Has a high degree of acceptance of self, others, and human nature
  3. Exhibits spontaneity
  4. Is problem-centered as opposed to self-centered
  5. Has need for privacy
  6. Demonstrates high degree of autonomy and independence

7. Has freshness of appreciation
8. Has frequent "mystic or peak" experiences
9. Shows identification with mankind
10. Shares intimate relationships with a few significant others
11. Has democratic character structures
12. Possesses strong ethical sense
13. Demonstrates unhostile sense of humor
14. Possesses creativeness
15. Exhibits resistance to conformity

Self-Perception/Self-Concept and Aging

A. Assessment
 1. Verbalizes fears or concerns
 2. Fears of a known or an unknown source
 3. Verbalizes loss of control over life
 4. Recently experienced significant losses
 5. Recently moved or been separated from significant others
 6. General appearance and posture
 7. Makes/avoids eye contact
 8. Verbalizes concerns regarding changes in appearance
 9. Negative comments regarding self
 10. Avoids looking in the mirror or at altered body parts
 11. Questions own worth
 12. Verbalizes feelings of failure
 13. Verbalizes hopelessness or despair
 14. Spends most of time alone
 15. Accepts directions from care givers passively, or expresses the desire to make own decisions
 16. Exhibit aggression, anger, or demanding behaviors
 17. Signs of autonomic nervous system stimulation (increased pulse or respiratory rate, elevated blood pressure, diaphoresis)
 18. Manifests any behaviors typical of emotional upset (pacing, hand-wringing, crying, repetitive motions, tics, aggressiveness)
 19. Changes in vocal quality, such as quivering
 20. Complains of headaches
 21. Difficulty focusing on activities, remembering things, or making decisions
 22. Changes in eating or sleeping patterns

B. Older adults likely to experience problems related to self-perception/self-concept
 1. Have conditions that result in change of body appearance (surgical removal of body parts, burns, obesity, skin lesions, chemotherapy, disfiguring endocrine disorders such as acromegaly or Cushing's syndrome)
 2. Have lost the ability to control bodily functions
 3. Have suffered significant losses (loss of significant others, possessions, social roles, financial status)
 4. Have recently relocated (particularly if involuntarily)
 5. Are experiencing chronic pain

C. Nursing interventions
 1. Visit daily for 10 to 15 minutes just to allow the resident to verbalize feelings and concerns
 2. Respect right to private space and belongings
 3. Actively include in care planning, present with options, and then follow through with choices
 4. Explain the reasons for any changes that must be made
 5. Keep call light handy and respond promptly when called
 6. Meet requests promptly
 7. Encourage participation in personal care
 8. Assist in identifying areas over which the resident can retain control

Psychologic Alterations (Normal Aging Process)

A. Intelligence
 1. Verbal ability and retained information remain unchanged
 2. Abstract thinking and performance response decline
 3. Performance of activities involving neuromuscular learning decline
 4. Attention span shortens
 5. Literal approach to problem-solving affects ability
 6. Fluid intelligence declines after adolescence

7. Crystallized intelligence continues to increase throughout life
8. Learning capacity continues
B. Memory
   1. Short-term: concentration and retention decline
   2. Long-term: minimal impairment
   3. Remote
      a. Remote memory is better than short-term memory
      b. Involved in reminiscence
C. Motivation
   1. Not risk takers
   2. Do not actively seek change
   3. Possess fear of failure
   4. Self-fulfilling prophecies
   5. Competitiveness declines
   6. Energy levels decline
D. Attitudes, beliefs, interests
   1. General attitude realignment
   2. Interests either narrow or expand
   3. Tend to keep lifelong beliefs amid rapidly changing society
E. Personality
   1. Basically unchanged
   2. Some exaggeration of behavioral responses is evident
   3. Adaptive capacities are diminished
   4. Reduced ability to handle stress

Theories of Aging
SOCIOLOGIC THEORIES

A. Disengagement
   1. Controversial
   2. Mutual withdrawal from social interaction by older individual or society
   3. Engagement meaning active occupation and devotion
   4. Supports leisure as a form of activity
   5. Respects individual-initiated withdrawal
B. Activity
   1. Individual remains active and interacts with society's events
   2. Pursues new interests, friends, and roles to substitute for lost roles
   3. Supports social activity as beneficial
C. Continuity or development
   1. Lifelong personality characteristics and coping strategies continue
   2. Sense of "inferiority" develops

   3. Supportive network of relationships established
D. Passages: life-cycle changes can be identified, predicted, planned for, and managed

BIOLOGIC THEORIES

A. Wear-and-tear
   1. Stress and use deplete the body cells of repair ability
   2. Coping mechanisms decline because of decrease in available energy
B. Collagen
   1. Most abundant body protein
   2. Collagen molecules held together by bonds
   3. Chemical reactions cause a switching of bonds between collagen molecules, resulting in structural changes characteristic of the aging process
C. Lipofuscin accumulation
   1. Lipofuscins or age pigments are insoluble end products of cell metabolism
   2. Accumulate in the cell, altering the cell's ability to function normally
D. Immunologic responses
   1. Aging is an autoimmune disease process
   2. Cells change, and the body does not recognize its own cells
   3. Autoimmune responses damage the cells, causing cell death
E. Cell death of genetic programming
   1. Cell reproduction is programmed
   2. The programming determines the rate and time a given species ages and dies
F. Stress adaptation
   1. Damage from stress accumulates
   2. System's resistance to stress steadily declines, leading to death
G. Free radical
   1. Molecules that have an extra electron are free radicals
   2. Free radicals attach to other molecules, altering function or structure
   3. There are internal and external sources of free radicals
   4. Believed that the free radicals do damage membrane function and structure
H. Mutation and error
   1. Cell division errors occur progressively over time

2. Mutated cells are altered in their function and effectiveness
3. Error theory expands mutation theory to include errors in interpretation of cell messages

Role and Relationship Changes

A. Types
   1. Crisis
      a. Sudden
      b. Not able to plan for appropriate replacement
      c. Substitute not readily available
      d. Stress producing
   2. Gradual
      a. Develops slowly
      b. Time available for preparation, which eases transition
      c. Control over whether to develop a substitute
B. Sufficient preparation and adequate support determine adjustment success or failure
C. Role changes that occur to the older adult are predominantly crisis oriented
   1. Forced retirement
   2. Alteration in income
   3. Loss of spouse
   4. Illness
   5. Friends move away or die
   6. Family members relocate, assume new roles, have increasingly less time for relationships
   7. Society's assigned role of decreased psychologic and physiologic functioning
D. Role losses
   1. Work
      a. No longer the breadwinner
      b. Job-related companionship
      c. Usefulness, competence, identity
      d. Income
      e. Sense of purpose
      f. Self-esteem
   2. Family
      a. Usually no longer the decision maker
      b. Not held in the same esteem
      c. Loss of independence
E. Role gains
   1. Grandparenthood or great-grandparenthood

   2. Family support roles assumed
      a. Economic
      b. Child care
      c. Caring role in illness
      d. House care
   3. Community activities
   4. Religious activities
   5. Recreational activities
   6. Clubs, organizations, and associations
   7. Advisory roles
   8. New friends
   9. Adult education
   10. Volunteerism
F. Assessment
   1. Marital status (single, married, widowed, divorced)
   2. Lost a spouse or significant other: When?
   3. Lives alone or with others
   4. If lives with others, who are they and in what way are they related? What is the family structure?
   5. Describes relationships within the family
   6. Family interactions observed
   7. Belongs to a social group
   8. Has close relationships with friends
   9. Employed? Relationships at work?
   10. Retired from work: How long ago? Feelings regarding retirement? What does the person do to occupy time?
   11. Feels a part of the community or neighborhood
   12. In a long-term care setting, has established relationships with other residents
   13. Recently relocated: From home to acute-care setting? From home to extended-care facility? From one unit or room to another?
   14. Spends a great deal of time alone
   15. Speaks with others or remain silent
   16. Exhibit signs of withdrawal, anger, depression, sorrow, fear, or shock
   17. Verbalizes concerns regarding losses of persons, jobs, abilities
   18. Sleep or eating patterns changed
   19. Ability to concentrate changed
G. Older adults likely to experience problems related to changes in roles and relationships
   1. Have recently lost a spouse, child, close friend, significant other, or cherished pet
   2. Have recently lost lifelong or valuable roles

3. Have recently made a major adjustment in environment
4. Are unable to perform familiar roles because of loss of functional abilities

H. Nursing interventions
1. Establish relationships and encourage verbalization of feelings
2. Identify source and acknowledge reality of loss
3. Encourage participation in ADLs
4. Spend time with individual (one-on-one)
5. Initiate referrals
6. Explore and access local resources

Alterations in Lifestyle
EMPLOYMENT

A. Society emphasizes the employed as valuable and the unemployed as useless
B. Increase in the number of older women working
C. Decrease in the number of older men working
D. Part-time employment more common
E. Trend toward early retirement
F. Serial careers emerging in keeping with interest changes
G. More women are joining the work force at a time when men are winding down their working lives
H. Older worker possesses involuntary limitations
1. Health problems
2. Sensory or perceptual alterations (e.g., visual and auditory acuity)
3. Decline in physical strength, endurance, and speed
I. Older workers possess innumerable strengths
1. Reliability
2. Dependability
3. Knowledge
4. Expertise
5. Experience

RETIREMENT

A. Mandatory retirement in federal employment eliminated
B. Mandatory retirement age raised to 70 in private employment
C. More people taking advantage of early retirement
D. Health problems are primary reason for voluntary retirement

E. Increase in leisure time
F. Stress-producing event at a time when one's ability to handle stress is diminished
G. Creates tremendous anxiety
H. Some derive an initial feeling of relief, but for most it's a loss that comes at a time of meaningful productivity
I. Adjustment depends on previously established patterns of adjustment, degree of financial security, state of health, and future outlook
J. For most it creates an additional series of losses and problems at a time in life when coping and problem-solving abilities are fragile
K. Job loss
1. Loss of daily routine
   a. Alters household routine
   b. Alters lifestyle
   c. Creates discouragement, depression, and loneliness
   d. Alters family relationships
2. Loss of income
   a. Relocation
   b. Daily decision making determined by economics
   c. Decreases self-esteem
   d. Increases fear and anxiety
   e. Increases insecurity
L. Welcome changes
1. New friends
2. New activities
3. New interests
4. Renewal of marriage
5. Seek new and different employment
6. Find purpose and opportunity
7. Rest and relaxation

ECONOMIC CHANGES

A. Most older adults live on fixed incomes
B. Of older adults, 1 out of 10 lives below the nation's poverty level
C. Independence declines as costs increase and buying power decreases
D. For many, Social Security is the sole source of income
E. Many older adults are not receiving the assistance to which they are entitled
1. Lack of resource knowledge
2. Inability to learn about resources
   a. Lack of mobility
   b. Health problems

F. Supplemental Social Security: may qualify for in addition to or instead of Social Security benefits
G. Economic penalties: limit on the amount a Social Security beneficiary can earn annually without losing some monthly payments
H. Income tax reforms: once-in-a-lifetime capital gains tax exemption on sale of personal residence for person over age 55
I. Income sources
   1. Public
      a. Social Security (Federal Old-Age, Survivors, and Disability Insurance)
      b. Supplemental Social Security income
   2. Private (e.g., pensions and investments)
   3. Other (e.g., Railroad Retirement System, Federal Employee's Retirement System, and Civil Service Retirement System)

HEALTH

A. Most older adults have more than one chronic disease
B. Health care needs increase with age
C. Cost of health care is increasing as financial income is either decreasing or fixed
D. Older adults account for one third of the nation's health care costs

RECREATION

A. Older adults have more time for recreation, but deterring factors exist
   1. Cost
      a. Transportation
      b. Special equipment
      c. Special clothing
      d. Fees for membership and use of facilities
   2. Health problems
   3. Diminished energy level
   4. Lack of incentive
   5. Sensory losses
   6. Lack of environmental aids
   7. Lack of conveniently located facilities (e.g., restrooms)
B. Most older adults depend on family as the major source of activity and interaction
C. Alternatives
   1. Religious activities
   2. Community activities (e.g., volunteerism)
   3. Daycare
   4. Senior citizen centers
   5. Clubs, organizations, and associations
   6. Recreation centers
   7. Adult education
   8. Shopping
   9. Cultural events

SOCIAL ISOLATION

A. Attitudinal: that which is self-imposed and that imposed by society
   1. Self-imposed aloneness, loneliness
   2. Society imposes myths about the older adults, perceptions of aging
B. Presentational: set apart or sets one apart
C. Behavioral: exhibits behaviors that are not acceptable to a youth-oriented society (e.g., confusion, eccentricity)
D. Geographic
   1. Lack of resources to relocate
   2. Psychologic safety and security at present location
   3. Fear of being victims of crime
   4. Distance from family and friends who have moved away

Stress

A. Selected events (situations) resulting in stress
   1. Death of a son or daughter
   2. Death of spouse
   3. Loss of ability to get around
   4. Illness or injury
   5. Moving to a long-term care setting
   6. Change in ability to perform personal care
   7. Hospitalization
   8. Fear of abuse from others
   9. Being judged legally incompetent
   10. Using savings for living expenses
   11. Death of a loved pet
   12. Change in sexual activity
B. Assessment
   1. Verbalizes feelings of tension, stress, frustration, or depression
   2. Complains of changes in eating habits
   3. Complains of changes in bladder or bowel elimination patterns
   4. Changes in sleep patterns
   5. Difficulty making decisions or solving problems
   6. Appears agitated, aggressive, angry, or hostile
   7. Depressed or withdrawn

8. Smokes or consumes alcohol excessively
9. Increased frequency of illness or accidents
C. Older adults likely to experience problems related to coping or stress tolerance
   1. Have suffered recent social, physical, emotional, or financial losses
   2. Are physically ill
   3. Are experiencing major life changes
D. Relocation stress syndrome
   Relocation stress is a common problem with aging:
   1. From a private home into the home of a family member
   2. From a home to an apartment or other shared living arrangement
   3. From one area of the city to another
   4. From home to the hospital
   5. From home to a long-term care facility
   6. From home to the hospital and then to a long-term care facility
   7. From one unit in the hospital or long-term care facility to another unit in the same facility
   8. From one room to another room in a hospital or long-term care facility
E. Nursing interventions
   1. Encourage verbalization of feelings
   2. Allow expressions of anger or frustration about family
   3. Encourage discussion of feelings with family
   4. Explain reasons
   5. Involve in decision making and care planning
   6. Maintain stable care assignment to build trust
   7. Encourage a positive attitude about change
   8. Offer opportunities to participate in social activities
   9. Encourage family to bring in more valued personal belongings
   10. Consult social worker or minister as appropriate to facilitate positive family interactions

Sexuality

A. Cultural stereotypes deny freedom of sexual expression for older adults
B. Lifelong sexual adjustment will determine how the older person deals with sexual needs

C. Partner availability is made difficult
   1. More older women than men
   2. Social and business roles change
D. Physiologic alterations affect self-image and foster nonparticipation
E. Families of older persons tend to discourage sexual relationships because of stereotypes and inheritance threats
F. Sexual focus shifts to companionship
G. Older persons continue to enjoy sexual activity; decrease is primarily a result of declining health or lack of available partner
H. Physiologic changes that impact sexuality in the older adult
   1. Female
      a. Decreased estrogen level results in decreased vaginal secretions
      b. Decreased tissue elasticity results in:
         (1) Decreased pubic hair
         (2) Increased vaginal tissue fragility
         (3) Increased tissue irritation
         (4) Decreased size of uterus
         (5) Decreased vaginal length and width
         (6) Decreased size of vaginal opening
         (7) Increased pain with intercourse (dyspareunia)
         (8) Decreased breast tissue mass
      c. Increased vaginal alkalinity results in increased risk of infection
   2. Male
      a. Decreased testosterone levels results in loss of facial, body, and pubic hair
      b. Decreased circulation results in:
         (1) Decreased rate of ejaculation
         (2) Decreased force of ejaculation
         (3) Decreased speed gaining erection
I. Assessment
   1. Discharge or drainage from the genitals
   2. If sexually active, any complaint of difficulty or discomfort during sexual activity
   3. Any diseases or disabilities that interfere with sexual activity
   4. Any medications that may interfere with sexual activity
J. Older adults likely to experience problems related to sexuality
   1. Have lost their partner

2. Have problems with physical mobility
3. Reside in a long-term care setting
4. Suffer from physical illness or a reaction to therapeutic medications
K. Nursing interventions
  1. Allow opportunities for both parties to verbalize feelings about continuing sexual contact
  2. Attempt to arrange for a shared room if this is agreeable to both parties
  3. Develop a method, such as a "Do Not Disturb" sign, for ensuring private time, while recognizing the need for access in case of emergency
  4. Assist with hygiene needs so that both parties are physically clean and attractive
  5. Verbalize understanding of the continued need for physical closeness throughout life
  6. Protect the dignity of the confused resident

Death and Dying

Loss and death are universal and individually unique events of the human experience. Illness and hospitalization frequently cause losses. The nurse works with many residents who experience types of loss. The nurse's role is to assist residents in understanding and accepting loss so that quality of life can continue.

Death in our culture is often difficult for the dying person, as well as for the person's family, friends and care givers.

A. Potential losses faced
  1. Former good health
  2. Independence
  3. Sense of control over life
  4. Privacy
  5. Modesty
  6. Body image
  7. Relationships
  8. Social status
  9. Sense of self-confidence
  10. Possessions
  11. Financial security
  12. Plans for future
  13. Fantasy of immortality
  14. Familiar daily routine
  15. Sleep
  16. Sexual functioning
  17. Leisure activities

B. Loss requires adaptation through the grieving process. The types of loss and the perception of the loss influence the degree of stress. Five types of losses include:
  1. Loss of external objects
  2. Loss of a known environment
  3. Loss of a significant other
  4. Loss of an aspect of self
  5. Loss of life

Grieving Process

The grieving process, with associated feelings and behaviors, can occur when individuals face their own death. Grief not only occurs in the persons experiencing the loss but also in family or friends. Important to remember is that while the resident passes through phases of grief, family and friends also experience grief in their own way and at their own pace.

A. Grieving process components
  1. Bereavement—the state of thought, feeling, and activity that follows loss; it includes grief and mourning
  2. Grief—a form of sorrow that follows the perception or anticipation of a loss; responses include helplessness, loneliness, hopelessness, sadness, guilt, and anger
  3. Mourning—the process that follows a loss and includes working through grief

FRAMEWORKS

The classic works of Engel (1964), Kubler-Ross (1969), and Martocchio (1985) provide frameworks for understanding the concept and dynamics of the grieving process. Each theory includes phases or stages experienced while resolving grief.

A. Engel
  1. Shock and disbelief—person denies reality of the loss, withdraws from family and friends; physical reactions may include fainting, diaphoresis, nausea, diarrhea, rapid heart rate, insomnia, and fatigue
  2. Development of awareness—person begins to feel loss acutely; experiences desperation; emotions of anger, guilt, frustration, depression, and emptiness; crying is common
  3. Restitution—guilt and remorse are common; person begins to reorganize life, and a new self-awareness develops

B. Kubler-Ross' stages of dying
   1. Denial—person acts as though nothing has happened; refuses to believe or understand that a loss has occurred
   2. Anger—person resists the loss and may strike out at everyone and everything in the environment
   3. Bargaining—attempts postponement of the reality of the loss; tries to prevent loss from occurring
   4. Depression—loss is fully realized; person feels overwhelmingly lonely and withdraws from personal interactions
   5. Acceptance—person finally accepts the loss
C. Martocchio's phases of grieving (these phases of grief have overlapping boundaries and no expected order)
   1. Shock and disbelief
   2. Yearning and protest
   3. Anguish, disorganization, and despair
   4. Identification in bereavement
   5. Reorganization and restitution

Resident Responses and Nursing Implications

A. Shock and disbelief/denial
   1. Resident response
      a. Denial is response to news of loss
      b. Mood swings common
      c. Physiologic response may include weakness, tremors, anorexia, cold, clammy skin
      d. Residents isolate themselves from sources of accurate information
      e. Reject offers of comfort and support
   2. Nursing implications
      a. Support emotional needs without reinforcing denial
      b. Offer to remain with resident without discussing reasons for behavior or need to cope unless resident addresses the subject
      c. Offer supportive care such as food, drink, safety
B. Yearning and protest/anger
   1. Resident responses
      a. Express anger and retaliation against family, staff, physician, Supreme Being
      b. Demanding and accusing

c. Resentful and jealous of others who still have loved one
   2. Nursing implications
      a. Provide guidance about feelings and intensity experienced
      b. Focus on anger
      c. Do not take anger personally
      d. Meet needs that cause angry response
C. Anguish, disorganization, despair/bargaining
   1. Resident responses
      a. Willing to do anything to avoid loss or change prognosis
      b. Bargains with Supreme Being
      c. Accepts new forms of therapy
   2. Nursing implications: provide information for decision making
D. Identification in bereavement/depression
   1. Resident responses
      a. Reality and permanence of loss recognized
      b. Confusion, indecision, crying common
      c. Resident quiet and withdrawn; loneliness surfaces
      d. Resident loses interest in appearance
      e. May become suicidal or begin behavior such as excessive drug use
   2. Nursing implications
      a. Provide support and empathy
      b. Support crying by offering touch
      c. Listen attentively
      d. Assess risk of harm to self
      e. Refer to physician for mental health professional referral if needed
E. Reorganization and restitution/acceptance
   1. Resident responses
      a. Accepts terms of loss
      b. Begins to plan for loss
      c. Shares feelings
      d. Reminisces about past
      e. Alternating periods of depression and well-being
      f. Life begins to stabilize
   2. Nursing implications
      a. Offer opportunity to share feelings verbally, in writing, through acting, or by tape recording
      b. Encourage review as often as resident wishes to talk
      c. Show acceptance of labile emotions
      d. Assist in discussing future plans

Additional Needs of Dying Person

A. Maintenance of independence
1. Allow resident to perform simple self-care tasks: washing face, putting on eyeglasses, eating
2. Help resident maintain dignity and sense of worth
3. Encourage decision making and sense of control
4. Observe for nonverbal cues suggesting unwillingness to participate
5. Do not force participation

B. Spiritual comfort
1. Ask clergy to visit
2. Support resident in expression of philosophy of life
3. Resident seeks to find purpose and meaning to life
4. Resident feels guilty if life perceived as unfullfilled
5. Resident asks forgiveness from Supreme Being
6. Nurse can pray with resident (if requested to do so), read inspirational literature, play music requested
7. Listen attentively to encourage resident to express feelings, clarify them, accept death

Support for the Grieving Family

A. Family members
1. Need to express own feelings
2. Must deal directly with resident's expressions of anger, denial, and fear
3. Are valuable resources in care of dying resident

B. Nursing actions
1. Assess family relationships
2. Determine family's desired role as observer, comforter, care giver
3. Show kindness, respect, and courtesy

C. Suggestions for involving family in care of dying resident
1. Assist in planning visitation schedule to prevent resident and/or family fatigue
2. Allow young children to visit if resident is able to communicate
3. Listen to family complaints about resident's care
4. Listen to family's negative or positive feelings about resident
5. Help family members learn to interact with dying resident
6. Relieve family from care activities so they can rest
7. Provide resources for meals and lodging
8. Provide privacy between resident and family
9. Encourage open expression of grief between resident and family
10. Provide information daily about resident's condition
11. Prepare family for sudden changes in appearance
12. Communicate news of impending death in private area—be willing to stay with family
13. At time of death, help family stay in communication with resident through short visits, caring silence, touch, and telling resident of their love
14. After death, assist family with decisions regarding mortician, family transportation, and resident's belongings

Review Questions

1. Which of the following statements is true about human sexuality?
   1. Children are essentially asexual
   2. There are sexual needs throughout life
   3. Homosexuality is a treatable illness
   4. Minor sexual dysfunctions are difficult to treat

2. The key factor in accurately assessing how a resident will cope with body image changes is the:
   1. Suddenness of the change
   2. Obviousness of the change
   3. Extent of body change present
   4. Resident's perception of the change

3. When planning care for an older adult the nurse is aware that normal aging has little effect on a resident's:
   1. Sense of taste or smell
   2. Gastrointestinal motility
   3. Muscle or motor strength
   4. Ability to handle life's stresses

4. The nurse's role in maintaining or promoting the health of the older adult should be based on the principle that:
   1. There is a strong correlation between successful retirement and good health
   2. Some of the physiologic changes that occur as a result of aging are reversible
   3. Thoughts of impending death are frequent and depressing to most older adults
   4. Older adults can better accept the dependent state chronic illness often causes

5. A female resident who has been told by her physician that she has untreatable metastatic carcinoma tells the nurse that she believes the physician has made an error and that she does not have cancer and is not going to die. The nurse evaluates that the resident is experiencing the stage of death and dying known as:
   1. Anger
   2. Denial
   3. Bargaining
   4. Acceptance

6. The grieving wife of a resident who has just died says to the nurse, "We should have spent more time together. I always felt the children's needs came first." The nurse recognizes that the wife is experiencing:
   1. Displaced anger
   2. Normal feelings of guilt
   3. Shame for past behavior
   4. Ambivalent feelings about him

7. The nurse encourages a terminally ill resident to make decisions about daily activities and care. The nurse would know that the resident, who had been extremely angry with everything and everybody, had resolved some of the anger when the resident states:
   1. "You've got a busy morning ahead of you! I'm really a mess."
   2. "What are you going to let me do this morning? You know I can help."
   3. "It's so hard to let someone do so much for me. It just doesn't seem right."
   4. "I can do my face, hands, arms, and chest today but I think you'd better do the rest."

8. The nurse recognizes that a characteristic behavior often demonstrated in the initial stage of a resident's coping with dying often includes:
   1. Criticizing medical care
   2. Sleeping for long periods
   3. Asking for additional medical consultation
   4. Ringing the call light as soon as the nurse leaves

9. A resident who is to have a segmental mastectomy for cancer of the breast tells the nurse that she is worried about what she will look like after the surgery. The nurse's most appropriate initial response is:
   1. "Try not to think about the surgery now."
   2. "Why don't you discuss this with your husband?"
   3. "I can understand that you'd be concerned."
   4. "Everyone having this surgery feels the same way."

ANSWERS AND RATIONALES FOR REVIEW QUESTIONS

1. **2** All persons have ongoing sexual needs.
   1 Children are sexual.
   3 Homosexuality is not considered a disease.
   4 Minor dysfunctions are relatively easy to treat.

2. **4** It is not reality, but the resident's feeling about the change, that is the most important determinant in the ability to cope.
   1 This is not relevant to the resident's ability to deal with a change in body image.
   2 This is not relevant to the resident's ability to deal with a change in body image.
   3 The extent of change is not relevant; it is whether the resident perceives the change as enormous or minuscule.

3. **4** An individual's ability to handle stress develops through experience with life; aging does not reduce this ability but often strengthens it.
   1 The senses of taste and/or smell are often diminished in older persons.
   2 Gastrointestinal motility is slowed in older persons.
   3 Muscle or motor strength is diminished in the older persons.

4. **1** The individual who can reflect back on life and accept it for what it was and is and who can adjust and enjoy the changes retirement brings is less likely to develop health problems, especially stress-related health problems.
   2 These changes are usually not reversible.
   3 This is untrue; most emotionally healthy older individuals do not focus on these thoughts.
   4 This is not true; dependency is often more threatening to this age-group.

5. **2** The resident has difficulty accepting the inevitability of death and attempts to deny the reality of it.
   1 In the anger stage the resident strikes out with "why me" and "how could God do this" type of statements; the resident is angry at life and still angrier to be removed from it by death.
   3 In this stage the resident attempts to bargain for more time; the reality of death is no longer denied, but the resident attempts to manipulate and extend the remaining time.
   4 In the acceptance stage the resident accepts the inevitability of death and peaceably awaits it.

6. **2** The spouse is expressing the normal feelings of guilt associated with the death of a loved one; there is always initial guilt over what might have been.
   1 No evidence supports this conclusion.
   3 The spouse is expressing guilt, not shame.
   4 No evidence supports this conclusion.

7. **4** This demonstrates the resident's diminished anger and is a realistic assessment and acceptance of present capabilities and limitations.
   1 This shows dependency; either the resident has given up or is being sarcastic.
   2 Anger is still apparent at loss of decision making; there is no real evidence of sharing.
   3 This shows dependency and suggests the resident has given up.

8. **3** Denial may be handled by seeking other opinions in an attempt to prove an unacceptable one incorrect.
   1 This occurs during the stage of anger, which is a later stage.
   2 This occurs during the stage of depression, which is a later stage.
   4 This is not associated with the initial stage; this behavior usually occurs after the resident recognizes the inevitable outcome and is fearful of being alone.

9. **3** Women facing breast surgery often have many feelings relating to their sexuality, change in body image, etc. The nurse plays a vital role in helping the resident verbalize feelings, and this response keeps channels of communication open.
   1 The resident's concerns are real, and such a statement will only block further communication.
   2 This can be interpreted as the nurse's reluctance to listen; the resident may not be able to talk with her husband about this.
   4 Does not focus on the importance of the resident as an individual; each person's feelings are different.

chapter eighteen

Communication

Communication

A. Definition: exchange of messages between two or more people, including information, thoughts, and feelings

B. Purposes in nursing
   1. To establish a meaningful, helping relationship between nurse and resident
   2. To transmit information between health care workers

C. Communication in nursing
   1. Communication: a complex activity consisting of a series of events, each interdependent on the other, which results in a negotiated understanding between two or more people in a given situation
      a. Communication is not merely the exchange of information
      b. Each message (input) generates an extremely complex reaction that eventually leads to a selective response (output), which in turn becomes a new input for the communicators
   2. Modes of communication
      a. The most apparent form is verbal (written or spoken language)
      b. Spoken communication is always accompanied by at least one of the following additional communication forms
         (1) Paralanguage: voice quality, tones, grunts, and other nonword vocalizations
         (2) Kinesis: facial expression, gestures, and eye and body movements
         (3) Proxemics: the spatial relationship between persons
         (4) Touch and messages to other sensory organs: aromas and cultural artifacts (jewelry, clothing, hair style)
      c. Effective communication is
         (1) Efficient: messages are simple, clear, and timed correctly
         (2) Appropriate: relevant to the situation
         (3) Flexible: open to alteration based on perceived response
         (4) Receptive: allows feedback (checking and correcting by either or both parties)
   3. Therapeutic communication
      a. Reflection: encourages continuation of the previous communication; for example, resident states, "I feel sad." Nurse responds, "You feel sad?"
      b. Encouraging comments; for example, "Go on."
      c. Open-ended statements; for example, "Say more..."
      d. Questioning: may block communication and should be used carefully
      e. Accepting: permitting resident to speak freely without fear of judgment, threats, or put-downs
      f. Giving recognition: calling by name, responding nonverbally such as leaning forward, nodding
      g. Placing events in sequence: helps resident to sort out confusing ideas
      h. Making observations; for example, "You look sad as you say that."
      i. Encouraging comparison; for example, "Was that how you were treated as a child?"

j. Restating: rearranging the resident's words (all or in part) to gain greater understanding

k. Focusing: helping resident keep to the subject

l. Exploring: helping to make logical connections

m. Giving information: concrete information, not advice

n. Seeking clarification; for example, "Do you mean . . .?"

o. Presenting reality; for example, "I know you believe that, but . . ."

p. Attempting to translate feelings; for example, "Are you feeling angry?"

q. Summarizing: concisely stating the overall meaning of the conversation

r. Paraphrasing: involves more active participation on the listener's part. The effort is to find the essence of what is said rather than simple mirroring the words.

s. Reflective feelings: similar to restatement, but you reflect the feeling the speaker expressed

t. Neutral: use noncommittal words; don't agree or disagree with person

u. Exploratory
   (1) Who
   (2) What
   (3) Where
   (4) Why
   (5) When

v. Nonverbal clues: responding to non-verbal cues shows understanding; technique involves observing the cue and making a comment or asking questions to clarify its meaning

w. Listening: deliberate use of nonverbal communication to indicate attention

x. Silence: adds importance to the other person's communication and allows time to formulate responses

4. Characteristics of listening
   a. Sensing
      (1) Focuses all attention on resident
      (2) Provides an appropriate setting in both physical/social terms
      (3) Tries to prevent outside interruptions
      (4) Allows others adequate time before questions or comments
      (5) Avoids wandering mentally or getting sidetracked
      (6) Avoids formulating responses while others are speaking
      (7) Refrains from taking overly detailed notes
      (8) Says, "I didn't hear that" or "Could you repeat" if necessary.
      (9) Uses appropriate nonverbal behavior to indicate message reception (e.g., eye contact, gestures, "uh-huh," nodding, facial expressions)
      (10) Does not allow resident's style, age, position, sex, looks, character, or positive or negative support affect sensing

   b. Interpreting
      (1) Determines the broad intent of resident (small talk, self-expression, information, persuasion)
      (2) Considers why this topic, at this time, at this place? Asks, "What does the resident want?" (specific intent)
      (3) Asks questions or rephrases to promote understanding and clarification; organization of content
      (4) Considers central ideas rather than isolated facts
      (5) Identifies supporting material and relates it to central ideas flexibly
      (6) Tries to reflect the resident's feelings to enhance understanding
      (7) Is aware of emotional barriers (e.g., red-flag words, deaf spots, stress, ego, bias)
      (8) Probes and uses restatement to check on potential semantic confusion such as connotation, context, personal meaning, grammatical structure

   c. Evaluating
      (1) Withholds judgment until resident is finished
      (2) Uses awareness of own filters,

          bias, or prejudice to help control or suspend judgment

    (3) Identifies own interference and assumptions while listening and tries to check them out, where possible

    (4) Uses appropriate nonverbal behavior to indicate ongoing evaluation (disagreement/agreement, like/dislike)

    (5) Looks for implications in what is being said and not being said; listens between the lines

    (6) Pays attention to voice tone, inflection, body language, or other nonverbal clues

    (7) Distinguishes carefully between facts, opinions based on fact, and opinions based on preferences

  d. Responding

    (1) Accepts obligation to respond in some way

    (2) Clarifies the expectations or wants of the resident through questions

    (3) Commits to respond to the resident

    (4) Reviews available resources

    (5) Reviews current priorities

    (6) Determines feasibility of and degree of response

5. Active listening
   a. Active listening is a constant search for meaning
   b. Analyzing what is being said
   c. Looking behind and through the words
   d. Mind racing
   e. Internal and external questioning
   f. Listening with the eyes, ears, and mind
   g. Being just as intellectually and emotionally active as the speaker
   h. A skill that can be developed
   i. Something you have to constantly work at
   j. Mirroring back feelings to the resident
6. Factors affecting listening
   a. The message and the occasion
      (1) Factual distractions occur because we tend to listen for facts instead of ideas

    (2) Semantic distractions occur when someone uses a word or phrase differently or one to which we react emotionally

    (3) Mental distractions occur when we engage in intrapersonal communication with ourselves while talking with others

    (4) Physical distractions include all the stimuli in the environment that interfere with our focusing on the resident

  b. Ourselves

    (1) Defensiveness occurs because one may feel threatened

    (2) Egocentrism is the tendency to view self as the center of any exchange or activity

  c. Perception of others

    (1) Status interferes when we accept what residents say easily rather than listening carefully and critically because of the status they may hold

    (2) Stereotyping affects our ability to listen when resident belongs to a group we respect or don't respect

7. Effective listening—the active listener:
   a. Seeks information of value
   b. Judges content
   c. Maintains control and concentrates on resident's points
   d. Listens for ideas upon which to thread facts
   e. Pays attention
   f. Is able to concentrate despite distractions
   g. Rapidly overcomes reaction to emotion-laden words
   h. Capitalizes on thought speed by making frequent mental recapitulations of what has been said
8. Ineffective listening—the inactive listener:
   a. Finds subject presented uninteresting and dry
   b. Criticizes
   c. Is emotionally overstimulated and thinks of arguments against what is being said

d. Listens only for facts
e. Fakes attention
f. Has low tolerance for distractions
g. Allows reaction to emotion-laden words
h. Thinks of unrelated topics during time available

The Nurse's Role
MAINTENANCE OF EFFECTIVE COMMUNICATION

A. The need to communicate is universal
B. People communicate to satisfy needs
C. Recognition of what is communicated is basic for the establishment of a therapeutic nurse-resident relationship
D. Clear and accurate communication among members of the health care team, including the resident, is vital to support the resident's welfare

NURSING RESPONSIBILITIES IN PROMOTION OF PRODUCTIVE COMMUNICATION

A. Be aware that effective communication requires skill in both sending and receiving messages
  1. Verbal (e.g., words and tone of voice)
  2. Written
  3. Nonverbal (e.g., facial expression, eye contact, and body language)
B. Recognize the high stress-anxiety potential of most health care settings created in part by:
  1. Health problem itself
  2. Treatments and procedures
  3. Exclusive behavior of personnel
  4. Foreign environment
  5. Change in lifestyle, body image, and self-concept
C. Recognize the intrinsic worth of each person
  1. Listen, consider wishes when possible, and explain when necessary
  2. Avoid stereotyping, snap judgments, and unjustified comparisons
  3. Be nonjudgmental and nonpunitive in response and behavior
D. Be aware that each individual must be treated as a whole person
E. Recognize that all behavior has meaning and usually results from the attempt to cope with stress or anxiety

1. Be aware of importance of value systems
2. Be aware of significance of cultural differences
3. Be sensitive to personal meaning of experiences to residents
4. Recognize that giving information may not alter the resident's behavior
5. Recognize the defense mechanisms that the individual is using
6. Recognize own anxiety and cope with it
7. Search for patterns of adaptation on which to base action
8. Recognize that resident's previous patterns of behavior may become inadequate under stress
  a. Health problems may produce a change in family or community constellations
  b. Health problems may lead to change in self-perception and role identity
9. Be aware that behavioral changes are possible only when the individual has other defenses to maintain equilibrium
F. Help the resident to accept the health problem and its consequences
G. Identify the individual's needs and determine priority for care
H. Maintain an accepting, open environment
  1. Be permissive rather than authoritarian
  2. Identify and face problems honestly
  3. Value the expression of feelings
  4. Be nonjudgmental
I. When possible, encourage resident participation in decision making
J. Recognize the resident is a unique person
  1. Use names rather than labels, such as room numbers or diagnoses, when referring to residents
  2. Maintain the resident's dignity
  3. Be courteous toward the resident, family, and visitors
  4. Protect the resident's privacy by use of curtains and avoidance of probing
  5. Permit personal possessions where practical (e.g., own nightclothes, pictures)
  6. Explain at the resident's level of understanding and tolerance
  7. Encourage expression of feelings

8. Approach the resident as a person with difficulties, not as a "difficult" person
K. Support a social environment that focuses on resident needs
   1. Use problem-solving techniques that focus on the resident
   2. Be flexible in carrying out routines and policies
   3. Be discreet in use of power
   4. Recognize that use of medical jargon can isolate the resident

INTERCHANGE BETWEEN RESIDENT AND NURSE

A. What residents bring to the nurse-resident relationship
   1. Cognitive
      a. Preferred ways of perceiving and judging
      b. Knowledge and beliefs about illness in general and their illness in particular
      c. Knowledge and beliefs about health promotion and maintenance in general and information about their own health care activities
      d. Ability to solve problems
      e. Ability to learn
   2. Affective
      a. Cultural values
      b. Feelings about seeking help from a nurse
      c. Attitudes toward nurses in general
      d. Attitudes toward treatment regimen
      e. Values toward preventing illness
      f. Willingness to take positive action about own health status at this time with this particular nurse
   3. Psychomotor
      a. Ability to relate and communicate with others
      b. Ability to carry out own health care management
      c. Ability to learn new methods of self-care
B. What nurses bring to the nurse-resident relationship
   1. Cognitive
      a. Preferred ways of perceiving and judging
      b. Knowledge and beliefs about illness in general
      c. Knowledge about their clinical specialty
      d. Knowledge and beliefs about health behaviors that prevent illness and promote, regain, and maintain health
      e. Ability to solve problems
      f. Knowledge about factors that increase resident compliance with treatment regimen
   2. Affective
      a. Cultural values
      b. Feelings about being a nurse-helper
      c. Attitudes toward residents in general
      d. Biases about nursing treatment regimen
      e. Value placed on being healthy
      f. Value placed on people actively preventing illness or enhancing well-being
      g. Willingness to help resident take positive action to improve their well-being
   3. Psychomotor
      a. Ability to relate and communicate with others
      b. Proficiency in administering effective nursing interventions
      c. Ability to teach nursing interventions to resident
C. Showing respect
   1. Acknowledging the resident
      a. Look at the resident
      b. Offer your undivided attention
      c. Maintain eye contact
      d. Smile if appropriate
      e. Move toward the other person
      f. Determine how the other person likes to be addressed
      g. Call the resident by name and introduce yourself
      h. Make contact with a handshake or by gently touching the individual
   2. For a first-time contact:
      a. Make it clear who you are and what your role is
      b. Wear your name pin or identification badge
      c. Ask what the other person needs or wants

d. Be clear about how you can be of help
e. Indicate how you will protect the resident's confidentiality
3. For an ongoing relationship:
   a. Ensure that the resident recalls who you are and what your role is
   b. Determine the resident's needs at this point.
   c. Indicate that you recall details about the individual
   d. Review the issue of confidentiality
   e. Refrain from gossiping about other residents
   f. If appropriate, suggest a referral so that the resident will receive the required assistance
D. The C.A.R.E. confrontation
   1. Clarify the behavior that is problematic. Be specific about the aspect of the resident's or your colleague's behavior that is self-destructive or destructive to others. The behavior to be changed should be the focus so that it is clear you are attaching no hurtful labels to others.
   2. Articulate why their behavior is a problem. Your articulation may include how their behavior is likely to hinder them or irritate others or how it makes you feel.
   3. Request a change in the resident's or your colleague's behavior. Your suggestions should be offered tentatively and respectfully.
   4. Encourage the resident or your colleague to change by emphasizing the positive consequences of changing or the negative implications if no change occurs
E. Feedback
   1. Giving
      a. Gain permission
      b. Be specific
      c. Convey your perspective
      d. Invite comments
      e. Be genuine
      f. Check how you are being received
   2. Receiving
      a. Get focused and ready to receive the feedback
      b. Arrange enough time
      c. Be specific
      d. Make sure you understand the communication

e. Request guidance on needed change if necessary
f. Thank resident for the feedback
g. Evaluate the content of the information
F. The nurse and unpopular residents
   1. Characteristics of unpopular residents
      a. Grumble or complain
      b. Indicate their lack of enjoyment at being in the facility
      c. Imply that they are suffering more than nurses believe
      d. Suffer from conditions nurses feel could be better cared for in other or in specialized facilities
      e. Take up more time and attention than are deemed warranted
      f. Are complaintive, uncooperative, or argumentative
      g. Have severe complications, poor prognoses, or difficult diagnoses
      h. Require extensive explanation, reassurance, or encouragement
      i. Are perceived to be of low social value
      j. Are perceived to be of low moral worth
      k. Have unchosen stigmata (such as sexual orientation, gender, race, or ethnicity)
      l. Have "own fault" diagnoses (such as alcoholism or lung cancer from heavy smoking)
      m. Have fear-causing conditions (such as highly contagious or incurable diseases, violent tendencies)
      n. Engender feelings of incompetence in nurses (have conditions about which nurses know little)
   2. Nurses' reactions to unpopular residents
      Nurses feel:
      a. Frustrated and impatient with "grumblers and moaners"
      b. Afraid of being trapped or "caught" by complainers
      c. Irritated that unpopular residents waste their time
      d. Incompetent to provide the necessary care for complicated cases and other residents
      e. Relief when "unmanageables" are transferred

f.   Dissatisfaction with their jobs

g.   Changes in their health (such as insomnia or anorexia)

Nurses act by:

a.   Ignoring or avoiding demanding residents

b.   Indicating to demanding residents that others need their attention more

c.   Labeling demanding residents as nuisances or hypochondriacs

d.   Showing reluctance to provide necessary care if residents are thought to be inappropriate

e.   Scolding and reprimanding

f.   Administering tranquilizers and sedatives to control their behavior

g.   Recommending transfer and discharge

h.   Requesting psychiatric consultation to manage unruly behavior

i.   Extending minimally adequate care

j.   Withdrawing from peers

k.   Becoming critical of the profession or the institution

l.   Withholding pain medication

m.   Ignoring residents' lights or call bells

n.   Being cool, detached, and insensitive

o.   Feeling guilty

3.   Characteristics of popular residents

a.   Able to converse readily with nurses

b.   Know the nurses' names

c.   Able to joke and laugh with the nurses

d.   Determined to get well again

e.   Cooperative and compliant with therapeutic regimen

f.   Manageable by routine methods

g.   Rarely complain of pain or discomfort

h.   Minimize the trouble they cause staff by being cooperative

4.   Nurses demonstrate the following reactions to popular residents:

a.   Enjoy interacting with residents who are "fun," have a good sense of humor, are easy to get along with, and are friendly

b.   Give superior care and do more for the popular resident in the long run

c.   Treat them more leniently

d.   Give them special favors and readily fill ordinary requests

5.   Overcome the negative attitudes about unpopular residents

a.   Perceive things from the resident's point of view

b.   To achieve an empathic perspective

c.   Put yourself in the resident's place

d.   Be aware of your feelings and their effect on the resident

e.   Identify for yourself the specifics that bother you

f.   Be more direct

g.   Solve problems

h.   Listen

i.   Be positive

j.   Focus on the present rather than the past or future

k.   Act responsibly and assertively

NOTE: The nurse should always try to identify the underlying feelings associated with behavior (e.g., anger, fear) by using these therapeutic communication techniques.

G.   Blocks to communication

1.   Excessive questioning or probing

2.   Using cliches that minimize resident's individuality

3.   Giving advice

4.   Avoiding emotionally charged topics (changing the subject)

5.   Missing important clues: verbal or nonverbal

6.   Rejecting: any open rejection will block communication

7.   Agreeing or disagreeing: adding your values about what is being said

8.   Testing or challenging; for example, "How could you prove that..."

9.   Defending: logically arguing your position

10.   Requesting explanation: residents usually do not have reasons for their behavior; reasons are not useful in their understanding of their behavior

H.   Nurse-resident relationship

1.   A one-to-one relationship between the nurse and a resident with a therapeutic goal or projected outcome

2.   The goal or outcome is based on the relief of symptoms or modification of the resident's behavior

3.   The relationship is composed of three phases

a. Orientation: initial mutual expectations are outlined

b. Working phase: the nurse and the resident work toward agreed-upon goals (e.g., activities of daily living)

c. Termination phase: the nurse and resident end the relationship in a satisfactory manner

Review Questions

1. To be most therapeutic when giving a 3-year-old toddler an intramuscular injection, the nurse should approach the child and say:
   ① "Act like a big child and we can be done real quick."
   ② "You are afraid of having a shot because of the pain."
   ③ "I know this might hurt, but it's important that you hold still."
   ④ "I brought another nurse along to help me give you your medicine."

2. A resident who has a hip prosthesis becomes depressed and says, "I'm never going to walk right again, am I?" The nurse's best response would be:
   ① "What makes you think you will never walk right again?"
   ② "Of course you will, it is just going to take time!"
   ③ "You will be up and walking before you know it."
   ④ "Why don't we see if there is something good on television?"

3. To encourage a professional relationship the nurse should:
   ① Call the resident by first name
   ② Offer sympathy to the resident
   ③ Identify self by name and title
   ④ Explain all medical procedures

4. For the past hour, the resident has been observed sitting in the corner of the room, staring out the window. A supportive nursing measure should include:
   ① Asking the resident if there is something the nurse can do
   ② Encouraging the resident to go to the day-room and interact with the other residents
   ③ Leaving the resident alone with his thoughts, but checking on him periodically
   ④ Taking a few minutes to sit with the resident in case he wishes to talk

5. A resident is depressed and is not eating or sleeping well. As the nurse approaches one morning, the resident is sitting on the side of the bed in nightclothes. The resident states, "I can't go on. I just can't go on." The best response by the nurse should be:
   ① "I understand how you feel. We all feel that way from time to time."
   ② "Let me help you shower and dress. It will make you feel better."
   ③ "You'll feel better once you are up and active."
   ④ "You're feeling hopeless and very sad."

6. At times a resident's anxiety level is so high it blocks attempts at communication and the nurse is unsure of what is being said. To clarify understanding, the nurse states, "Let's see whether we both mean the same thing." This is an example of the technique of:
   ① Reflecting feelings
   ② Making observations
   ③ Seeking consensual validation
   ④ Attempting to place events in sequence

7. A resident with expressive aphasia becomes frustrated and upset when attempting to communicate with the nurse. To help alleviate this frustration the nurse should:
   ① Face the resident and speak loudly so that the resident can see and hear better
   ② Limit the resident's contact with others to limit the frustration
   ③ Anticipate needs so that the resident does not have to ask for help
   ④ Allow plenty of time so that the resident does not have to respond under pressure

8. A resident is diagnosed as having expressive aphasia. The nurse anticipates that the resident will have difficulty with:
   ① Following specific instructions
   ② Recognizing words for familiar objects
   ③ Speaking and/or writing
   ④ Understanding speech and/or writing

ANSWERS AND RATIONALES FOR REVIEW QUESTIONS

1. **3** This is a truthful statement; the nurse recognizes the fact that this might hurt and requests expected behavior.
    1 This puts unrealistic expectations on the child.
    2 This puts a thought in the mind of the child.
    4 This would be too threatening for the child.
2. **1** This statement allows the resident to express feelings.
    2 This statement provides false assurance.
    3 This statement provides false assurance.
    4 This statement avoids the resident's feelings and does not allow self-expression.
3. **3** Best response based on resident's rights and expectations of nurse. Resident should know who you are and what your position is.
    1 Not considered a professional attitude.
    2 Empathy, not sympathy, encourages a good nurse-resident relationship.
    4 The nurse should explain all nursing procedures; however, in some cases may be called on to explain some medical procedures. Such explanation is the responsibility of the physician.
4. **4** Taking the time to sit with the resident indicates care and concern for the resident as an individual.
    1 This is the nurse's need; it demonstrates that the nurse is uncomfortable with the resident's behavior.
    2 This fails to acknowledge the resident's feelings and ability to make his own decisions.
    3 In some circumstances this might be appropriate, but it is not supportive.
5. **4** Use of reflection will help the resident identify feelings and encourage verbalization of them.
    1 This response is nontherapeutic; it does not acknowledge the resident's feelings.
    2 This response is nontherapeutic; it does not acknowledge the resident's feelings.
    3 This response is nontherapeutic; it does not acknowledge the resident's feelings.
6. **3** This is a technique that avoids misunderstanding so that both the resident and the nurse can work toward a common goal in the therapeutic relationship.
    1 This would not provide for clarification or understanding.
    2 This would not provide for clarification or understanding.
    4 This would not provide for clarification or understanding.
7. **4** Giving adequate time to respond and employing a calm, accepting, deliberate, and interested manner will reduce the resident's anxiety and tension and will increase self-esteem.
    1 Sensory pathways are unaffected; the resident can see, hear, and understand.
    2 Isolation is not therapeutic; the resident must be encouraged to remain in contact with others.
    3 The resident should continue to speak so that new pathways can develop and speech can gradually improve.
8. **3** Damage to Broca's area, located in the posterior frontal region of the dominant hemisphere, causes problems in the motor aspect of speech.
    1 This would be associated with receptive aphasia, not expressive aphasia; receptive aphasia is associated with disease of Wernicke's area.
    2 This would be associated with receptive aphasia, not expressive aphasia; receptive aphasia is associated with disease of Wernicke's area.
    4 Although difficulty writing may be associated with expressive aphasia, understanding speech would be associated with receptive aphasia.

chapter *nineteen*

Cognitive and Emotional Considerations

Cognitive Functioning

Cognitive functioning is the means by which individuals perceive and react to the world around them, based on the knowledge and skills they learned and developed after birth, and which most persons continue to acquire throughout their lives.

Even though it is normal for individuals to continue to learn from new and changing experiences, some changes in cognitive functioning occur over time. These changes or declines do not develop uniformly, either across all areas of cognitive functioning, or at the same rate in all individuals. Some cognitive abilities are stable for many decades and decline late in life, while other abilities show change in middle age and then remain stable or show less decline with advancing age.

Anxiety

A. Definition: a state of alertness or apprehension, tension, or uneasiness; a major component of all mental disturbances. Anxiety is an internal state experienced by the individual when there is a perceived threat to the physical body or to the psychologic integrity of the person. It interferes with concentration, focusing attention on the perceived threat. In its mild form anxiety serves to alert the person to danger and to prepare the body to react to danger; in its severe form it is debilitating and may immobilize the person and interfere with activities. Anxiety is usually described in degrees or levels.
B. Levels of anxiety
   1. Alertness level: awareness of danger; ready for action
   2. Apprehension level: individual feels uncomfortable and prepares to face imminent danger
   3. Free-floating: generalized sensation of discomfort; a feeling of impending danger or disaster
   4. Panic level: a total uncontrolled response dominates perceptions and distorts reality; great discomfort
C. Signs of anxiety
   1. Vocal changes
   2. Restlessness
   3. Rapid speech
   4. Fatigue
   5. Palpitations
   6. Perspiration
   7. Nausea
   8. Frequent urination
   9. Diarrhea
   10. Vomiting (occasionally)

Prevalent Cognitive Disorders

A. Dementia—an organic disorder with symptoms progressing along a continuum from forgetfulness to a total lack of capacity for self-care, incontinence, and failure to recognize family and friends.
   1. Symptoms and behaviors: short- and long-term memory impairment; impairment in abstract thinking; impaired judgment; aphasia; apraxia; agnosia; and personality changes
   2. Levels of dementia: mild, moderate, and severe

3. Categories of dementia: primary result from pathologic changes taking place within the cerebral cortex or subcortical structures of the brain; secondary result from factors external to the brain stemming from metabolic or nutritional disorders and prescribed medications acting alone or in combination

4. Primary dementias
   a. Alzheimer's disease—slow, insidious onset; loss of olfaction; lack of specific focal neurologic signs; rigidity, slowing of movement, abnormal gait (later stages); deterioration in all areas of cognitive functioning along with changes in personality, mood, and behavior
   b. Multiinfarct dementia—resident has history of hypertension; recurrent strokes or emboli; rapid onset; a fluctuating course with stepwise deterioration; relative preservation of personality; nocturnal confusion; neurologic signs such as weakness of extremities, defects in visual fields, and diminished reflexes

5. Secondary dementias
   a. Myxedema (hypothyroidism)—may lead to progressive cognitive impairment, which may not be totally reversible even following treatment
   b. Alcoholism
   c. Metabolic and nutritional disorders
   d. Prescribed medications such as antihistamines, antispasmodics, antidepressants, and anti-Parkinsonism drugs have been shown to produce neuropsychiatric side effects (anxiety, hallucinations, or cognitive impairment)

6. Nursing implications
   a. Recognition of symptoms and behaviors
   b. Monitor all drug use for adverse effects
   c. Support for residents and families

B. Delirium—an acute organic disorder with impaired cognitive function and change in level of consciousness; closely related to the dementias; frequently associated with hallucinations and delusions

1. Symptoms and behaviors—reduced ability to maintain attention to external stimuli; disorganized thinking; reduced level of consciousness; memory impairment; disorientation to person, place, time; disturbance of the sleep cycle; increased or decreased psychomotor activity

2. Nursing implications
   a. Monitoring adequacy of hydration, nutrition, and oxygenation
   b. Monitoring for drug interactions that may adversely affect mental status
   c. Provide environmental support
   d. Protect resident from self-injury

C. Depression—a functional disorder characterized by loss of interest or pleasure in usual activities or pastimes; a disorder of mood occurring at any age

1. Symptoms and behaviors—depressed mood; significant weight loss or gain; insomnia or hypersomnia; fatigue or loss of energy; low self-esteem; decreased ability to concentrate and make decisions; psychomotor agitation or retardation; recurrent thoughts of death, thoughts of suicide, or suicide attempt

2. Nursing implications
   a. Observe for sudden or progressive change in appearance, speech, movement, and behavior
   b. Assess changes in cognitive functioning
   c. Observe for physical disorders that may induce depressive symptoms
   d. Clarify distinction between somatic complaints that are emotional in origin and those having a treatable underlying pathology

Violent Behavior

A. Indications
   1. Substance abuse (e.g., alcoholism)
   2. Hypoglycemia
   3. Epilepsy
   4. Mental subnormality
   5. Psychiatric disturbance/personality disorder, schizophrenia
   6. Space occupying lesions (e.g., brain tumors)

7. Organic brain conditions (e.g., Alzheimer's disease, Korsakoff's psychosis)
8. Presence of/or withdrawal from mood-altering chemicals
9. History of assaultive behavior

B. Severity index—stage 0: at risk, but no physical or laboratory evidence of violence
   1. Assessment
      a. Assess level of agitation:
         (1) Clenched fists
         (2) Increased voice volume
         (3) Angry facial expressions
         (4) Grimacing
         (5) Gritting teeth
         (6) Frowning or glaring, hostile stare
      b. Assess intellectual dimension:
         (1) Understanding of instructions
         (2) Attentiveness
      c. Assess social dimension: ability to interact with health care team and significant other(s)
      d. Collect information regarding the resident's/significant other's knowledge about violence
      e. Monitor therapeutic effects of prescribed medications
   2. Planning
      a. Establish mutually agreeable outcomes with resident and significant other(s)
      b. Design actions to prevent precipitating events
      c. Design an anger-release plan with resident
      d. Modify the interventions outlined in this stage as indicated by resident condition or physician order
      e. Modify resident education outlined in this stage based on resident's/significant other's knowledge of violence and readiness to learn
      f. Modify the outcomes in this stage based on assessment data
   3. Interventions
      a. Do not touch resident without permission
      b. Speak in a calm, firm manner
      c. Reduce environmental stimulation
      d. Implement anger-release plan as indicated

4. Evaluation
   a. Analyze resident progress toward outcomes
   b. Evaluate effectiveness of teaching
   c. Analyze response to interventions, treatment, and medications
   d. Analyze degree of understanding and cooperation with plan of care

C. Severity index—stage 1: mild or argumentative
   1. Assessment
      a. Assess level of agitation:
         (1) Fists clenched
         (2) Increased voice volume
         (3) Angry facial expressions
         (4) Grimacing
         (5) Gritting teeth
         (6) Frowning or glaring, hostile stare
         (7) Verbal threats
      b. Assess intellectual dimension:
         (1) Understanding of instructions
         (2) Attentiveness
      c. Assess social dimension: ability to interact with health care team and significant other(s)
      d. Collect information regarding resident's/significant other's knowledge about violence
      e. Monitor therapeutic effects of prescribed medications
   2. Planning
      a. Design activities to correct/control/prevent precipitating event and diffuse verbal assault
      b. Design a conflict-resolution approach
      c. Design an anger-release plan
      d. Modify the interventions outlined in this stage as indicated by resident condition or physician order
      e. Modify resident education outlined in this stage based on resident's and significant other's knowledge of violence and readiness to learn
      f. Modify the outcomes in this stage based on assessment data
   3. Interventions
      a. Do not touch resident; accept resident's arguments as legitimate
      b. Speak in a calm, firm manner
      c. Seek immediate help to diffuse the situation

d. Administer medication if ordered and if possible
e. Reduce environmental stimulation
f. Provide alternative means for release of anger; distract resident if possible
g. Maintain physical distance; do not invade personal space
h. Do not approach resident from rear
i. Alert security, physician, house supervisor
j. Remove other residents from immediate area
k. Face the resident at all times; stand between resident and the door
l. Implement anger-release plan
m. Implement conflict-resolution approach

4. Evaluation
a. Analyze progress toward outcomes
b. Evaluate effectiveness of conflict-resolution approach
c. Analyze response to interventions, treatment, and medications
d. Analyze effectiveness of teaching
e. Analyze degree of understanding and cooperation with plan of care

D. Severity index—stage 2: moderate or physically threatening
1. Assessment
a. Assess level of agitation:
(1) Increased voice volume
(2) Angry facial expressions
(3) Grimacing
(4) Gritting teeth
(5) Clenched fists
(6) Frowning or glaring, hostile stare
(7) Verbal threats
(8) Physical threats
b. Assess intellectual dimension:
(1) Understanding instructions
(2) Attentiveness
c. Assess social dimension: ability to interact with health care team and significant other(s)
d. Collect information regarding resident's/significant other's knowledge about violence
e. Monitor therapeutic effects of prescribed medications

2. Planning
a. Meet stat with at least one other staff member competent to manage stage 2 behaviors and plan appropriate approaches to resident
b. Plan an immediate referral to psychiatric liaison division
c. Design activities to control/correct/prevent precipitating events and defuse potential for physical assault
d. Prepare quiet room
e. Prepare for chemical or physical restraint according to procedure
f. Modify the interventions outlined in this stage as indicated by resident condition or physician order
g. Modify resident education outlined in this stage based on resident's and significant other's knowledge of violence and readiness to learn
h. Modify the outcomes in this stage based on assessment data

3. Interventions
a. Remove other residents/staff from immediate area
b. Initiate restraining holds according to plan if necessary
c. At least two competent staff members remain with resident until physician determines resident is no longer violent
d. Remain between the resident and the door at all times
e. Face the resident at all times
f. Administer medication if ordered and if possible
g. Speak in a calm, firm manner
h. Reduce environmental stimuli
i. Provide alternative means for release of anger; distract if possible
j. Maintain physical distance; do not invade personal space
k. Do not approach resident from rear
l. Observe resident at all times; do not be lulled into false sense of security
m. Escort resident to designated quiet room
n. Call security to the scene as back-up

4. Evaluation
   a. Analyze progress toward outcomes
   b. Evaluate effectiveness of seclusion
   c. Analyze response to interventions, treatment, and medications if administered
   d. Evaluate effectiveness of teaching
   e. Analyze degree of understanding and cooperation with plan of care

E. Severity index—stage 3: advanced or assaultive behavior
   1. Assessment
      a. Assess level of agitation as evidenced by:
         (1) Increased voice volume
         (2) Angry facial expressions
         (3) Grimacing
         (4) Gritting teeth
         (5) Clenched fists
         (6) Frowning or glaring, hostile stare
         (7) Verbal threats
         (8) Physical demonstration of violence
      b. Assess intellectual dimension:
         (1) Understanding instructions
         (2) Attentiveness
      c. Assess social dimension: ability to interact with health care team and significant other(s)
      d. Monitor therapeutic effects of prescribed medications
   2. Planning
      a. Choose crisis team leader
      b. Design aggression-management plan
      c. Prepare seclusion room: follow policy and procedure
      d. Schedule crisis team debriefing
      e. Obtain an order for locked seclusion and renew q24h based on evaluation of resident status
      f. Obtain an order for restraints
      g. Plan to have the same sex staff member escort resident to seclusion room
      h. Prepare for chemical or physical restraint according to procedure
      i. Modify the interventions outlined in this stage as indicated by resident condition or physician order
      j. Modify resident education outlined in this stage based on resident's and significant other's knowledge of violence and readiness to learn
      k. Modify the outcomes in this stage based on assessment data
   3. Interventions
      a. Remove your glasses, rings, earrings, pins, watches, keys, or anything else that could cause injury to you or the resident
      b. Remove furniture and objects that can be used as weapons
      c. Remove other residents and staff
      d. Approach the resident as a team
      e. Initially two team members approach resident from the front, taking control of arms to lead resident to seclusion room
      f. If resident struggles, other team members take control of legs and head and carry resident to seclusion room
      g. One team member opens doors, moves obstacles, and brings restraint bag
      h. Apply physical restraints if ordered or necessary
      i. Provide range of motion, skin care, and change of position q2h
      j. Reduce environmental stimuli
      k. Always approach the resident with a minimum of two staff members
      l. Do not threaten, argue, or respond with hostility
      m. Watch resident's eyes; resident will usually focus on body part to be attacked
      n. Do not leave resident alone
      o. Remove restraints one at a time for 10 minutes each, q1h
      p. Offer food and fluids every 15 to 30 minutes
      q. Use paperware and plastic eating utensils (no knives)
      r. Termination of restraints/seclusion: contract with resident to maintain control of behavior
   4. Evaluation
      a. Analyze progress toward outcomes
      b. Analyze resident's response to interventions, treatment, and medications
      c. Evaluate any resident injuries sustained during incident

d. Evaluate any injuries to others sustained during incident
e. Evaluate any property damage sustained during incident
f. Evaluate readiness for restraint release as evidenced by signs of:
    (1) Self-control
    (2) Decreased anxiety and agitation
    (3) Stabilization of mood
    (4) Increased attention span
    (5) Reality orientation and judgment
    (6) Regulation of sleep and normalization of sleep patterns
g. Analyze response to release of restraints
h. Evaluate how incident was handled

F. Severity index—stage 4: severe or hostage situation
 1. Assessment (while waiting for law enforcement/security to arrive)
    a. Monitor hostage-taker for evidence of:
        (1) Alcohol/drug use if possible
        (2) Psychiatric disorder
        (3) Organic and/or medical disorder
        (4) Domestic dispute
        (5) Grudge against institution
        (6) Political cause
    b. Monitor anxiety level of crisis team
 2. Planning
    a. Select which staff remains on scene with crisis team
        (1) May be someone familiar with hostage-taker if hostage-taker is resident
        (2) If hostage-taker is family member or acquaintance of staff or resident, do not have that family member or acquaintance on scene
    b. Have someone at outside entrance to meet police and expedite their arrival
    c. Plan communication with administration and law enforcement
 3. Interventions (as a member of the crisis team)
    a. Assist in communication to others when delegated by leader
    b. Follow instructions of law enforcement

c. Relieve leader if lengthy hostage situation
d. Assist with evacuation of area if ordered
e. Position self in place of safety (e.g., behind a barrier, in outer room)
f. Avoid heroics
 4. Evaluation
    a. Critique incident within 24 hours
    b. Consider an evaluation framework to measure all future incidents against:
        (1) Policy appropriateness
        (2) Timeliness of response
        (3) Training for future incidents
        (4) System's difficulties to overcome
        (5) Working with security
        (6) Delegating to team
        (7) Role of administration
        (8) Communication to media and to others
        (9) Effectiveness of facilities control (heat/light/phones)

Review Questions

1. The family of an Alzheimer's disease resident asks the nurse how long it will take the resident to recover. What is the best answer?
   ① "With proper treatment and care, not that long."
   ② "There is no way to tell how long he will be ill."
   ③ "He will not be able to regain what was lost."
   ④ "He will continue to get progressively worse."

2. A 90-year-old widow is experiencing forgetfulness, confusion, and bouts of disorientation that are worse at night. A medical diagnosis of Alzheimer's disease has been made. The nurse serves the meal and later returns to find the tray untouched. On the basis of the nurse's understanding of this resident's condition, the nurse believes the most likely cause of refusal to eat is that the resident:
   ① Does not care for hospital food
   ② Is too forgetful to remember to feed herself
   ③ May believe the food is poisoned
   ④ Is too depressed to eat

3. A resident has Alzheimer's disease. To support the resident's nutritional needs, the nurse's priority nursing intervention should be to:
   ① Have a staff member feed the resident
   ② Have the nutritionist come to talk with the resident about food preferences
   ③ Have a staff member or a family member remain with the resident while eating
   ④ Talk with the resident about nutritional needs

4. The nurse observes a resident naps during the day but tends to become agitated and wander during the night. This behavior, called sundowning, is common to residents who have organic mental disorders. The best nursing intervention for sundowning is to:
   ① Request a sleeping medication from the physician that will enable the resident to get some rest
   ② Interrupt the resident's napping in the daytime so that he can rest better at night
   ③ Ask the resident the next morning if anything had bothered him the night before
   ④ Have the resident sleep in a room that is well lit

5. Which of the following questions would most effectively allow the nurse to judge the emotional changes that a resident with Alzheimer's disease is experiencing as a result of the illness?
   ① "Have you noticed any forgetfulness?"
   ② "Are you still able to care for yourself?"
   ③ "Is it difficult for you to make decisions?"
   ④ "Have you been feeling depressed lately?"

6. A confused and disoriented resident is unable to remember the location of his room and is constantly approaching nursing staff members and asking, "Where do I live?" The most appropriate nursing approach to this problem is:
   ① Color coding
   ② Reminiscence therapy
   ③ Reality orientation
   ④ Remotivation therapy

7. A resident has just been diagnosed with Alzheimer's disease. With which of the following would the resident experience the most difficulty in stage I of Alzheimer's disease?
   ① Getting dressed
   ② Remembering telephone numbers
   ③ Walking up and down stairs
   ④ Brushing his teeth

8. Which of the following is most appropriate when the nurse is aware that a resident is hallucinating?
   ① Tell the resident that there is no one there
   ② Ask the resident to describe his or her feelings at this time
   ③ Use simple statements in communicating with the resident
   ④ Encourage the resident to participate in self-care

9. The nurse can minimize agitation in a disturbed resident by:
   ① Ensuring constant resident and staff contact
   ② Increasing appropriate sensory stimulation
   ③ Discussing the reasons for suspicious beliefs
   ④ Limiting unnecessary interactions with the resident

10. When caring for the depressed resident the nurse usually has the most difficulty dealing with the:
    ① Resident's lack of energy
    ② Negative nonverbal responses
    ③ Resident's psychomotor retardation
    ④ Contagious quality of depression

11. A resident becomes increasingly agitated and screams at, curses at, fights with, and bites other residents. The physician orders a stat injection of haloperidol decanoate (Haldol). The nurse should carry out the order to administer the Haldol:
    ① Quickly, with an attitude of concern
    ② After the resident agrees to take the injection
    ③ Before the resident suspects what is happening
    ④ Quietly, without any explanation of the reason for it

12. The older, confused person with socially aggressive behavior needs an environment that:
    1. Allows freedom of expression
    2. Is mainly group oriented
    3. Provides control by setting limits
    4. Can be manipulated

13. When a continent bedridden resident with a chronic illness expresses anger through urinary incontinence, the nurse should:
    1. Frequently ask if the resident needs the bedpan to void
    2. Create an environment that prevents sensory monotony
    3. Limit the resident's fluid intake in the evening
    4. Provide television or radio for the resident when alone

14. In working with residents using manipulative, socially acting-out behaviors, the nurse should be:
    1. Sincere, cautious, and consistent
    2. Strict, punishing, and restrictive
    3. Accepting, supportive, and friendly
    4. Sympathetic, motherly, and encouraging

15. When planning care for a confused or delusional resident, it is most important for the nurse to:
    1. Maintain quiet, dim surroundings to minimize stimuli
    2. Encourage realistic activity considering the resident's ability
    3. Recognize that the resident is completely unable to differentiate fantasy from reality
    4. Provide physical hygiene and comfort to demonstrate the resident is worthy of receiving care

16. The nursing care plan for the resident with organic brain deterioration should include:
    1. An extensive reeducation program
    2. Details for protective and supportive care
    3. The introduction of new leisure time activities
    4. Plans to involve the resident in group therapy sessions

ANSWERS AND RATIONALES FOR REVIEW QUESTIONS

1. **4** This is the most accurate answer. Alzheimer's disease progresses at a different rate in different people, although the end result is always the same.
   1 This is untrue. He will not recover from his deficits.
   2 This is true, although it does not really explain anything to his family.
   3 This is not necessarily true because the nurse has only seen him under stress. This can make his deficits appear more pronounced than they are.

2. **2** The resident's short-term memory is too impaired to allow her to feed herself.
   1 This is unlikely.
   3 There is no indication that the resident is delusional.
   4 The resident is at risk for becoming depressed, which is characteristic of stage I of Alzheimer's disease. Depression is probably not the cause of her not eating.

3. **3** The resident needs support and encouragement to perform self-feeding. The nurse should help the resident maintain independence as much as possible.
   1 This is indicated only if the resident is physically weak or impaired.
   2 The nutritionist will be helpful, but this measure is not the priority.
   4 This will not address the resident's difficulty in performing self-feeding.

4. **4** A well-lit room will help the resident to remain oriented when he awakens in the night.
   1 Any sleeping medication will further compromise the resident's brain functioning. If the resident receives any medication such as a benzodiazepine or a barbiturate, he will be significantly more disoriented for several days. It takes much longer for an older person to clear these drugs from the body.
   2 This is a good intervention for a younger person. It is not especially effective in an older person.
   3 Even if the resident had been markedly agitated during the night, he may not recall it.

5. **4** This will elicit information about his feelings, especially because depression is a common secondary symptom of Alzheimer's disease.
   1 This is important, but does not address emotional changes.
   2 This is important, but does not address emotional changes.
   3 This is important, but it addresses judgment.

6. **1** Color coding has been successful in helping older residents identify locations they cannot remember.
   2 Reminiscence therapy assists one with adaptation to the aging process.
   3 Reality orientation emphasizes orientation to time, place, and person.
   4 Key components of remotivation therapy are stimulating participation and interest in the environment and the reinforcement of normal behavior.

7. **2** Memory losses are the most common symptom of stage I of this disease.
   1 Gradual loss of motor function is characteristic of stage II of the disease.
   3 Loss of gross motor coordination is seen in stage II.
   4 Loss of fine motor coordination is seen in stage II.

8. **2** This allows the resident to describe what he sees so that the nurse can further discuss what he is experiencing.
   1 Denying what the resident sees does not help him deal with what he believes he sees.
   3 The nurse should introduce conversation gently, but there is no indication in the situation that simple statements need to be used.
   4 Changing the subject is not therapeutic.

9. **4** Limiting unnecessary interactions will decrease stimulation and thus agitation.
   1 Constant resident and staff contact increases stimulation and thus agitation.
   2 This bombards the resident's sensorium and increases agitation.
   3 Not all disturbed residents are suspicious.

10. **4** Depression is contagious; it affects the nurse as well as the resident.
   1 The resident's lack of energy does not make nursing care difficult.
   2 These residents usually do not offer negative responses; they offer no response.
   3 The resident's lack of energy does not make nursing care difficult.

11. **1** Quickness is used for safety; an attitude of concern may help to reduce the resident's anxiety.
   2 A resident this upset would never agree; the resident may harm self or others and must be sedated.
   3 The resident must be told why sedation is being used.
   4 The resident must be told why sedation is being used.

12. **3** Having poor superego control, these individuals cannot set limits for themselves and require an environment in which appropriate limits for behavior are set for them.

  1 This person has too much freedom of expression and is unable to control impulses.

  2 This would be too stimulating for a person with socially aggressive behavior.

  4 An environment that can be manipulated teaches the resident nothing; it encourages a continuation of maladjustive behavior.

13. **2** For psychologic equilibrium the resident's environment must be one of novel and changing stimuli, promoting physical activity and effective interaction with others.

  1 Since the resident has been able to control elimination, frequent toileting is not the problem.

  3 To prevent urinary stasis and dehydration, fluid intake should be encouraged.

  4 Although stimulation is important, it should be varied and the resident's preferences taken into consideration; radio and television do not promote interaction.

14. **1** A sincere, cautious, and consistent attitude limits this individual's ability to manipulate both situations and staff members.

  2 An attitude such as this would allow the resident to rationalize the manipulative behavior to deal with the response of the nurse.

  3 In accepting the person, the nurse should not support negative behavior; a friendly attitude may encourage further problem behavior.

  4 This would only encourage residents to continue in their lifestyle rather than learn better ways to relate to their environment.

15. **2** These residents need sensory stimulation to maintain orientation and should be encouraged to do as much as possible for themselves, depending on their ability.

  1 Surroundings should be bright to minimize confusion of stimuli.

  3 Residents are usually not completely out of contact with reality; it is important to differentiate fantasy from reality, but this would not take top priority in care.

  4 Although it is important to make certain that residents receive physical hygiene and comfort, they should be encouraged to help themselves as much as possible.

16. **2** Damaged brain cells do not regenerate. Care is therefore directed toward preventing further damage and providing protective and supportive care.

  1 The deterioration of the brain cells makes an extensive reeducation program unrealistic.

  3 A resident with this disorder may not be able to grasp, understand, or enjoy new leisure activities.

  4 It is beyond the scope of the resident's ability to function in a group therapy session.

Specialty Practice Issues

chapter *twenty*

Education Issues

Establishment Of A Teaching-Learning Environment

A. Teaching is communication that is specially structured and sequenced to produce learning

B. Learning is the activity through which knowledge, attitudes, and skills are acquired, resulting in a change in behavior

C. All problems in learning and identified knowledge deficits should be addressed when establishing the appropriate nursing diagnoses for a resident

D. Goals of learning
   1. Understanding or acquiring knowledge: cognitive learning (e.g., What is diabetes, and how does it affect me?)
   2. Feeling or developing attitudes: affective learning (e.g., What does this health problem mean to me?)
   3. Performing or developing psychomotor skills: conative learning (e.g., How do I give myself an injection?)

Principles of Teaching-Learning Process and Related Nursing Approaches

A. Learning occurs best when there is a felt need or readiness to learn
   1. Identify the resident's emotional or motivational readiness: whether the person is ready to put forth the effort necessary to learn
   2. Identify the resident's experiential readiness: whether the person has the necessary background of experience, skills, attitudes, and ability to learn

   3. Determine the resident's level of adaptation: different teaching strategies may be necessary during the various stages of adaptation because the resident is expressing denial, anger, and/or depression; once the initial defensive compensatory reactions have passed, the individual is more receptive to teaching
   4. Assess the resident's level of human needs; the resident whose physical and safety needs are not met will not be concerned with interpersonal and intrapersonal needs
   5. Specific signs of the resident's readiness to learn
      a. The resident is adapting to the initial crisis
      b. The resident has a developing awareness of the health problem and its implications
      c. The resident is asking direct questions
      d. The resident is presenting clues that indicate indirect seeking of information
      e. The resident's physical condition or behavior invites the nurse to intervene through teaching
   6. Once a need has been recognized, readiness has been determined, and the time and place are appropriate, develop a plan and teach

B. The method of presentation of material influences the resident's ability to learn
   1. A tentative teaching plan should be developed with the resident and/or the resident's significant others and communicated to all members of the health care team

2. Information presented should be organized, accurate, and concise (e.g., presented in a format of simple to complex, general to specific)
3. Appropriate teaching methods should be instituted
   a. Concepts are best taught with lectures, audiovisual materials, and discussion
   b. Attitudes are taught by exploring feelings, role playing, discussions, and an atmosphere of acceptance
   c. Skills are taught by illustrations, models, demonstration, return demonstration, and practice
4. Teaching tools should be used when indicated (e.g., models, filmstrips, illustrations)
5. The resident and family should be encouraged to ask questions, which should be answered directly
6. Repetition enhances learning; periodic practice will stabilize the learning
7. Opportunities should be provided for evaluation

C. Consider the resident's background when preparing teaching materials
   1. Vocabulary level should be carefully chosen to suit the resident
   2. For older residents, use larger, bolder, and plainer letters

D. Learning is made easier when material to be learned is related to what the learner already knows
   1. Find out what the resident knows about the problem
   2. Begin the teaching program at the resident's level of understanding
   3. Avoid the use of technical terminology; use simple terms or ones with which the resident feels comfortable

E. Learning is purposeful; short- and long-term goals are important because they identify the behavior to be attained
   1. With the resident, set short- and long-term goals
   2. Goals should meet the following criteria:
      a. Resident centered
      b. Specific: state exactly what is to be accomplished
      c. Measurable: set a minimum acceptable level of performance
      d. Realistic: must be potentially achievable
      e. Have a time frame

F. Learning is an active process and takes place within the learner
   1. Use a teaching approach that includes the learner (e.g., programmed instruction books, discussion, questions and answers, return demonstration)
   2. Provide opportunities for the resident to practice motor skills
   3. Encourage self-directed activities

G. Every individual has capabilities and strengths (e.g., physical strengths, emotional maturity, a supportive family) that can be used to help the resident learn
   1. Identify the resident's personal resources
   2. Build on the identified strengths
   3. Use these personal resources when and where appropriate

H. Energy and endurance levels affect the resident's ability to learn and perform
   1. During instruction, balance teaching with sufficient rest periods
   2. Provide teaching at opportune times (e.g., earlier in the day rather than at night, after periods of rest)
   3. Present instruction in a manner the resident can comprehend and at a pace that can be maintained
   4. Be flexible and adjust the plan according to the resident's rest and activity needs

I. Aging may affect the resident's ability to learn and perform
   1. Pace the learning, focus on a single topic at a time, and limit environmental distractions to accommodate changes in cognitive ability
   2. Ensure adequate lighting, a quiet room, large print, and bright colors for written material to accommodate sensory impairments

J. Learning does not always progress in a straight forward-and-upward manner; the resident may experience plateaus and remissions with a resulting change in adaptation and needs
   1. Accept the resident's feelings regarding lack of progress
   2. Point out progress that has been made
   3. Be patient and do not cause additional stress for the learner

4. Try alternative approaches for achieving goals
5. Identify short-term objectives for meeting goals
6. Alter long-term goals as necessary

K. Learning from previous experience can be transferred to new situations
   1. When teaching something new, relate the commonalities or similarities of previously learned experiences
   2. Base the plan of instruction on the foundation of the resident's knowledge
   3. Once the known is reinforced, the unknown can be explored and the differences taught

L. Accurate and prompt feedback enhances learning
   1. Prompt feedback provides a feeling of satisfaction if the resident is successful
   2. Even when correction is necessary, feedback can reduce resident's tension because then the learner knows what is learned and what has not yet been mastered

Motivation

A. Definition: motivation is the process of stimulating a person to assimilate certain concepts or behavior

B. Principles of motivation and related nursing approaches:
   1. People are complex products of self, family, and culture; the nurse must care for the resident as a unified being
      a. Respect the resident as a person
      b. Accept the resident's feelings without minimizing them
      c. Assist the resident and family in accepting that the person's individuality and wholeness continue despite the changed physical or emotional state
      d. Involve the resident in deciding what to do and how to do it
      e. The resident must take precedence over the purpose of the lesson
   2. Learning is fostered when the plan of instruction is designed to operate within the individual's personal attitude and value system
      a. Provide an atmosphere that allows for acceptance of differing value systems
      b. Let the resident explore personal values, attitudes, and feelings concerning the health problem and its implications
      c. Explore with the family the possibilities of carrying out instruction and how to individualize it so it is acceptable and practical for the resident and family
   3. A motivated learner assimilates what is learned more rapidly than does one who is unmotivated
      a. The resident needs an opportunity to explore and discover personal learning needs and feelings concerning them
      b. Awareness of a need to know can cause mild anxiety, which in itself is motivating
      c. Motivation that is too intense may reduce the effectiveness of learning
      d. Determine the resident's readiness for learning
   4. Intrinsic motivation (stimulated from within the learner) is preferable to extrinsic motivation (stimulated from outside the learner)
      a. Identify factors that are essential for the individual to have a feeling of meaningful achievement (e.g., being able to care for own health needs, respect and appreciation from others, acquiring new knowledge, receiving a reward)
      b. Satisfaction with learning progress promotes additional learning; therefore, design nursing care that will assist the resident in attaining a feeling of meaningful achievement
      c. Encourage the resident to participate as a member of the health care team and to be self-directed
   5. Information is learned more readily when it is relevant and meaningful to the learner
      a. Help the resident interpret why the information is important and how the information gained will be useful
      b. Relate the information by building the teaching plan on the resident's foundation of knowledge, experience, attitudes, and feelings

6. Learning motivated by success or rewards is preferable to learning motivated by failure or punishment
   a. Help the resident set realistic goals within the motivation zone (goals set too high may be too challenging, whereas goals set too low may lead to no action)
   b. Focus on the resident's strengths and abilities rather than on failures and disabilities
   c. Select learning tasks at which the resident is likely to succeed
   d. Assist the resident to master or feel successful at one stage of instruction before moving on to the next
   e. Errors must be accepted as part of the learning process
   f. Tolerance for failure is best taught through providing a backlog of success that compensates for experienced failure

7. Planned reinforcement is essential for learning; operant conditioning is based on the theory that satisfaction motivates learning and that those events that occur together are associated
   a. For each resident, identify and use factors that are stimulants or incentives for action (e.g., praise, smile, rewards, rest, specific privileges, being able to care for self)
   b. Provide visible reinforcements (e.g., progress charts, graphs)
   c. Repetition is a form of reinforcement; therefore repeated activities tend to become habitual
      (1) Provide opportunities for the resident to practice old and new skills
      (2) Review information previously taught before introducing new information
   d. Involve the resident in groups of people who have the same health problems but are at various stages of convalescence
      (1) To be successful, it is helpful for the resident to associate with successful people
      (2) Individuals can often learn more by teaching others

8. Evaluation of performance aids in learning
   a. Purpose
      (1) To measure and interpret results with regard to what degree the set goals are attained
      (2) To reinforce correct behavior
      (3) To help the learner realize how to change incorrect behavior
      (4) To help the teacher determine the adequacy of the teaching
   b. Together the teacher and learner should observe and evaluate the learner's response in light of the desired behavior
   c. Identify factors that may have contributed to attainment or nonattainment of goals
   d. Value judgments, especially "poor" or "inadequate," must relate to the performance rather than to the individual

Teaching Methodologies

A. Lecture
   1. Preparation
      a. Clarify your objectives: what you hope the listeners will gain
      b. Assess the resident's education level, diversity of the group being addressed, socioeconomic characteristics, and cultural belief system
   2. Organization
      a. Group your ideas to make them easier to grasp and recall
      b. Tailor the lecture content to fit the assessed needs and characteristics of the residents
   3. Delivery
      a. Your language and pace should be appropriate for the residents
      b. Break up straight lecture by use of audiovisuals or handouts
      c. Talk from your notes but do not read your paper; maintain eye contact
      d. Consider the need for a microphone

B. Discussion
   1. Get the discussion underway by asking an open-ended question
   2. Get the group back on topic when discussion strays
   3. When no new information or ideas are forthcoming, move on to the next topic
   4. End the discussion by summarizing ideas

C. Demonstration
  1. Assemble and pretest before residents arrive
  2. Advance knowledge of the general procedure to be followed helps residents develop a mindset that will facilitate their learning
  3. Use a positive approach: emphasize what to do rather than emphasizing what not to do
  4. Ensure a good view for everyone watching the demonstration
  5. Offer running comments that focus resident's attention
  6. Use a true-to-life setting if possible
  7. Hold a discussion period following the demonstration
  8. Have residents practice
D. Modeling: you are teaching, whether or not you are aware of your effect as a role model

Review Questions

1. A stroke resident has an order for turning q2h. When the nurse goes into the room to turn the resident, the family refuses and states that the resident has "had enough" and needs to rest. The nurse should:
   ① Call for assistance and turn the resident; instruct the family that physician orders must be followed
   ② Wait an hour or so and hope the family members will change their mind; if not, insist that the resident be turned
   ③ Explain that the physician's order must be followed; family members will need to speak to the physician on his next rounds
   ④ Explain the importance of turning to the family and arrange for the resident to rest uninterrupted for the next 2 hours

2. Learning occurs best when there is a felt need or readiness to learn. Which of the following responses by the resident indicates a readiness to learn about diabetes?
   ① "I'll go to another doctor; I just can't have diabetes. No one else in my family has it."
   ② "Will the insulin I take be sufficient to cover my needs for a full day?"
   ③ "As long as I take my pills I really don't have to worry about doing anything special."
   ④ "Why does this always happen to me?"

3. To be most effective when teaching colostomy care to a resident, the nurse must first:
   ① Wait until a family member is present
   ② Assess barriers to learning ostomy care
   ③ Begin with simple written instructions concerning the care
   ④ Wait until the resident has accepted the change in body image

4. The nurse is teaching a newly diagnosed diabetic resident to administer insulin. Which of the following responses by the resident is most indicative of the resident's knowledge of the procedure?
   ① The resident is able to state the signs and symptoms of hypoglycemia.
   ② The resident is able to prepare and administer the insulin correctly.
   ③ The resident identifies verbally the correct steps for the procedure.
   ④ The resident is able to identify the importance of diet in his medication regimen.

5. An older long-term care resident is a newly diagnosed diabetic. The nurse has given the resident a diabetic diet sheet and discussed the diet. The resident expresses interest by telling the nurse she understands what she has been taught. The nurse has also shown the resident a syringe and the type of insulin that will be used. What barriers to change may be present in this situation?
   ① Unclear short-term goals
   ② Lack of support system
   ③ Insufficient skill to follow plan
   ④ Lack of motivation

ANSWERS AND RATIONALES FOR REVIEW QUESTIONS

1. **4** An explanation of the need to prevent pressure ulcers will help the family to understand and cooperate with the plan; it also recognizes their concern for the resident's need to rest.
   1 This option ignores the family's concerns and could evoke anger, especially if the family is fearful of the resident's deteriorating condition.
   2 The nurse could choose to wait another hour if concern was not high for the resident developing a pressure ulcer; however, an explanation to the family would be best.
   3 This also ignores the family's concern. The nurse can independently explain the purpose of the treatment.

2. **2** The resident is asking a direct question.
   1 The resident is in denial and therefore is not ready to learn.
   3 The resident has not yet developed an awareness about his condition or its implications.
   4 The resident is exhibiting anger and therefore is not ready to learn.

3. **2** Before a teaching plan can be developed, the factors that interfere with learning must be identified.
   1 Although family members can be helpful, resident involvement in care is important for promoting independence and self-esteem.
   3 This is premature; assessment comes before intervention; written instructions may not be the most appropriate teaching modality.
   4 This may be an unrealistic expectation; the resident may never accept the change but must learn to manage care.

4. **2** By demonstrating the procedure correctly, the resident has shown knowledge of insulin administration.
   1 Although this is important information for diabetics to know, it does not convey understanding of insulin administration.
   3 The resident must be able to actually demonstrate correct insulin administration.
   4 Although this is important information for diabetics to know, it does not convey understanding of insulin administration.

5. **3** The resident has not had the training to use the insulin and syringe.
   1 No evidence that goals were ever set.
   2 Nursing staff also serve to function as part of the resident's support system.
   4 The resident is interested to begin the health maintenance plan.

chapter *twenty-one*

Ethical and Legal Considerations

The term *ethics* indicates what a person should do and how one should behave in relation to others. It is concerned with questions of good and bad, right and wrong conduct, character, and motives. A code of ethics provides a standard of behavior that serves as a guide for nurses in education and practice, legislation affecting nurses, licensing of nurses, and public participation of nurses.

Ethical Concepts and Nursing

A. Nurses and people
1. A nurse's primary responsibility is to the residents
2. The nurse promotes an environment in which values, customs, and beliefs of individuals are respected
3. A nurse holds in confidence personal information and uses judgment in sharing this information
B. Nurses and practice
1. Personal responsibility for nursing practice
2. Personal responsibility for continued education and competence
3. Maintains highest standard of nursing care possible
4. Uses judgment in relation to individual competence when accepting and delegating responsibilities
5. Maintains high standards of personal conduct that reflect credit on the profession
C. Nurses and society: as a citizen the nurse shares responsibility for initiating and supporting actions to meet health care and social needs of the public

D. Nurses and co-workers
1. Maintains cooperative relationship with co-workers in nursing and other areas
2. Takes appropriate action to safeguard resident when care is endangered by co-worker or any other person
E. Nurses and the profession
1. Plays major role in determining and implementing desirable standards of nursing practice
2. Active in developing core of professional knowledge
3. Participates in establishing and maintaining equitable social and economic working conditions in nursing
4. Acts through professional organization

Maintaining Professional Accountability

A. Self
1. Report personal conduct that endangers residents
2. Stay informed of current nursing practice theory and issues
3. Make judgments based on facts
B. Resident
1. Provide resident with accurate information about care
2. Ensure resident safety and well-being
C. Profession
1. Maintain ethical standards in practice
2. Encourage peers to follow same
3. Report a colleague's unethical behavior

D. Employing institution—follow policy and procedures defined by the institution

E. Society—maintain ethical conduct in care of residents in all settings

Federal and State Legislation Affecting Residents in Long-Term Care

A. Medicare—a federally funded health insurance program for people who are over age 65 and for some disabled persons.
   1. The Health Care Financing Administration (HCFA) of the U.S. Department of Health and Human Services (USDHHS) is responsible for this program
   2. Part A—hospital insurance portion; helps pay for in-hospital care, care in skilled nursing facilities, home health care, and hospice care
   3. Part B—medical insurance portion; helps pay for physician services for out-patient care, durable medical equipment, and prostheses; partially financed through monthly premium paid by Medicare beneficiaries

B. Medicaid—a state-operated and state-administered program for the medically indigent
   1. The program is partially federally aided
   2. Medicaid becomes the secondary payor for those residents who have exhausted their Medicare benefits and meet the current criteria for eligibility imposed by the state that administers the program

C. The Omnibus Budget Reconciliation Act of 1987 (OBRA)
   1. Definition: major federal legislative reform known as Nursing Home Reform Amendments (NHRA); passed by U.S. Congress as part of OBRA
   2. Significant provisions include:
      a. Abolition of the distinction between skilled nursing facilities (SNFs) and intensive care facilities (ICFs) under the Medicaid program in favor of a single classification called a *nursing facility*
      b. A single set of more stringent requirements based on current SNF conditions of participation
      c. New requirements for a uniform resident assessment

d. The recognition of residents' rights as a critical aspect of residents' psychosocial health, including the right to pretransfer and predischarge notice

e. Preadmission screening and annual resident reviews for residents who are mentally ill or mentally retarded

f. Required training and certification of nurses' aides, as well as the establishment of a nurse's aide registry to record the names of aides who have neglected or abused residents or misappropriated residents' property

g. Provisions to outlaw discrimination against Medicaid recipients

h. Strengthening of social service requirements

i. Development of a survey protocol designed to measure outcomes and the actual care provided to residents

j. Enhanced enforcement authority, including mandated intermediate sanctions for facilities that fail to comply with the regulations

Quality Assurance
CONTINUOUS QUALITY IMPROVEMENT

A. Definition: a method used to ascertain the extent to which nursing practice meets particular indicators based on predetermined standards; monitoring mechanisms have two dimensions: focus and time frames of indicators

B. Focus of indicators
   1. Definition: refers to the different approaches that can be monitored in terms of what contributes to the provision of quality care
   2. Types of approaches
      a. Structure indicators: include the organizational framework, level of financial support to nursing service, and physical and functional characteristics of facility
      b. Process indicators: measure nursing actions used to reach expected and desired outcomes in a resident
      c. Outcome indicators: measure resident's status on discharge against desired outcomes in residents with the same diagnosis

C. Time frame of indicators
1. Definition: time frame is related to when data is collected during the length of stay
2. Time frames
   a. Prospective: refers to the identification of a sample before care is given (e.g., the next 10 residents who are treated for a fall injury will be monitored for quality of emergency care delivered)
   b. Concurrent: permits assessment of what is presently occurring (e.g., monitoring of nursing care in the process of being delivered)
   c. Retrospective: refers to comparing documentation from the past (found in the clinical record) against established indicators
D. Improves nursing care by:
1. Providing accountability to the resident
2. Identifying the need for additional services, personnel, or equipment
3. Identifying deficiencies in policies and procedures
4. Improving interdisciplinary and intradisciplinary communication and coordination of resident services
5. Promoting individual growth of staff members
6. Providing direction for development of educational programs
7. Meeting the requirements of regulatory agencies
8. Improving interagency and intraagency health care systems

Abuse and Neglect

A. Definition: an act or omission that results in harm or threatened harm to the health or welfare of a person
B. Abuse
1. Intentional infliction of physical or mental injury
2. Sexual abuse
3. Withholding of necessary items (e.g., food, clothing)
4. Withholding of medical care necessary to meet physical and mental health needs
5. Verbal abuse
C. Neglect
1. Failure to provide some degree of minimal care
2. The deliberate or unintentional withholding of assistance vital to the performance of activities of daily living or necessary for the avoidance of physical harm, mental anguish, or mental illness
D. Financial abuse—assets of the resident are misappropriated
E. Characteristics of abused
1. Over age 60
2. Parent of abuser (most often)
3. Widowed
4. Repeated victimization
5. Not employed
6. Possibly physically or mentally impaired
F. Characteristics of abuser
1. Age 40 to 60
2. Son/daughter or care giver of victim
3. Married
4. Possible history of own childhood physical/sexual abuse
5. Socioeconomic status not a factor
6. May be professional or semiretired
7. Education may be high school or college level
G. Nursing assessment
1. Unexplained bruises or burns
2. Poor skin care
3. Severe dehydration or malnutrition
4. Fear response to the care giver by the resident
5. Conflicting histories from caregiver and the resident
6. Inappropriate explanation of an injury
7. Long delay in treatment of an injury
F. Nursing intervention
1. Provide an interim safe environment
2. Provide access to protective devices
3. Report suspicions to the appropriate supervisor or community agency according to policy outlined by your facility

Informed Consent

A. According to *Black's Law Dictionary*, consent is "an act of reason accompanied by deliberation wherein the mind weighs, as a balance, the good or evil on either side"

B. Types of consenting behaviors include inferred consenting, implied consenting, and expressed consenting

C. Purposes of informed consent
1. Makes possible a contract between two individuals with each sharing equally
2. Makes a competent decision possible for resident, who has the final decision

D. Consent is essential for any treatment, except in an emergency in which failure to institute treatment may constitute negligence

E. In an emergency situation, two physicians may sign consent for the resident when failure to intervene may cause death or the common law permits administration of health care to unconscious or mentally incompetent persons in an emergency situation as long as the resident does not express nonconsent while conscious or mentally competent

F. Essential elements of legally effective consents are that the consent:
1. Is voluntary
2. Authorizes the specific treatment or care and the person giving the treatment or care
3. Is given by a person with the legal capacity to consent
4. Is given by a mentally competent person
5. Is an informed decision

G. The informed consent includes:
1. An explanation of treatment to be administered, with a presentation of advantages and disadvantages
2. Description of possible alternatives
3. Time for decision making
4. Absence of undue pressure
5. Decision making occurs before sedation is given

H. Problems arise in determining:
1. What constitutes adequate information
2. Who should give explanation
3. Whether to give alternatives when one treatment is clearly preferable
4. What constitutes mental incompetency in a resident from whom consent is sought

I. The resident has a right to know, agree to, or refuse, and this right is reflected in literature of the residents' rights associations and legislation

J. The nurse's responsibility is to respect the rights of the individual resident, thus avoiding legal action

K. The nurse is a resident/family advocate when the resident cannot function in this role and when all elements of an informed consent are not in place

Advanced Directives, Power of Attorney and DNR Status

In October 1990 Congress enacted the Patient-Self Determination Act, which empowers residents to receive necessary information concerning health care decisions. At this time 41 states and the District of Columbia have living will statutes. Nurses should become knowledgeable concerning the law in the state where they practice

A. Advanced directive—living will
1. Signed and witnessed documents providing specific instructions for health care treatment if person is unable to make a decision personally when one is needed
2. Details how much medical care person wants to receive if terminally ill
3. Document can assist family and health care providers in carrying out resident's wishes
4. Based on right to self-determination—right to refuse or accept recommended medical treatment
5. Resident may revoke advanced directive at any time and through any method of communication

B. Durable power of attorney
1. Document that appoints another person to make decisions in event of resident's incompetence
2. Some states have enacted statutes known as *medical durable power of attorney*
3. Must be signed and dated in the presence of two witnesses who are not blood relatives and to whom no property is being left
4. Person's signature must be notarized

C. Do not resuscitate (DNR) status
1. DNR status determination continues as an important issue and includes dilemmas in any health care environment, including the home
   a. All health care institutions are required to have DNR procedures to meet accreditation standards
   b. Standards for home care from the Joint Commission on Accreditation of Health Care Organization includes "a statement regarding the need to docu-

ment discussions with patients and significant others about life sustaining measures"

    c. Documentation of DNR status includes progress notes of all DNR discussions and decisions and DNR orders in the resident's cumulative medical record and on the problem list, if the resident wishes not to be resuscitated; it may also be on the resident's wristband

2. Most important factors considered in determining a resuscitation order are the resident's wishes, the prognosis, the resident's ability to cope, and whether cardiopulmonary resuscitation (CPR) will provide benefits sufficient to make it worthwhile to endure the "burdens" of resuscitation

3. Reasons expressed by residents who choose not to be resuscitated are that the CPR will provide no benefit for them because of widespread terminal or debilitating disease, that their present quality of life is unacceptable to them, that CPR would only prolong suffering, and that the further deterioration caused by CPR would be unacceptable to them

4. In New York State, the right to request a DNR status is maintained by law within the Patient's Bill of Rights, and hospitals must provide education on the issue of DNR to residents and families

5. A DNR order must be a team decision; the family and, if possible, the resident must be included in the decision-making process

6. A DNR order, although legal, is still not clear in implementation

Community Resources

A. Factors to consider when assessing needs for referral:
1. Physical status
2. Mental status
3. Motivation of resident
4. Health conditions and related care requirements
5. Capacity of activities of daily living (ADLs) and independent activities of daily living (IADLs)
6. Family resources
7. Financial resources

B. General services available
1. Information and referral—includes local libraries, office on aging, health department
2. Financial aid—local offices of the Social Security Administration and Department of Social Services
3. Banks—offer free checking for older persons; some assist with balancing checkbooks and managing bills
4. Recreation—local bureaus of recreation, religious groups, senior centers
5. Transportation—local chapters of the Red Cross, public transit agencies, and hospital social work departments may be able to provide transportation for doctor visits

Review Questions

1. The nurse auscultates a resident's lungs and notes a fine crackling sound in the left lower lung during respiration. If crackles and rhonchi in the left lower lung were charted on the nurse's notes, the notation would be:
   ① A nursing diagnosis
   ② A correct nursing notation
   ③ An inaccurate interpretation
   ④ Correct if palpation ruled out crepitus

2. If the nurse leaves a supply of nitroglycerin tablets at the resident's bedside, the nurse should:
   ① Count the tablets left in the bottle and record the amount taken by the resident each time
   ② Check and record the resident's blood pressure q6h
   ③ Discourage the resident from taking too many pills, which could lead to drug dependency
   ④ Realize that nurses have no responsibility for residents regarding nitroglycerin

3. In most agencies the use of a pencil to record resident information is acceptable on which of the following documents?
   ① Flow sheet
   ② Discharge summary
   ③ Medication record
   ④ Kardex

4. The resident has the right to:
   ① Refuse treatment
   ② Choose own physician
   ③ Receive a proper standard of care
   ④ All of the above

5. The purpose of Good Samaritan laws is to:
   ① Mandate nurses and physicians to stop and render care at accident sites
   ② Encourage emergency aid at accident sites
   ③ Prevent any liability arising from care rendered at accident sites
   ④ Have universal laws mandating emergency aid at accident sites

6. It is determined that a staff nurse has a drug abuse problem. As an initial intervention the staff nurse should be:
   ① Counseled by the staff psychiatrist
   ② Dismissed from the job immediately
   ③ Forced to promise to abstain from drugs
   ④ Referred to the employee assistance program

7. On admission to nursing homes, residents designate a person as having durable power of attorney. This means that the resident legally appoints a person on his behalf to:
   ① Make decisions regarding his finances
   ② Make health care decisions for him even when he is able
   ③ Make decisions regarding how he will spend his money for health care
   ④ Make health care decisions for him when he is unable to do so

8. Nursing assessment must be accurately documented. The charted observation states that a resident had "tachypnea." The nurse knows that respirations were:
   ① Increased in rate and depth
   ② Slow and regular in rate
   ③ Deep and fast, then shallower and slower with apneic periods
   ④ Increased in rate and decreased in depth

9. OBRA requires that each assessment be conducted or coordinated by:
   ① Any staff members directly caring for the resident
   ② Any licensed persons
   ③ Only registered nurses
   ④ Any staff members caring indirectly for the resident

10. Of the following methods of charting, which one best describes the recording of events as they occur throughout the day?
    ① Narrative charting
    ② SOAP charting
    ③ Focus charting
    ④ PIE charting

11. A resident is placed on a stretcher and restrained with Velcro straps while being transported to the x-ray department. A Velcro strap breaks, and the resident falls to the floor, sustaining a fractured arm. Later the resident states, "The Velcro strap was worn just at the very spot where the strap snapped." The nurse is:
    ① Completely exonerated, since only the hospital, as principal employer, is primarily responsible for the quality and maintenance of equipment
    ② Exempt from any lawsuit because of the doctrine of *respondeat superior*
    ③ Normally liable, along with the employer, for misapplication of equipment or use of defective equipment that harms the resident
    ④ Totally and singly responsible for the obvious negligence because of failure to report defective equipment

ANSWERS AND RATIONALES FOR REVIEW QUESTIONS

1. **3** Rhonchi are coarse sounds heard over the larger airways; including rhonchi in the notation makes it inaccurate.
   1 Crackles and rhonchi are resident adaptations, not a nursing diagnosis.
   2 It would be incorrect to use the term rhonchi to refer to crackling sounds in the lower lung.
   4 Crepitus, which indicates subcutaneous emphysema, is a condition unrelated to the breath sounds heard on auscultation.

2. **1** Although the resident should take the nitroglycerin as needed, the amount taken must be documented on the record.
   2 It is not necessary to take the blood pressure q6h.
   3 This is not necessarily a dependency drug.
   4 It is the nurse's responsibility to monitor nitroglycerin use.

3. **4** A Kardex is not a permanent part of the record and is altered frequently; therefore, using a pencil is appropriate.
   1 The flow sheet is part of the permanent record, and the use of a pen is legally required for making entries.
   2 The discharge summary is a permanent part of the chart and therefore requires the use of a pen.
   3 The medication record is part of the permanent record, and the use of a pen is required.

4. **4** All are included in the Patient's Bill of Rights.
   1 The right to refuse treatment to the extent permitted by the law.
   2 To know by name the physician responsible for coordinating care.
   3 To considerate and respectful care.

5. **2** Many states have Good Samaritan laws to encourage medical aid at the scene of an accident by limiting the legal liability that might arise.
   1 It is not mandatory for nurses or physicians to render emergency aid.
   3 It is expected that the person rendering aid will act as a reasonable, prudent person would act under similar circumstances. A higher standard of medical aid would be expected of a nurse, physician, or member of a first-aid squad than of the general public.
   4 Laws vary in each state.

6. **4** This is a nonpunitive approach that attempts to salvage the nurse as an individual and as a professional.
   1 This may be necessary for long-term therapy but would not be the initial approach.
   2 This is a punitive, nontherapeutic response that offers no chance for rehabilitation.
   3 The nurse is addicted; promises will not keep a person from abusing drugs.

7. **4** A recently enacted law requires residents to have a legally designated person to make decisions about health care in the event that they are not able to do so.
   1 This does not pertain to financial decisions.
   2 This is not intended to take away the decision-making power from residents who are able to make such decisions.
   3 This does pertain to health care financing.

8. **4** Correct.
   1 Hyperventilation.
   2 Bradypnea.
   3 Cheyne-Stokes.

9. **3** Assessments must be conducted or coordinated by RNs and involve appropriate participation of other health care professionals.
   1 All health care personnel can participate, but the RN is the designated coordinator.
   2 All health care personnel can participate, but the RN is the designated coordinator.
   4 All health care personnel can participate, but the RN is the designated coordinator.

10. **1** Narrative charting describes events in sequence throughout the course of a nursing shift.
    2 SOAP charting is problem-oriented in nature; S stands for subjective data, O for objective data, A for assessment or analysis of the problem; and P for the plan of care.
    3 Focus charting is a modification of the SOAP charting method and uses a DAR format; D stands for data, A for action, and R for response.
    4 PIE is a problem-oriented form of charting; PIE is the acronym for problem, intervention, and evaluation.

11. **3** The nurse was negligent in using a stretcher with worn straps. Such oversight did not reflect the actions of a reasonably prudent nurse.
    1 The nurse is responsible for determining the safety of hospital equipment.
    2 Nurses are responsible for their own actions and must ascertain the adequate functioning of equipment.
    4 The hospital shares responsibility for safe, functioning equipment.

Leadership and Management

chapter twenty-two

Interdisciplinary Team

The resident's needs are addressed through an interdisciplinary approach, using such tools as the Minimum Data Set (MDS) and the Care Plan. Both the resident and family are included in the problem-solving process.

Rationale: an interdisciplinary approach of the resident permits more indepth evaluation of needs and permits greater problem-solving ability.

Tools Utilized

A. MDS
B. Interdisciplinary Team Conference
C. Care Plan

MINIMUM DATA SET (MDS)

A. A standardized assessment tool developed to make the process of assessment more consistent and reliable throughout the country
  1. Triggers—clues to the problems identified on the MDS
  2. Raps—guidelines that help the health care team develop the resident's Care Plan

INTERDISCIPLINARY TEAM CONFERENCE

A. Physicians
B. Nurses
  1. RN
  2. LPN
  3. Nursing assistant
C. Social Service
D. Activity
E. Dietary
F. Resident
G. Family members

COMPREHENSIVE CARE PLAN

A written guide that gives direction about the care a resident should receive—plan consists of:
  1. Identification of resident problem
  2. Goals for care
  3. Action to be taken to help resident solve problems

Review Questions

1. The purpose of the team-nursing method of delivering resident care is to:
   1. Maximize abilities of all nursing personnel
   2. Challenge all nurses to provide good nursing care
   3. Teach student nurses to give orders, make assignments, and administer treatment
   4. Lessen the workload of all employees

2. When discussing the team's best approach for a resident whose behavior is characterized by pathologic suspicion, one of the key goals of care should be to:
   1. Help the resident realize the suspicions are unrealistic
   2. Remove as much environmental stress as possible
   3. Help the resident to feel accepted by the staff on the unit
   4. Ask the resident to explain the reason for the feelings

3. A terminally ill resident is furious with one of the staff nurses. Over the next several days the resident refuses the nurse's care and insists on performing self-care. A different nurse is assigned to care for the resident. The nurse's initial step in

revising the nursing care plan to meet the resident's needs would be to:

① Obtain a full report from the first nurse and adjust the plan accordingly

② Ask the physician for a report on the resident's condition and plan accordingly

③ Speak with the resident about the change in staff responsibilities and assess the resident's reaction

④ Assess the resident's present status and capabilities and include the resident in a discussion of revisions

4. The husband of a resident who is dying tells the nurse that he knows that his wife is asking the nurses to leave her pain medication on her bedside table and expresses his fear that she is saving it up for a suicide attempt. The nurse knows that many of the staff members have mixed feelings about the resident's terminal status and prolonged pain. The nurse uses an approach that is ethically sound by:

① Speaking to all the nurses and telling them not to leave the medication at the bedside

② Reporting the information and concern to the supervisor and letting the supervisor handle it

③ Asking the head nurse to handle the problems of the resident's medication and the staff's feelings

④ Suggesting a nursing conference be held to discuss both staff feelings and the medication problem

5. At a staff meeting the question of a staff nurse returning to work after a drug rehabilitation program is discussed. The nursing supervisor helps the staff to decide that the best way to handle the nurse's return would be to:

① Offer the nurse support in a direct, straightforward manner

② Avoid mentioning the problem unless the nurse brings up the topic

③ Assign another staff member to keep the nurse under close observation

④ Make certain the nurse is assigned to administer only nonnarcotic medications

ANSWERS AND RATIONALES FOR REVIEW QUESTIONS

1. **1** Most practical method of rendering effective and efficient resident care, because nursing personnel work to the maximum of their ability.
   2 Nurses are accountable to give good nursing care no matter what type of care system the hospital utilizes.
   3 Student nurses are under the direction of a registered nurse instructor, who may use method for student to gain leadership skills.
   4 Assigning team members to tasks best suited for their individual capabilities provides quality care for residents.

2. **3** Delusions are protective and can be abandoned only when the individual feels secure and adequate. This response is the only one directed at building the resident's security and reducing anxiety.
   1 This would be a nursing action to help the resident develop trust; the goal is to have trust.
   2 This is helpful more in regard to hallucinations than delusions.
   4 The resident is unable to explain the reason for the feelings.

3. **4** Because the resident feels a loss of control, it would be important to include the resident in revision of the plan.
   1 This does not consider changes in the resident or the resident's feelings.
   2 This is unnecessary; planning nursing care is within the nurse's function and judgment, not the physician's.
   3 This is very authoritarian and places total control with the nurse.

4. **4** This approach is positive because it attempts to deal with the staff's feelings and the problem without singling out people for blame; the nurse therefore is taking ethically sound action without being moralistic or authoritarian.
   1 This abdicates the nurse's responsibility and may create anger and guilt in the staff.
   2 This abdicates the nurse's responsibility and may create anger and guilt in the staff.
   3 This abdicates the nurse's responsibility and may create anger and guilt in the staff.

5. **1** This allows the nurse to use the staff as a support system and removes the opportunity to deny the problem.
   2 This supports and permits denial; both the nurse and the staff know a problem exists, and the nurse must admit it.
   3 This is a nonprofessional approach that would be nontherapeutic for the nurse.
   4 This is a nonprofessional approach that would be nontherapeutic for the nurse.

chapter twenty-three

Leadership and Management Issues

Leadership

Leadership is a process used to move a group toward goal setting and goal achievement. The leadership process may be used by any person; therefore, any person can theoretically be a leader at any given time. Leadership can also be learned.

Learning about leadership begins with an understanding of what constitutes a leader and a group. There are three requirements for being a leader: (1) one must have a goal or an idea to which one is strongly committed; (2) one must have at least one follower to lead; and (3) one must employ the leadership process.

STYLES OF LEADERSHIP

A. Three basic styles
   1. Autocratic: leader does not seek input from the group but sets the goals, plans, makes the decisions, and evaluates the action taken
   2. Democratic: leader seeks input from the group, and responsibilities for action taken are shared between the leader and the group
   3. Laissez-faire: leader's input and control of the group are minimal, permitting individuals to set independent goals
B. Leadership styles influenced by the leader, the environment, and the cultural climate of the organization
C. The effective leader modifies leadership style to fit changing circumstances, problems, and people (e.g., autocratic style of leadership is appropriate in an emergency situation)

PRINCIPLES OF LEADERSHIP

A. Interpersonal influence depends on a knowledge of human behavior and a sensitivity to others in terms of feelings, values, and problems
   1. Explore and understand attitudes, feelings, and personal values about self
   2. Project self into the place of those being led
   3. Know how you appear to subordinates
B. Communication is an essential component of leadership
   1. Effective communication depends on use of the appropriate medium
      a. Communication may be verbal, written, and/or nonverbal
      b. Communication may be formal or informal
      c. Communication should have two directions: up and down the chain of command and among equals
   2. Communication style can affect the person or persons with whom the leader communicates
      a. Meanings or ideas communicated should be received or intended without distraction
      b. People react to communication differently
      c. Written communication should be in language that is understood by the person or persons intended (e.g., ancillary personnel should have a written assignment that does not require them to make judgments)

d. Verbal communication can be influenced by facial expressions, body movement, and tone of voice

3. Effectiveness of communication can be influenced by inappropriate timing; the information communicated may be correct, but the time may be wrong (ascertain readiness)

C. Leader's success is influenced by how the leader's ability to respond to group needs effectively is perceived by those being led

1. A role is composed of a number of expectations for the behavior of an individual in a specific position or status classification

   a. Any individual's role consists of a number of expectations and relationships

   b. The nurse leader, by virtue of behavior and status, can influence the perceptions of peers, residents, and colleagues

2. Power is a leader's source of influence

3. Power may be positional or professional

   a. Positional power: acquired through the position the leader has in the hierarchy of the organization

   b. Professional power: acquired through the knowledge or expertise displayed by the leader and/or perceived by the followers

D. Leadership moves from one person to another as changes occur in the work situation

1. The nurse's expertise about a specific resident care problem, along with the availability of other resources, can place the nurse in the position of providing leadership for a group

2. A member of another discipline may assume the role of leadership in specific situations (e.g., the physician leads the cardiac arrest team; the nurse coordinates physical rehabilitation and nutrition for the resident)

E. Leadership process requires the use of actions associated with problem solving: decision making, relating, influencing, and facilitating

1. Decision making requires knowledge about and skill in solving the problem; participatory decision making lends itself to the quality of the decision made, improves relationships, and influences the readiness of an individual or group to accept change (e.g., the resident or the family should have the opportunity to participate in the development of the resident's plan of care; unit staff may decide which primary nurse or team leader should care for a newly admitted resident)

2. Effective delegation of responsibilities is inherent in effective leadership; delegation of work requires matching the task with the appropriate position (e.g., a nursing assistant should not provide care that requires the expertise of a licensed nurse; using a licensed nurse for housekeeping duties is wasteful)

F. Need for change should be understood by those effecting the change as well as by those affected by the change

1. Movement from goal setting to goal achievement involves change

2. Process of changing includes communication, planning, participation, and evaluation by the individual or group affected

3. Change is more acceptable when:

   a. It has not been dictated, but instead follows a sequence of impersonal principles

   b. Individuals or groups affected have participated in its creation

   c. It has been planned

   d. It follows a number of successful rather than unsuccessful series of changes

   e. It is initiated after other changes have been absorbed, not during the confusion of a major change

   f. It does not threaten security

G. Effective use of leadership is conducive to accomplishing the goals of the group; an evaluation process is necessary if the results of efforts to attain the goals are to be interpreted accurately

1. Goals should be identified as short-term and long-term

2. Evaluation process should be ongoing

3. Climate in which the evaluation process occurs influences its success

GUIDELINES FOR EFFECTIVE LEADERSHIP

A. Orient the team you will be working with. Members should be aware of their job descriptions. The workplace will be less stressful if everyone is familiar with any uniqueness you or others may have concerning the nursing care given.

B. Keep notepad and pencil with you.

C. Develop your own system of abbreviations for your information—use only standard abbreviations on legal documents.

D. Make rounds as soon as report is over. Note on your "pocket notes" date and time, and briefly state what you observe or hear. This is helpful if the resident's condition changes.

E. Check all equipment and supplies that you will be responsible for during your shift. You may assign these duties to another responsible person if one is available. These checks can become part of the routine and will assist in the proficiency of the staff.

F. Provide individual staff recognition when appropriate.

G. Keep informed of the events within the facility.
1. Attend necessary meetings.
2. Become familiar with rules and regulations of the facility in which you are employed.
3. Learn what surveys or inspections will be conducted.
4. Learn where the policy and procedure documents are kept; ensure that they are located in a central area and that they are updated.

GUIDELINES TO EFFECTIVE TIME MANAGEMENT

A. Set goals, plan, and evaluate feedback relative to your goals.

B. Set priorities—know what you want, how you want it, and when you want it.

C. Use "to do" lists daily, weekly, and monthly. Mark off tasks as completed.

D. Do not procrastinate. Identify and confront underlying problems that lead to procrastination, and resolve them.

E. Be organized. Avoid time wasters, and learn to delegate.

F. Stay focused.

G. Be self-disciplined—it generates pride and satisfaction.

H. Do one of four things with paperwork: complete it, act on it, save it (if it is important), or destroy it (if it is of no value).

I. Keep motivated—think in a positive manner.

J. Learn to use computers efficiently—thoroughly learn a computer program.

K. Learn your peak time, when energy and attention levels are optimal; match your energy level with complexity of tasks to be completed.

Management

Management is achieving outcomes through others. Management involves supervision, direction, and evaluation of other members of the health care team.

SELECTED MANAGEMENT ISSUES

A. Transcribing orders
1. Physician orders (precautions)
   a. Check that orders are written on the correct chart.
   b. If there is more than one order, read through all orders before beginning.
   c. Process stat orders first. (A stat order signifies that a single dose of medication is to be given immediately and only once.)
   d. If there is some confusion during a telephone order, have another nurse listen in on the line for clarification.
2. Basic guidelines (may vary from one facility to another; check the agency's policy)
   a. The medication needed should be ordered from the pharmacy: include the date, resident's name, room number, time, medication, route of administration, dosage, and frequency.
   b. Record the orders in the required areas, such as Kardex, Medex, or medication card. Be certain to include the date.
   c. A stat medication may need to be written on a card of a different color. Write *stat* on the card, and also write the room number, resident's name, drug dose, route, and time. Pay special attention to stat orders—the card should be destroyed after the order is given and recorded. Stat orders are to be carried out immediately, not at the next routine time for medication administration or procedure performance.

d. Make very certain that all orders have been carried out and recorded in the proper record. (Have a second nurse verify for accuracy until you gain experience.)

e. Each order should be checked off on the physician's order sheet and signed with your name or initials.

f. Those nurses responsible for administering medications should be notified of any new order.

g. Most facilities use a sign that indicates a new order (e.g., red flag may be placed on each chart; or the physician may place the chart in a specific place, such as on the unit secretary's desk).

h. Preferably the charge nurse should be assigned to examine all residents' charts for new orders. This should happen during each shift.

B. Procedure for discontinuing or changing a medication

1. Mark old medication order off the Kardex or Medex by crossing through with a highlighter marking pen. If it is an order change, write a new order.

2. Notify the nurse responsible for carrying out new orders about discontinued and newly ordered medications.

3. If a medication card is issued, ensure that the old medication card is destroyed.

4. Check off on the physician's order sheet.

C. End-of-shift report

1. The purpose of the end-of-shift report is to provide the next shift with pertinent information about the resident. The quality of nursing care the resident receives is contingent on how well each shift communicates with the other.

2. Before beginning the report, plan your communication. Be cognizant of what you want to express. Consider your choice of words. Be precise. Use accepted medical/nursing terminology.

3. Once all appropriate data is compiled, use Kardex and begin the report. Be systematic and report the following:

a. State resident's room and bed number, name, age, physician, all diagnoses, and date of surgery if postoperative.

b. Summarize resident's day/evening/night.

c. Report all pertinent nursing care.

d. Describe change in resident's condition. Most facilities report only abnormal vital signs except first postoperative day, and then last vital signs are given.

e. Report special medications, intravenous solutions, infusion rate, IV credits. State time, method, and dosage of analgesics given and the effect.

f. Report all intake and output.

g. Report status of lungs and bowel sounds.

h. Report mental status and level of consciousness.

i. Report circulatory checks, pedal pulses, and skin abnormalities in turgor or color.

j. State diagnostic procedure, such as CT scans, x-ray studies, MRI, endoscopy, proctoscopy, thoracentesis, and surgery. Report diet changes, special permits, preoperative procedures, daily weights, activity status, Accuchecks, Hematest for stools, clean catch urine for analysis and/or C&S, sputum specimen for C&S, respiratory therapy, and physical therapy orders. Report all nursing interventions, such as dressings, packs, ostomy care, and oxygen.

k. Discuss resident and family education.

l. Note other services, such as social services, pastoral care, and discharge planning.

m. State any pertinent information helpful in resident care.

n. Report "no code" status.

o. Present the report in an unbiased, nonjudgmental manner.

D. Conflict management

1. Conflict is a part of everyday life. A conflict exists when two or more parties (individuals, groups, or organizations) differ with regard to facts, opinions, beliefs, feelings, drives, needs, goals, methods, values, and so on. Anything may be a source of conflict. Conflict produces a feeling of tension, and most people wish to do some-

thing to relieve the discomfort that results from tension.

2. Five characteristics of a conflict situation:
   a. At least two parties are involved in some form of interaction
   b. Difference in goals and/or values either exists or is perceived to exist by the parties involved
   c. The interaction involves behavior that will either defeat, reduce, or suppress the opponent or will gain a victory
   d. The parties come together with opposing actions and counteractions
   e. Each party attempts to create an imbalance or favored power position

3. Types of conflict
   a. Interpersonal—arises between two individuals
   b. Intergroup—arises between two small groups, two large groups, or a large group and a small group
   c. Personal-group—arises between an individual and a large group
   d. Intrapersonal—arises within an individual

4. Common approaches to conflict
   a. Denial
   b. Ignore or suppress
   c. Win-lose approach
   d. Bargain or compromise
   e. Mediation or arbitration
   f. Problem solve or collaborate

5. Strategies for managing conflict
   a. Attain or maintain a balance of power between the conflicting parties
   b. Employ good communication skills
   c. Define the conflict or problem exactly as each party involved views it
   d. Recognize the human needs of those involved in the conflict or problem

E. Key points of performance appraisal
   1. The purpose of a performance appraisal is to encourage the development of employees who will meet the organization's objectives.
   2. The performance appraisal provides a profile of the employee's strengths and weaknesses. The weaknesses, or performance discrepancies, can then be analyzed so that they may be eliminated, corrected, or altered to benefit both the employee and the organization.
   3. To conduct a productive performance appraisal, the nurse-leader should use a format that promotes discussion between the nurse-leader evaluator and the group member being evaluated.
   4. It is usually best to focus first on the positive aspects of performance because this is more comfortable for both parties.
   5. The discussion concludes with the development of a plan to help the group member improve performance, which includes methods to accomplish the established goals.
   6. The nurse-leader evaluator writes a summary of the discussion, documenting the group member's strengths and weaknesses, goals, and plans for accomplishing the goals, and gives an overall rating of the group member.
   7. The nurse-leader conducting an evaluation can prepare herself for a performance appraisal by reviewing the appraisal procedure and her observations either with her supervisor or with another nurse-leader.
   8. When possible, the nurse-leader evaluator should have the group member do a self-evaluation, which provides a basis for discussion and usually results in a more objective, fair, and complete evaluation of the group member.

Review Questions

1. The nurse has been observing a resident for some time. The resident is quite delusional, talking about people who are plotting to do harm. The nurse assistant reports that the resident is pacing more than usual. The nurse decides that the resident is beginning to lose control and directs the assistant to:
   ① Allow the resident to use a punching bag
   ② Move the resident to a quiet place on the unit
   ③ Allow the resident to continue pacing under supervision
   ④ Suggest that the resident sit down for a while

2. If a resident is dissatisfied with the physician, the staff nurse may:
    ① Report the matter to the charge nurse or team leader
    ② Suggest three other physicians to the resident
    ③ Report the matter to the medical director
    ④ Report the matter to the resident's family

3. A nursing assistant complains to the nurse that an older female resident with senility will perform tasks, but only when she feels like doing them; the assistant wonders how to deal with this. The nurse's response to the assistant should be based on the understanding that in addition to this resident's senility, older persons:
    ① Lose their ability to cooperate
    ② Are ambivalent toward authority
    ③ Lose ego flexibility
    ④ Utilize strong superego control

4. A resident is placed on suicide precautions. The charge nurse knows that the most therapeutic way to provide these precautions would be to:
    ① Remove all sharp or cutting objects
    ② Not allow the resident to leave his room
    ③ Give the resident the opportunity to ventilate feelings
    ④ Assign a staff member to be with the resident at all times

5. During the acute phase following a myocardial infarction, the nurse should instruct the nurse assistant to make the resident's bed by:
    ① Changing the top linen and only the necessary bottom linen
    ② Changing the linen from top to bottom without lowering the head of the bed
    ③ Sliding the resident onto a stretcher, remaking the bed, then sliding the resident back to the bed
    ④ Lifting rather than rolling the resident from side to side while changing the linen

6. An agitated, acting-out, delusional resident is receiving large doses of haloperidol (Haldol), and the charge nurse is concerned because this drug can produce undesirable side effects. The nurse should alert the staff that the drug will be immediately stopped if the resident exhibits:
    ① Dizziness
    ② Sleepiness
    ③ Extrapyramidal symptoms
    ④ Jaundice

7. A manifestation of conflict that the charge nurse might observe in staff is:
    ① Anxiety
    ② Homeostasis
    ③ Panic
    ④ Motivation

ANSWERS AND RATIONALES FOR REVIEW QUESTIONS

1. **2** Residents losing control feel frightened and threatened. They need external controls and a reduction in external stimuli.
   1 This is helpful for pent-up aggressive behavior but not for agitation associated with delusions.
   3 The resident may get completely out of control if allowed to continue pacing.
   4 The resident would be unable to sit in one place at this time; agitation is building.

2. **1** The nurse must bring the matter to the attention of the supervisor, since the supervisor is responsible for the resident's welfare.
   2 The nurse must inspire the resident to have confidence in the physician and must never advocate dismissal or replacement of a physician.
   3 Not the staff nurse's responsibility.
   4 Not the staff nurse's responsibility.

3. **3** Fears and anxieties about themselves and their possessions are common in older persons because of decreased self-concept and altered body image.
   1 Aging does not necessarily result in an inability to cooperate.
   2 The attitude of older persons about authority or others in their environment is set; indecision about life situations may be due to insecurity.
   4 Older persons fear the loss they must face in almost every aspect of their lives; this leads to lowering of their self-esteem and faulty reality testing.

4. **4** Emotional support and close surveillance can demonstrate the staff's caring and their attempt to prevent acting out of suicidal ideation.
   1 This would be routinely done; not necessarily therapeutic by itself.
   2 This would be punishment for the resident, who still may find a way to carry out a suicide attempt in the room.
   3 This is not a suicide precaution.

5. **1** Until the resident's condition has reached some degree of stability after myocardial infarction, routine activities such as changing sheets are avoided so the resident's movements will be minimized and the cardiac workload reduced.
   2 Changing all the linen causes unnecessary movement, which increases oxygen demands and makes the heart work harder.
   3 Activity is contraindicated because it increases oxygen consumption and cardiac workload.
   4 Any activity is counterproductive to rest; rest must take precedence so the cardiac workload will be reduced.

6. **4** Jaundice signifies liver function interference and requires stopping the medication.
   1 This symptom usually subsides after several weeks of treatment.
   2 This symptom usually subsides after several weeks of treatment.
   3 These symptoms usually require that the dose be reduced; if symptoms do not subside, the drug is stopped.

7. **1** Anxiety is a manifestation of conflict.
   2 Homeostasis is a steady state unrelated to conflict.
   3 Panic is usually not seen in conflict unless anxiety is extreme.
   4 Conflict may result in motivation, but this is not always present.

chapter *twenty-four*

Safe and Effective Care Environment

A safe environment is one in which basic needs are achievable, physical hazards are reduced, exposure to carcinogens is reduced, transmission of pathogens and parasites is reduced, sanitation is regulated, and pollution is controlled.

Ill, disabled, poor, illiterate, or older adult residents often require the nurse's help in achieving a safe environment. To do this the nurse needs to understand factors contributing to a safe environment and then thoroughly assess the environment and the resident for threats to safety.

Basic Types of Risks to Safety

A. Falls
B. Resident-inherent accidents
C. Procedure-related accidents
D. Equipment-related accidents

Factors Influencing Safety

The accident-prone resident: vulnerability to accidents is caused by losses, both physical and psychosocial, noted in the course of aging

A. Slowed reaction time
B. Unsteady gait—poor muscular coordination, poor balance mechanism
C. Blindness or poor vision
D. Faulty hearing
E. Decrease in sense of touch—lessens response to pain or temperature (heat or cold)
F. Responses to medications taken—multiple medication interaction
G. Bone density decreases
H. Compromised immune system

Assessment and Interventions for Residents At Risk for Falling

A. History of previous falls: assess previous pattern of falling and establish safety guidelines with resident and family
B. Orient to environment—free environment from obstacles
C. Demonstrate nurse call system
D. Explain location and use of bathroom

MENTAL STATUS

A. Assessment
　　1. Disoriented-repeatedly reinforce activity limits and safety needs to resident
　　2. Confused—unable to make purposeful decisions
B. Interventions
　　1. Move resident closer to nurses' station
　　2. Involve family as much as possible
　　3. Recommend safety belt if needed
　　4. Recommend use of personal electronic security system if available
　　5. Alert staff to resident's confusion

MOBILITY DEFICITS

A. Assessment
　　1. General debility
　　2. Hemiparesis
　　3. Paraparesis
　　4. Hemiplegic
　　5. Ataxia
　　6. Use of cane
　　7. Use of crutches
　　8. Amputee

B. Nursing intervention requires provision for safe environment
  1. Bed in low position; brakes locked
  2. No unnecessary furniture
  3. Side rails up if applicable
  4. Nightlights at bedside and in bathroom
  5. Nonskid footwear
  6. Call light working and within easy reach
  7. Assistive device within reach

COMMUNICATION DEFICITS

A. Assessment
  1. Dysarthric
  2. Aphasic
  3. No verbal response
  4. Foreign language
B. Nursing intervention
  1. Assess resident's communication pattern
  2. Establish effective communication system with resident (e.g., use of visual aids, bells)
  3. Make frequent rounds
  4. Provide interpreter for foreign language resident if possible

VISUAL DEFICITS

A. Assessment
  1. Blind O.S.
  2. Blind O.D.
  3. Blind O.U.
  4. Use of glasses or contacts
  5. Postoperative eye
B. Nursing intervention
  1. Assess vision in nonaffected eye
  2. Check effectiveness of eyeglasses (include frequent cleaning of lenses)
  3. Label eyeglasses with resident's name
  4. Hang poster above resident's bed, indicating sensory deficit

MEDICATIONS

A. Assessment
  1. Diuretics
  2. Laxatives
  3. Barbiturates
  4. Tranquilizers
  5. Pain medications
  6. Hypnotics
  7. Eyedrops
  8. Sleeping medications
B. Nursing intervention

  1. Evaluate resident's medication (appropriate dosages)
  2. Assess risk of side effects, particularly drug-associated hypotensive episodes; alert resident to side effects
  3. Check for use of laxatives and diuretics
  4. Be particularly aware of drug side effects in older residents
  5. Be aware of potential drug interactions for those residents requiring multiple medications

URINARY ALTERATIONS

A. Assessment
  1. Urgency
  2. Frequency
  3. Incontinence
B. Nursing intervention
  1. Assess usual pattern of urination
  2. Plan individualized toileting schedule
  3. Assess need for bedside commode, Texas catheter, bedpan

AUDITORY DEFICITS

A. Assessment
  1. Use of hearing aid
  2. Deaf in right ear
  3. Deaf in left ear
B. Nursing intervention
  1. Assess resident's ability to hear
  2. Check effectiveness of hearing aid; make batteries available
  3. Speak as loudly as needed to communicate
  4. Place poster in room, indicating sensory deficit, according to agency policy

IMPROPERLY FITTING FOOTWEAR—check shoes and slippers for fit, safety, and nonskid soles

PRESENCE OF ORTHOSTATIC HYPOTENSION

Nursing interventions
A. Determine history of problem
B. Teach resident to ambulate in stages
C. Apply elastic stockings as ordered
D. Teach resident to make position changes slowly

Burns and Fire

A. Control of smoking
  1. Most state or local fire regulations prohibit unattended smoking in bed; residents must

be assisted in confining their smoking to smoking areas, where proper ashtrays and supervision are provided

    a. For the resident who is unable to cooperate, tobacco and matches or lighters should be stored by staff

    b. Family or visitors should be advised of smoking safety rules

B. Administration of oxygen

  1. Unless confined to an air-tight area, oxygen is not explosive. However, objects that burn in the presence of oxygen-enriched air burn so rapidly they appear to explode

  2. Nursing intervention when resident is receiving oxygen

    a. Be certain matches and lighters are not available

    b. Inform resident and visitors that smoking is prohibited

    c. Post "No Smoking—Oxygen in Use" signs

    d. Do not use flammable liquids such as oils, nail polish remover, or alcohol in the room

    e. Avoid use of electrical equipment such as radios and electric razors

    f. Turn off electrical equipment before unplugging it to prevent sparks

C. Electrical burns and shock

  1. Electrical burns or shock may result from faulty electrical equipment or improper handling

  2. Nursing intervention

    a. Observe for defective plugs, outlets, or wiring

    b. Do not permit or use overloaded electric outlets—using extension cords to permit many plugs can create a fire hazard

    c. Carefully assess those residents with brain-cell damage for possible need to provide devices that limit access to electrical outlets

    d. Do not pull plug using the cord—grasp plug firmly and pull

    e. Report shocks experienced while using equipment—have equipment checked

D. Sunburn

  1. Residents whose skin is unaccustomed to strong sun rays may get severe sunburns when enjoying outdoor activities

  2. Nursing intervention—sunscreen lotions applied to exposed skin prevent accidental burning; a physician's order to use sunscreen may be required

E. Scalding

  1. Burns from hot liquids are a frequent occurrence among older residents

  2. Nursing intervention

    a. Assess resident for ability to see and handle cup of hot liquid; place within reach; assist when necessary

    b. Scalding accidents can occur in the shower or bath; bath water must be checked to make sure it is within acceptable range designated by each state's regulations—many states require range between 105° F and 110° F

    c. Hot water bottles and electric heating pads are discouraged (and are illegal in some states); application of heat or cold is done only by physician's order

Suffocation

Suffocation results when a resident cannot breathe in an adequate supply of oxygen to supply the lungs. If this period extends longer than 3 minutes, the result can be death or severe brain damage. Suffocation may be caused by choking, drowning, or pollution of the air supply by fire or other gaseous substances.

A. Nursing intervention

  1. Have staff member present during meal times; group residents together

  2. Cut food into bite-size pieces

  3. Make certain residents needing dentures have them in their mouths at mealtime

  4. Request chopped or pureed food for those residents unable to chew properly

  5. In event of vomiting, quickly turn resident to side-lying position

  6. Never leave resident unattended in bathtub or whirlpool

  7. Evaluate residents in rooms containing smoke or gas-polluted air during fire or disaster; follow fire drill instructions to prevent spread of these noxious gases to other areas

  8. Never give food or fluid to resident who is not alert or has a nasogastric tube in place

  9. Know how to safely administer the Heimlich maneuver to dislodge foreign objects from the throat

Poisoning

Poisoning is a threat to the safety of vision-impaired residents who cannot read labels and confused residents who do not understand the use of many substances.

Nursing interventions:

1. Chemical substances such as cleaning supplies and medical disinfectants must be stored in locked area
2. Excessive alcoholic beverage consumption can also cause toxic effects; alcoholic beverages found at a resident's bedside should be reported to the supervisor
3. The nurse should be aware of the possible interaction of resident's medications and alcoholic beverages

Incident Reports

Any accident necessitates the filing of an incident report, a confidential document that completely describes any resident accident occurring on the premises of a long-term care facility.

In addition to completing the incident report, the nurse must document the incident in the resident's medical record and describe its effect on the resident's health status. Do not write "incident report completed" in the medical record. Follow the established policy in your long-term care facility.

Infection Control

A. Infection: a disease state that results from the invasion and growth of microorganisms in the body; major safety and health hazard
   1. Area affected
      a. May be localized
      b. May be generalized, involving entire body
   2. Symptoms
      a. Fever
      b. Pain or tenderness
      c. Fatigue
      d. Loss of appetite
      e. Nausea
      f. Vomiting
      g. Diarrhea
      h. Rash
      i. Sores on mucous membrane
      j. Redness
      k. Swelling
      l. Discharge or drainage from affected area
   3. Causes
      a. Invasion of body by microorganisms
      b. Decline in efficiency of resident's immune system
   4. Prevention: single, most important precaution is frequent hand washing
B. Microorganisms: living plant or animal that cannot be seen without microscope
   1. Where found:
      a. In the air
      b. Food
      c. Mouth
      d. Nose
      e. Respiratory tract
      f. Stomach
      g. Intestines
      h. On the skin
      i. Soil
      j. Water
      k. Animals
      l. Clothing
      m. Furniture
   2. Pathogens: cause infections and are harmful
   3. Nonpathogens: do not usually cause infections
   4. Types of microorganisms
      a. Bacteria
      b. Fungi
      c. Protozoa
      d. Rickettsieae
      e. Viruses
   5. Requirements of microorganisms
      a. Reservoir (host) containing water, nourishment, oxygen, warmth, and darkness
      b. Some microorganisms cannot live where there is oxygen
C. Universal precautions—issued in 1987 by CDC
   1. Developed to prevent spread of AIDS
   2. AIDS virus spread through contact with blood and body fluids
   3. Hepatitis B, AIDS, other infections possibly undiagnosed
   4. Universal precautions—to be used for all residents

a. Gloves are worn when touching blood, body fluids, body substances, and mucous membranes
b. Gloves are worn when there are cuts, breaks, or openings in the skin
c. Gloves are worn when there is possible contact with urine, feces, vomitus, dressings, wound drainage, soiled linen, or soiled clothing
d. Masks, goggles, or face shields are worn when splattering or splashing of blood or body fluids is possible (this protects the eyes and the mucous membranes of the mouth); gowns or aprons are worn when splashing, splattering, smearing, or soiling from blood or body fluids is possible
e. Hands and other body parts must be washed immediately if contaminated with blood or body fluids
f. Hands are washed immediately after removing gloves
g. Hands are washed after contact with the resident
h. Avoid nicks or cuts when shaving residents
i. Handle razor blades and other sharp objects carefully to avoid injuring the resident or yourself
j. Use resuscitation devices when mouth-to-mouth resuscitation is indicated
k. Avoid resident contact when you have open skin wounds or lesions; discuss the situation with your supervisor

Review Questions

1. A resident has been placed on one-to-one observation for suicidal intentions. Which of the following items should the nurse remove from the resident's possession?
   ① Daily newspaper
   ② Hairbrush
   ③ Metal nail file
   ④ Shoes
2. Before intramuscular injection of medication, the nurse should aspirate for blood. If blood returns in the syringe, the nurse should:

① Proceed with the injection of medication
② Withdraw needle and prepare a new syringe
③ Slowly inject medication and massage the site
④ Withdraw the needle and give the injection in another site

3. To ensure that the right resident is receiving a prescribed medication, it is essential that the nurse take which of these actions?
   ① Check the name on the resident's wristband
   ② Call the resident by name
   ③ Read the name of the resident on the bed card
   ④ Check the medication record for the resident's room number

4. What special precaution will the nurse take in caring for a resident with hepatitis?
   ① Use gloves when removing the bedpan
   ② Wear a mask when entering the room
   ③ Prevent droplet spread of the infection
   ④ Sterilize equipment used in the room with a disinfecting agent

5. Nosocomial refers to infections that:
   ① Are acquired in the hospital
   ② Are confined to a specific area
   ③ Have spread throughout the body
   ④ Have spread shock-causing toxins throughout the body

6. Before leaving the isolation unit, the last thing you would do is:
   ① Reach into dirty linen hamper to push down the piled linen
   ② Remember to wash and sterilize the thermometer before taking the next resident's temperature
   ③ Remove the dietary tray from the bedside table
   ④ Remove the gown and gloves

7. A resident develops a wound infection and is placed in an isolation unit. You would explain to the resident that the purpose of isolation is to:
   ① Cure the resident's infection
   ② Help prevent spread of microorganisms to others
   ③ Be sure that nursing personnel do not become infected
   ④ Protect the resident from further infection

8. While changing a resident's sterile dressing, you spill normal saline solution on the sterile field. The area that becomes wet should:
   ① Be a good place to put the sterile sponges for cleaning the wound
   ② Be considered contaminated
   ③ Be dried before continuing the procedure
   ④ Be removed or covered with a dry towel

9. When the nurse is administering medications, the resident informs the nurse that the tablet usually received is a different color. The nurse should:
   ① Insist that the resident take the tablet she poured
   ② Have the resident take the tablet and then recheck the order
   ③ Leave the medication at the bedside and recheck the order
   ④ Recheck the order before giving the drug

10. The nurse's initial approach to creating a therapeutic environment for any resident should give priority to:
    ① Accepting the resident's individuality
    ② Promoting the resident's independence
    ③ Providing for the resident's safety
    ④ Explaining everything that is being done for the resident

11. During the day a nurse puts side rails up on the bed of a 73-year-old resident who was admitted with a fractured hip, because:
    ① This action is a standard safety measure because of the resident's age
    ② All residents over age 65 should use side rails
    ③ Older persons are often disoriented for several days after anesthesia
    ④ The side rails serve as handholds and facilitate the resident's mobility in bed

12. While assisting a resident with a repaired fractured hip to transfer from the bed to a wheelchair, the nurse should remember that:
    ① During a weight-bearing transfer the resident's knees should be slightly bent
    ② Transfers to and from the wheelchair will be easier if the bed is higher than the wheelchair

③ The transfer can be accomplished by pivoting while bearing weight on both upper extremities and not on the legs
④ The appropriate proximity and visual relationship of wheelchair to bed must be maintained

13. When assisting a resident to ambulate following repair of a fractured right hip, the nurse should be standing:
    ① In front of the resident
    ② Behind the resident
    ③ On the resident's left side
    ④ On the resident's right side

14. The nurse should provide a confused resident with an environment that is:
    ① Challenging
    ② Nonstimulating
    ③ Variable
    ④ Familiar

15. A resident with a spinal cord injury resulting in paraplegia is placed on a CircOlectric bed primarily to:
    ① Promote mobility
    ② Prevent calcium loss from long bones
    ③ Prevent pressure sores
    ④ Promote orthostatic hypotension

16. A resident is admitted with a diagnosis of chronic adrenocortical insufficiency. Because of this condition, it would be unwise to place this resident in a room:
    ① With an older resident who has a CVA
    ② With a middle-age resident who has pneumonia
    ③ That is private and away from the nurses' station
    ④ Next to a 17-year-old resident with a fractured leg

17. In creating a therapeutic environment for a resident who has just had a myocardial infarction, the nurse should provide for:
    ① Daily papers in the morning
    ② Telephone communication
    ③ Short family visits
    ④ Television for short periods

ANSWERS AND RATIONALES FOR REVIEW QUESTIONS

1. **3** Sharp items should be removed.
   1 There is no need to deny the resident this item.
   2 There is no need to deny the resident this item.
   4 Shoe laces should be removed from the shoes, but there is no need to remove the shoes.
2. **2** If blood is aspirated, a new needle and syringe should be prepared and an alternative site used.
   1 The nurse should never proceed, because there is danger of injecting the medication directly into the bloodstream.
   3 The nurse should never inject because of the danger of giving medication directly into the bloodstream.
   4 The needle and syringe are contaminated and must be changed before injecting in an alternative site.
3. **1** The wristband check is the most accurate means of resident identification.
   2 Calling the resident by name is not a method to ensure accuracy, because the resident may respond to any name.
   3 Bed cards may not be updated; this method does not ensure accuracy.
   4 Residents are frequently moved from room to room, and their medication record may not reflect this occurrence.
4. **1** Spread through the fecal-oral route.
   2 Mask alone will not stop the spread.
   3 Spread through the fecal-oral route primarily.
   4 Will not destroy the virus.
5. **1** Nosocomial infections are acquired in the hospital.
   2 Local infections are confined to a specific location.
   3 Systemic infections have spread throughout the body.
   4 Infections producing septic shock are those generally caused by gram-negative organisms.
6. **4** Contaminated gown and gloves cannot be worn outside the isolation unit.
   1 Would need to be done before removing gown and gloves so that hands and arms are not exposed to contaminated linens.
   2 Thermometer would be left in the resident's room until resident is discharged or isolation discontinued.
   3 Tray would be handled while the nurse was still gowned and gloved.

7. **2** Isolation keeps pathogens confined to a specific area, thus reducing transmission to others.
   1 Mere isolation does nothing to destroy or reduce the numbers of microorganisms.
   3 Isolation helps protect other residents and all members of the health care team.
   4 Would be provided only by reverse isolation.
8. **2** Moisture carries organisms by capillary action, thus rendering the field contaminated.
   1 Sterile sponges placed on a wet area of the field would be contaminated.
   3 Drying would be impossible.
   4 Removing would be impossible. Whatever would be used to cover the area would also become moist, thus contaminated.
9. **4** To promote safety and prevent errors.
   1 Inappropriate nursing action; residents usually know their medications, especially if they have been taking them over a period of time.
   2 Inappropriate action; medication may be incorrect and action could be harmful to resident.
   3 *Never* leave medication at the bedside; this is essential to good nursing practice relative to administration of medications.
10. **1** Each person is unique. The nurse should avoid making the resident feel dehumanized.
   2 This would be a later nursing action.
   3 Although safety is a priority, it is not the initial need.
   4 It is important that the resident understand what is happening; however, individuality must be considered first.
11. **4** Devices such as side rails can help residents increase their mobility by facilitating movement in bed. Side rails are immovable objects and provide a handhold for leverage when changing positions.
   1 The need to use side rails for safety must be evaluated for each individual based on the mental and physical status and hospital regulations.
   2 The need to use side rails for safety must be evaluated for each individual based on the mental and physical status and hospital regulations.
   3 The need to use side rails for safety must be evaluated for each individual based on the mental and physical status and hospital regulations.

Chapter Twenty-four Answers

12. **4** The wheelchair should be angled close to the bed so the resident will have to make only a simple pivot on the stronger leg. When the wheelchair is within the resident's visual field, the resident will be aware of the distance and direction that the body must navigate to transfer safely and avoid falling.

1 If the knees are flexed, the resident may be unable to support the weight on the unaffected leg.

2 Moving a resident back to bed in this situation would encompass moving against gravity.

3 The large muscles of the legs rather than the arms should be used to prevent muscle strain.

13. **3** When ambulating a resident, the nurse walks on the resident's stronger or unaffected side. This provides a wide base of support and therefore increases stability during the phase of ambulation that calls for weight bearing on the affected side as the unaffected limb moves forward.

1 This tends to change the center of gravity from directly above the feet and may cause instability.

2 This tends to change the center of gravity from directly above the feet and may cause instability.

4 The nurse should stand on the resident's stronger or unaffected side (left side).

14. **4** Sameness provides security and safety and reduces stress for the resident.

1 A challenging environment would increase anxiety and frustration.

2 A nonstimulating environment would add to the resident's diminishing intellect.

3 Confused residents do not do well in a constantly changing environment.

15. **3** The CircOlectric bed facilitates frequent vertical turning of the resident to prevent decubiti, which can form within 24 hours because of pressure.

1 The resident with paraplegia is immobile, and the special bed does not increase mobility.

2 Because of the lack of weight bearing on bones, calcium is generally lost in residents confined to bed; this bed limits but does not prevent this from occurring.

4 Orthostatic hypotension is not desired; the movement of the bed may allow for gradual changes of position that would prevent it from developing.

16. **2** Exposure to infection, cold, or overexertion in a resident with chronic adrenocortical insufficiency (Addison's disease) can cause circulatory collapse.

1 This would be an appropriate room assignment.

3 This would be an appropriate room assignment.

4 This would be an appropriate room assignment.

17. **3** Visits by family members can allay anxiety and consequently reduce emotional stress, an important risk factor in cardiovascular disease.

1 The resident may be disturbed by current news. This would raise the metabolic rate, increasing oxygen demands on the heart.

2 Family, community, or work problems conveyed by phone may cause anxiety; only social communications with family should be permitted.

4 Television programs can cause anxiety or excitement, which would increase the metabolic rate and cardiac output.

Comprehensive Examination

1. An 80-year-old resident has recently moved into a nursing home. While visiting with him, a nurse notes that he is depressed. The geriatric nursing assistants have expressed frustration working with him because of his depression. The nurse may need to explain to the assistants that it may be difficult to maintain an effective relationship with this resident when he is depressed primarily because:
   ① People who are depressed are very lazy
   ② His poor personal grooming results in disgust from others
   ③ Independence and pride prevent him from asking for any kind of assistance
   ④ His pessimism arouses frustration and anger in others

2. When caring for a dying resident who is in the denial stage of grief, the *best* nursing approach is to:
   ① Agree with and encourage the resident's denial
   ② Reassure the resident that everything will be okay
   ③ Allow the denial but be available to discuss death
   ④ Leave the resident alone to confront feelings of impending loss

3. The nurse is assisting the physician with a procedure requiring a sterile field and sterile tray. The nurse notices that the sterile drape has been soiled with povidone iodine (Betadine), because it was poured into the cup on the sterile tray. The *most appropriate* nursing action should be to:
   ① Prepare another sterile field with a new sterile tray
   ② Say nothing and watch to be sure that the physician does not use the contaminated part of the field
   ③ Inform the physician that he contaminated the field and will have to start over; provide the new sterile tray
   ④ Remove the soiled drape; place a new one onto the field while the tray is held with gloved hands

4. A resident with a long history of alcohol abuse who has been in the long-term care facility for a week tells the nurse, "I feel much better and will probably not require any further treatment." When evaluating the resident's progress the nurse should recognize that:
   ① The resident has accepted the illness and now needs to use willpower to resist the alcohol
   ② As long as the resident's family remains supportive, the resident will probably not use alcohol again
   ③ The resident lacks insight about the emotional aspects of the illness and most likely needs continued supervision
   ④ The physician must be notified of the resident's statement so that aversion therapy can be started before the resident's discharge

5. A resident's diagnosis is diabetes ketoacidosis. The nurse should carefully assess this resident for:
   ① Profuse diaphoresis
   ② Lethargy
   ③ Tremors
   ④ Tachycardia

6. When preparing to administer medications to geriatric residents, the nurse knows that as a general rule, medications for older adults should be given in:
   ① Smaller doses, closer together
   ② Larger doses, closer together
   ③ Smaller doses, farther apart

④ Larger doses, farther apart

7. Theophylline (Theo-Dur) therapy was started for a resident with emphysema. The *main* pharmacologic action of this drug is:
① Relaxation of bronchial smooth muscle
② Bronchial constriction
③ Liquefying and thinning secretions
④ Vasoconstriction of major vessels

8. A resident has been in a coma for 2 months and is maintained on bedrest. The nurse understands that to prevent the effects of shearing force the head of the bed should be at an angle of:
① 30 degrees
② 45 degrees
③ 60 degrees
④ 90 degrees

9. An 86-year-old resident is admitted to a nursing home following hospitalization for a fractured left wrist sustained from a fall in her garden. Her medical diagnoses are chronic brain syndrome, arteriosclerotic heart disease, and status-post left wrist fracture. The nurse observes the resident to be withdrawn, frequently nonresponsive to conversation directed to her, complaining that everyone mumbles, and believing that others are talking about her. The nurse should suspect that the resident is experiencing:
① Psychosis
② Presbycusis
③ Presbyopia
④ Presbyophrenia

10. A resident who is receiving mechanical ventilation begins to "fight" the respirator and the physician orders atracurium (Tracrium). The *most important* nursing action for a resident receiving Tracrium is to:
① Decrease anxiety
② Monitor skin integrity
③ Promote urinary output
④ Maintain mechanical ventilation

11. While observing a resident for signs of increased intracranial pressure, the nurse notes that the blood pressure changes from 110/70 to 130/60, and the pulse rate is now 120. What would be the *appropriate* nursing action?
① Report the vital-sign changes to the physician making rounds
② Recheck vital signs and report immediately to the charge nurse
③ Wait 1 hour, recheck vital signs, and document immediately

④ These changes are not necessary to report because they are insignificant

12. Anticonvulsants are used in treating seizure disorders and are considered:
① Cholinergic blocking agents
② Central nervous system (CNS) stimulants
③ Antispasmodics
④ CNS depressants

13. A resident has an inoperable brain tumor and is in the terminal phase of the illness. While being helped with the morning bath, the resident begins to talk about dying. The *best* response by the nurse should be to:
① Ask if the resident would like to see a member of the clergy
② Say little and listen to what the resident has to say
③ Act as if the resident was not heard and excuse oneself from the room
④ Encourage the resident to keep his hope up and think positively

14. In planning nursing care for a resident with underwater-seal drainage, the nurse should remember that the *primary* goal for using this procedure is to:
① Allow expansions of the affected lung by draining secretions and air by gravitation
② Restore the negative pressure within the thoracic cavity
③ Restore the atmospheric pressure within the thoracic cavity
④ Equalize the pressure within the thoracic cavity by allowing expansion of both lungs

15. Fluid and electrolyte balance need to be maintained for residents with congestive heart failure by which of the following?
① Maintaining strict input and output and daily levels
② Limiting fluid intake and maintaining daily levels
③ Limiting activity and maintaining a salt-free diet
④ Limiting activity and maintaining a low-sodium diet

16. A resident is on a ventilator. One of the nurses asks what should be done when condensation as a result of humidity collects in the ventilator tubing. The best response to this question would be to:
① "Notify the respiratory therapist."
② "Empty the fluid from the tubing."

③ "Decrease the amount of humidity."
④ "Measure the fluid and record it on the intake and output sheet."

17. A female resident's osteoporosis has progressed dramatically in the last 5 years, and she is especially prone to falling. The statement that *best* reflects the resident's understanding of why there is a greater risk for falls would be:
① "I do not have the stamina that I used to have."
② "At my age, I'm more prone to dizziness and falling."
③ "Because of the curvature of my spine, it is hard to keep my balance."
④ "Because I am bent over, I look down instead of up while I'm walking."

18. When caring for a resident who has open-angle (chronic) glaucoma the eye drops the nurse should expect to administer would be:
① Tetracaine (Pontocaine)
② Cyclopentolate (Cyclogyl)
③ Atropine sulfate (Atropisol)
④ Pilocarpine hydrochloride (Pilocarpine)

19. The position that would provide for the greatest respiratory capacity for a resident with dyspnea would be the:
① Sims' position
② Supine position
③ Orthopneic position
④ Semi-Fowler's position

20. Levodopa is prescribed for a resident with Parkinson's disease. The sign or symptom that would be unrelated to the administration of levodopa would be:
① Nausea
② Anorexia
③ Bradycardia
④ Mental changes

21. When the nurse discovers a reddened area on the coccyx, an *appropriate* nursing intervention is to:
① Rub the area with alcohol
② Keep the resident in a semi-Fowler's position
③ Massage the surrounding area gently with lotion
④ Apply warm compresses four times a day

22. The nurse is preparing to change a resident's dressing. The statement that *best* explains the basis of surgical asepsis that the nurse will follow in this procedure is:

① Keep the area free of microorganisms
② Protect self from microorganisms in the wound
③ Confine the microorganisms to the surgical site
④ Keep the number of opportunistic microorganisms to a minimum

23. A side effect of a cholinergic drug may be:
① Increase in peristaltic action and urine output
② Decrease in peristaltic action and urine output
② Increase in peristaltic action and a decrease in urine output
④ Decrease in peristaltic action and a decrease in urine output

24. For a resident with rheumatoid arthritis, instructions to *best* decrease pain and stiffness would include:
① Taking a cool bath or shower on arising
② Active exercises to all joints using weights
③ Taking aspirin 20 minutes before arising
④ Aerobic exercise for 30 minutes three times a week

25. Anticholinergic drugs are usually contraindicated in residents with:
① Hypertension
② Diabetes mellitus
③ Cardiac failure
④ Glaucoma

26. The licensed practical nurse/vocational nurse (LPN/VN) is a secondary nurse in a primary hospice team. The LPN/VN's functions and responsibilities include:
① Providing physical assistance for the resident, and emotional and spiritual support for the resident and family
② Providing instruction to the resident, and family about health care management and the effects of medication and illness
③ Providing companionship, respite care for family relief, and emotional support
④ Providing opportunities for spiritual reconciliation and healing, as well as prayer

27. In caring for a resident with CVA who has exhibited dysphagia, it is most important that the nurse *first*:
① Gear verbal communication techniques to compensate for the resident's deficits
② Assess the gag reflex

③ Use simple pictures to retrain the resident in the identification of objects

④ Offer small sips of water and progress as tolerated

28. A female resident who is dying jokes about the situation even though she is becoming sicker and weaker. The nurse's *most* therapeutic response would be:
① "Why are you always laughing?"
② "Your laughter is a cover for your fear."
③ "Does it help to joke about your illness?"
④ "She who laughs on the outside, cries on the inside."

29. Drug levels are routinely monitored for which of the following medications?
① Cephalothin sodium; clindamycin
② Cephalexin (Keflex); aspirin
③ Gentamicin sulfate; theophylline
④ Meperidine hydrochloride (Demerol); morphine sulfate

30. Residents who have had a CVA with resulting expressive aphasia will benefit most if the nurse:
① Speaks more slowly and louder
② Uses gestures and facial expressions
③ Provides the residents with a tablet and pencil
④ Removes unnecessary items from the environment

31. The *priority* nursing action to be initiated for a child admitted with a diagnosis of salmonellosis should be to:
① Weigh the child
② Set up enteric isolation
③ Obtain a recent food history
④ Establish a skin care routine

32. The physician decides to treat a resident with a history of chronic renal failure with continuous ambulatory peritoneal dialysis (CAPD). When assessing the resident before the institution of CAPD, the nurse should be alert for the presence of:
① Motivation
② Dysrhythmias
③ Emotional lability
④ Pulmonary problems

33. Which of the following is an example of a communication technique that best expresses the nurse's interest in what the resident has to say?
① Maintaining direct eye contact with the resident during the interaction

② Sharing several personal experiences with the resident
③ Smiling throughout the interaction
④ Providing privacy so that the resident's concerns will not be overheard

34. A resident's respiratory status necessitates endotracheal intubation and positive pressure ventilation. The *most* immediate nursing intervention for this resident at this time would be to:
① Prepare the resident for emergency surgery
② Facilitate the resident's verbal communication
③ Assess the resident's response to the equipment
④ Maintain sterility of the ventilation system the resident is using

35. A major nursing consideration that the nurse must deal with during the early years of a cerebral palsy resident's life is:
① Seizure activity
② Increased muscle tone
③ Decreased muscle tone
④ Sensory impairment

36. Positioning of an unconscious resident includes:
① Elevating the head slightly to promote venous return
② Elevating the feet to promote circulation to the brain
③ Placing the resident on his or her side to prevent aspiration
④ Placing the resident flat to allow the diaphragm to expand

37. Which of the following statements regarding glycerin suppository insertion is the nurse expected to know to be true?
① Glycerin suppositories should be warmed to room temperature before insertion
② It is not necessary to lubricate glycerin suppositories before insertion
③ Glycerin suppositories should be inserted into a bolus of stool
④ Glycerin suppositories should be inserted before an attempt is made to toilet a resident in a bowel-retraining program

38. To obtain a urine culture and sensitivity from an indwelling catheter, the nurse should:
① Attach a sterile drainage bag and obtain the specimen from the outlet spout
② Protect the end of the drainage tubing while letting urine drip from the catheter into a sterile specimen tube

③ Use a needle and syringe, inserting the needle directly into the catheter

④ Use a needle and syringe, inserting the needle into the port

39. The Health Care Financing Administration (HCFA) mandates comprehensive assessment as a basis for developing a plan of care to assist nursing home residents in attaining the highest physical, mental, and psychosocial functioning possible. To meet this requirement, nursing homes throughout the country have developed the Minimum Data Set (MDS) for Nursing Home Resident Assessment and Care Screening, and 18 Resident Assessment Protocols (RAPs) for problem identification. The MDS is a tool regarding resident care that:

① Has added a great deal of paperwork to caring for older adults

② Provides a simple list of problems that a nurse uses to assess each resident

③ Is a functionally based assessment tool identifying pertinent information needed to develop a comprehensive care plan

④ Is the same for all states

40. Which of the following barriers to communication is being demonstrated by a nurse who says to a resident, "There, there . . . don't worry. Everything will turn out for the best."

① Disagreeing with the resident

② Offering a cliché as an expression of reassurance

③ Belittling the resident's feelings

④ Giving approval

41. While in the playroom, a 7-year-old child has a myoclonic seizure of the right arm and leg that almost immediately progresses to a tonic-clonic seizure with clenched jaws. The nurse's *best initial* action would be to:

① Take the other children to their rooms

② Put a plastic airway into the child's mouth

③ Place a large pillow under the child's head

④ Move the toys and furniture away from the child

42. Bulk-forming laxatives, such as psyllium husk (Metamucil), should be administered:

① At bedtime

② With meals

③ With a full glass of fluid

④ With an antacid

43. A 64-year-old resident has a 7-year history of Parkinson's disease. Which of the following

goals are *most appropriate* and realistic in planning nursing care?

① Preparing for terminal care

② Stopping progression of disease

③ Maintaining optimal body functioning

④ Curing the disease

44. Nursing home administrations developed 18 Resident Assessment Protocols (RAPs) for problem identification. The RAPs specify "trigger" definitions that:

① Have added a great deal of paperwork to caring for older adults

② Provide a simple listing of problems that a nurse uses to assess each resident

③ Are the same as the MDS

④ Explicitly suggest specific care that requires implementation

45. The nurse is teaching a resident with type II diabetes about the mechanism of action of oral hypoglycemic agents. Which of the following statements made by the resident would indicate understanding of the teaching plan?

① "The medication will replace my insulin."

② "The medication will help me digest glucose better."

③ "The medication will help me lose weight."

④ "The medication will help my pancreas produce more insulin."

46. In planning care for a 60-year-old resident with congestive heart failure, the nurse should observe for which of the following signs and symptoms?

① Fatigue

② Restlessness

③ Excessive thirst

④ Respiratory difficulty

47. If the nurse is instructing the resident on factors that predispose someone to hypertension, which of the following would be identified in the teaching plan?

① Obesity, heavy salt intake

② Smoking, heavy calcium intake

③ Age, intake of polyunsaturated fat

④ Age, passive personality

48. The nurse begins teaching the resident with angina about the use of nitroglycerin (NTG) sublingual. Which statement indicates that the resident understands how to use the medication?

① "I'll take it after doing any exercising."

② "I'll take it at bedtime to prevent nighttime attacks."

③ "I'll take it every 6 to 8 hours to prevent any chest pain."

④ "I'll take it as soon as I notice any sign of chest pain."

49. A resident is placed on a ventilator. Because hyperventilation can occur when mechanical ventilation is used, the nurse should monitor the resident for signs of:
① Hypoxia
② Hypercapnia
③ Metabolic acidosis
④ Respiratory alkalosis

50. HCFA received a federal mandate through the Omnibus Budget Reconciliation Act (OBRA) to ensure that the MDS and RAPs systems are implemented. These requirements are for:
① All long-term care facilities participating in Medicare or Medicaid programs
② All long-term care facilities participating in Medicare programs
③ All long-term care facilities participating in Medicaid programs
④ For everyone covered by Medicare, Medicaid, and private insurance plans

51. A resident with a diagnosis of angina asks, "How does the nitroglycerin relieve my chest pain?" The *best* response by the nurse is:
① "It improves the pumping action of the heart."
② "It increases cardiac output."
③ "It constricts coronary vessels."
④ "It dilates the coronary arteries."

52. Doses of warfarin sodium (Coumadin) are ordered on the basis of measurement of the resident's:
① Fibrinogen level
② Prothrombin time (PT)
③ Bleeding time
④ Capillary refill time

53. Which of the following nursing behaviors *best* indicates that the nurse is meeting a resident's need for emotional support?
① The nurse spends time listening to the concerns of a resident scheduled for surgery
② The nurse assists an older resident with eating a meal
③ The nurse accompanies a resident having a x-ray examination
④ The nurse avoids disturbing a resident who is praying

54. At a team conference, the nurse would contribute which of the following toward the development of a care plan for a resident with ulcerative colitis?
① Bed rest with bedside commode privileges
② No restriction of visitors or phone calls
③ Attention given to the resident's emotional state, rest, and a private room with a bathroom
④ Semiprivate room, bedside commode, and restriction of visitors

55. The physician has diagnosed a coronary occlusion in a resident. When planning this resident's nursing care, the nurse knows this diagnosis means the resident has:
① A seizure
② A spasm of the muscles
③ A stationary blood clot
④ An obstruction or cutting-off

56. The husband of a resident with aphasia as a result of a cerebrovascular accident asks if his wife's speech will ever return. The nurse should respond:
① "You will have to ask your doctor."
② "It should return to normal in 2 or 3 months."
③ "It is hard to say how much improvement will occur."
④ "This will probably be the extent of her speech from now on."

57. A bowel-retraining program requires the nurse to do which of the following *first*:
① Assess the resident's bowel habits
② Obtain a bowel history
③ Implement the program at first sign of incontinence
④ Plan an individualized program

58. In maintaining safe practice procedures, which of the following is the *best* nursing method for preventing an accidental puncture from a contaminated needle?
① Remove the needle from the syringe and discard in special container
② Recover the needle with its cap and discard in regular containers
③ Leave the needle uncapped after use and discard entire syringe in a special container
④ Bend or break the needle from the syringe and discard in regular container

59. The nurse must turn a resident from the left side to the right side. What is the most important safety measure to use when moving the resident?

① Maintain the bed in a low position
② Keep the opposite side rail up
③ Remove the pillow from under the resident's head
④ Ensure that the bed is in a locked position

60. Objective evidence of the therapeutic effects of antianxiety drug therapy would be:
① Crying, facial grimaces, rigid posture
② Anger, aggressive behavior
③ Decreased blood pressure, pulse, respiration
④ Verbal statements of worry, feeling ill, resting poorly

61. A resident develops a nonhealing ulcer of the right lower extremity and complains of leg cramps after walking short distances. The resident asks the nurse what causes these leg pains. The nurse's *best* response would be:
① "Muscle weakness occurs in the legs because of a lack of exercise."
② "Edema and cyanosis occur in the legs because they are dependent."
③ "Pain occurs in the legs while walking because there is a lack of oxygen to the muscles."
④ "Pressure occurs in the legs because of vasodilation and pooling of blood in the extremity."

62. The nurse is aware that a resident understands the instructions about an appropriate breathing technique for chronic obstructive pulmonary disease (COPD) when the resident:
① Inhales through the mouth
② Increases the respiratory rate
③ Holds each breath for a second at the end of inspiration
④ Progressively increases the length of the inspiratory phase

63. A resident with a history of chronic obstructive pulmonary disease (COPD) develops cor pulmonale. When teaching about nutrition, the nurse should encourage this resident to:
① Eat small meals six times a day to limit oxygen needs
② Lie down after eating to permit energy to be used for digestion
③ Drink large amounts of fluids to help liquefy respiratory secretions
④ Increase protein intake to decrease intravascular hydrostatic pressure

64. Kidney stones most often occur in persons who:

① Drink large amounts of fluids
② Eat foods high in fats and proteins
③ Are not following a regular exercise schedule
④ Are on long-term bed rest

65. When planning nursing care for a resident with angina pectoris, which of the following should be considered a *primary* goal?
① Administering vasodilating drugs promptly
② Restricting dietary fat and cholesterol
③ Relieving the resident's anxiety
④ Monitoring the resident's weight daily

66. A resident worries about a diagnosis of essential hypertension. The resident exhibits signs of anxiety and apprehension. The *best* nursing intervention is to:
① Teach the resident about hypertension
② Let the resident express his or her feelings
③ Explain that everybody has the same feelings
④ Avoid subject of the resident's disease

67. A nursing colleague had a Mantoux test performed after being notified that a resident has an active case of tuberculosis. The nurse is aware that this test is read after:
① 24 hours
② 36 hours
③ 48 hours
④ 96 hours

68. The physician orders a stationary (nonrolling) walker for a resident to aid in ambulation. The nurse plans to teach the resident to:
① Place the back legs of the walker about 10 inches in front of the feet, shift the body weight to the walker, and step forward
② Move the walker about 8 inches forward while stepping forward to the walker with body weight on the walker and both legs
③ Place the walker flat on the floor with the front legs about 12 inches in front of the feet, shift the body weight to the walker, and step forward
④ Move the walker about 10 inches in front of the feet with only the front legs of the walker on the floor, then step forward and put the walker flat

69. A resident refuses to go to the twice-a-day prescribed sessions in physical therapy. The nurse might *best* approach this problem by:
① Having the resident observe the progress of a more cooperative resident with the same problem

② Being the resident's advocate and asking the physician if therapy can be decreased to once daily

③ Planning a conference with the resident, the physical therapist, and the nurse to discuss the resident's feelings

④ Assuring the resident that analgesic medication will be administered before the scheduled physical therapy sessions

70. The nurse should recognize that a genitourinary factor that may contribute to urinary incontinence in older adults is:
① A sensory deprivation
② A urinary tract infection
③ The frequent use of diuretics
④ The inaccessibility of a bathroom

71. Foods to avoid when residents are receiving an MAO-inhibitor drug include:
① Aged cheeses, coffee, chocolate
② Poultry, bananas, eggs
③ Green, leafy vegetables, raisins, milk
④ Pork, pickles, whole wheat bread

72. The nurse should recognize that the sequence of events that occurs in the respiratory response to acidosis is:
① Hypoventilation; increased CO_2 elimination; decreased blood H ions; increased pH
② Hypoventilation; decreased blood H ions; increased CO_2 elimination; decreased pH
③ Hyperventilation; increased CO_2 elimination; decreased blood H ions; increased pH
④ Hyperventilation; decreased CO_2 elimination; decreased blood H ions; decreased pH

73. The first choice of treatment for ventricular fibrillation is:
① Emergency administration of IV atropine
② Immediate defibrillation
③ Endotracheal intubation
④ Cardioversion

74. Oxygen by nasal cannula is prescribed for a resident. The nurse plans to use safety precautions in the room because oxygen:
① Is flammable
② Supports combustion
③ Has unstable properties
④ Converts to an alternate form of matter

75. During a teaching session about insulin injections, a resident asks the nurse, "Why can't I take the insulin in pills instead of taking shots?" The nurse should respond:

① "Insulin cannot be manufactured in pill form."
② "Your doctor will order oral hypoglycemics when you are ready."
③ "The route of administration is decided on by the physician."
④ "Insulin is destroyed by gastric juices, rendering it ineffective."

76. While leading a self-help group of individuals with seizure disorders, the nurse informs them that not everyone has an aura before a seizure. The nurse should describe an aura as a:
① Postseizure amnesia state
② Generalized feeling of relaxation
③ Hallucination during a seizure
④ Warning of impending seizure

77. Digitalis preparations must not be given without the specific direction of the physician whenever:
① The systolic blood pressure is above 100 mm Hg
② The rectal temperature is subnormal
③ The pulse rate is 60 beats/min or below
④ A resident is flushed and perspiring

78. Resident education is an important aspect of resident care, and the nurse must remember to:
① Have answers to anticipated questions written out in order to read them to the resident
② Involve the resident in decision making concerning his or her care
③ Identify community resources available to the resident
④ Encourage involvement of family and significant others

79. It is determined that a resident will require implantation of a permanent pacemaker to assist heart function. In response to the resident's inquiries as to why this is necessary, the nurse's *best* response would be:
① "It shocks the AV node to contract."
② "It will cause a normal heartbeat to occur."
③ "It will work the valves of your heart better."
④ "It will slow down the heart to a more normal rate."

80. A resident with chronic renal failure is on a restricted protein diet and is taught about high biologic value protein foods. An understanding of the rationale for this diet is demon-

strated when the resident states that high bio-logic value protein foods are:
- ① Needed to increase weight gain
- ② Necessary to prevent muscle wasting
- ③ Used to increase urea blood products
- ④ Responsible for controlling hypertension

81. Preoperative care for a resident scheduled for a left midthigh amputation should include:
- ① Elevation of the affected leg to decrease the need for blood to circulate to the area
- ② Repeated blood work to determine the amount of blood flow to the lower extremity
- ③ Bed rest to decrease movement of the affected leg
- ④ Palpation of bilateral pedal pulses

82. To appropriately assess a resident's symptoms related to angina pectoris, the nurse understands that the factor distinguishing angina pectoris from myocardial infarction is that the pain:
- ① Usually lasts longer than 15 minutes
- ② Usually occurs during periods of exertion
- ③ Is accompanied by diaphoresis and tachy-cardia
- ④ Does not radiate to the upper extremities

83. As the nurse prepares to change the dressing for a resident with a mastectomy for the first time, the resident begins to cry and says, "I can't bear to look at my ugly body." The nurse's *best* response should be:
- ① "Even though you feel disfigured now, you can always have reconstruction surgery."
- ② Say nothing, and change the dressing.
- ③ "Everyone feels that way after a mastec-tomy. You'll get used to it."
- ④ "You're having a difficult time right now."

84. To promote measures directed at reversing inappropriate health behaviors in the resident, the nurse should:
- ① Inform the resident that unhealthy behav-iors can harm other people
- ② Ask the resident to explain why he or she still engages in this unhealthy practice
- ③ Supply the resident with educational mate-rials aimed at reducing the unhealthy prac-tice
- ④ Realize that the resident may resist chang-ing a behavior that has become a habit

85. To provide for the safety of a resident who is restrained in a chair in his room, how should the nurse position the resident?
- ① Close to the door
- ② Differently every 3 hours
- ③ Next to a roommate
- ④ Near a call bell

86. At lunch time, a resident appears to have diffi-culty swallowing and appears to choke. The nurse should:
- ① Feed the resident at a slower rate
- ② Note the episode on the chart
- ② Suction the secretions as needed
- ④ Perform the abdominal thrust maneuver

87. To promote comfort and optimal functioning to a child who is placed in a Croupette, which of these actions would be *most appropriate* for the nurse to take?
- ① Change the bed linens and the resident's gown as often as necessary to keep the res-ident dry and comfortable
- ② Establish continuous drainage from the ice chamber as the ice melts
- ③ Restrain the child to prohibit changing position in bed
- ④ Maintain child in a prone position

88. Before administering medication through a nasogastric tube, the nurse must make sure the:
- ① Tube is in the esophagus
- ② Tube is in the stomach
- ③ Pill will dissolve
- ④ Pill is enteric-coated

89. One of the most common myths associated with aging is that:
- ① The majority of older adults reside in their own homes
- ② Most older adults have at least one chronic condition
- ③ All people become senile when they become older
- ④ Most older adults are isolated and alone, averaging one weekly contact with family

90. Which of the following statements is consid-ered a correct, factual recording of resident data in the nurse's notes?
- ① "Resident is aggressive and obnoxious today."
- ② "Resident stated something about wanting to die."
- ③ "Resident is hard to please and refusing any efforts to make him comfortable."
- ④ "Resident refused lunch and did not engage in conversation. Observed staring blankly at wall."

91. Which of the following is the position of choice when caring for a resident with increased intracranial pressure (ICP)?
    ① Supine, with the bed flat
    ② Prone, with the head of the bed flat
    ③ Sims' position, with foot of the bed elevated 30 degrees
    ④ The supine position with the head elevated 30 degrees

92. A 68-year-old resident with severe arteriosclerosis, is scheduled for a left midthigh amputation. Preoperative teaching should include making the resident aware:
    ① Of the adjustment period needed when using an artificial limb
    ② Of the need to turn frequently
    ③ That he will not experience phantom limb pain
    ④ Of the need to lie on his back without too much movement

93. A resident, who has been diagnosed as having peripheral vascular disease, tells the nurse that before hospitalization exercise resulted in severe cramplike pain in both legs. The nurse should include in the teaching plan specific measures the resident can use to increase arterial blood flow to the extremities. These measures should include:
    ① Exercises that promote muscular activity
    ② Meticulous care of minor skin breakdown
    ③ Elevation of legs above the level of the heart
    ④ Daily cleansing of feet by soaking in hot water

94. A resident states, "It's such a beautiful day; will my new dog learn to sit up; give me some fruit." The resident is exhibiting:
    ① Confusion
    ② Flight of ideas
    ③ Delusions
    ④ Hallucinations

95. When planning care for a resident who is ill, the nurse is aware that dehydration can occur when:
    ① The body is unable to excrete sufficient amounts of sodium
    ② There is inadequate food or fluid intake
    ③ The kidneys are unable to excrete wastes normally
    ④ The bladder is unable to hold urine

96. A 5-year-old child has eczema. Nursing care for the child should include which of the following nursing interventions?

    ① Maintaining the child in one position
    ② Keeping the child fully clothed
    ③ Maintaining skin integrity
    ④ Applying warm moist dressings

97. When caring for a resident with an underwater-seal drainage system, the nurse should make sure the bottles remain:
    ① Higher than the resident
    ② Lower than the resident
    ③ At the same level of the resident's chest
    ④ The level of the bottles is not important

98. The nurse is sitting with a resident one day when the resident turns and says, "Isn't that singing beautiful!" The nurse does not hear anything and concludes that the resident is probably experiencing a hallucination. The *best* response by the nurse should be:
    ① "I understand you think you hear singing; however, I don't hear anything."
    ② "Tell me the words to the song."
    ③ "What are you talking about? I don't hear any singing."
    ④ "Yes, I'm enjoying the song."

99. The resident is to receive 50 mg of meperdine hydrochloride (Demerol) with 25 mg of hydroxyzine hydrochloride (Vistaril) at 7:30 PM. The charge nurse states that she drew up the medication for you and hands you the syringe. Which of the following actions is the *most appropriate*?
    ① Place the syringe in the medication drawer for the resident
    ② Recheck the physician's order before administering
    ③ Check drug compatibility chart for drug interactions
    ④ Refuse to give the injection

100. A resident is scheduled for a chest x-ray examination tomorrow morning. The resident is in respiratory isolation due to constant coughing and suspected tuberculosis. The nurse would initiate which of these plans?
    ① Place a mask and gown on the resident as he or she travels to the radiology department
    ② Notify the charge nurse about scheduling a portable chest x-ray examination
    ③ Contact the infection control nurse about the scheduled test
    ④ Contact the radiologists and suggest that the technicians wear a mask during the procedure

101. A resident is scheduled for a below-the-knee amputation of the right leg. Legally, the resident may not sign the operative consent if:

① Ambivalent feelings regarding the operation are present

② Any sedative type of medication has recently been administered

③ A discussion of alternatives with two physicians has not occurred

④ A complete history and physical have not been performed and recorded

102. Before administering digoxin (Lanoxin) to a resident with congestive heart failure, the nurse will hold giving the medication and report to the charge nurse if the resident:

① Complains of nausea and vomiting and has a pulse rate of 52

② Complains of nausea and vomiting and has a pulse rate of 80

③ Has a regular and strong pulse

④ Complains of nausea and vomiting

103. During the evening visiting hours, the family remains out in the hall across from a resident's room. The nurse hears the family arguing, "This is your fault, you didn't take care of her well enough," "No, this is your fault, you are only concerned with yourself." The family continues bickering for 10 minutes before entering the resident's room. What would be an appropriate nursing diagnosis for this family?

① Anxiety related to the resident's medical diagnosis

② Hopelessness related to resident illness

③ Family processes, altered, to inadequate coping behaviors

④ Social isolation as a result of many hospital visits and length of the resident's illness

104. The physician orders Lanoxin (digoxin) 5 mg for residents. Recognizing this to be a high dose for the resident, the nurse's *most appropriate* action should be to:

① Transcribe the order as digoxin 0.5 mg, because this is a normal dosage for your resident

② Transcribe the order as written

③ Seek clarification now from the physician regarding the required dosage

④ Hold the medication until the physician makes rounds

105. The nurse observes a coworker using the following techniques in caring for a resident on respiratory isolation. Which technique is in error?

① Leaving the glass thermometer in the resident's room

② Washing hands before entering the resident's room

③ Wearing a mask while applying antiembolic (TED) stockings

④ Wearing a gown while obtaining a sputum specimen

106. When assessing a resident with Parkinson's disease, a common adaptation the nurse would expect to find is:

① Leaning toward the affected side

② Blank facies or lack of expression

③ Tremors of the hand on movement

④ Hyperextension of the affected extremity

107. An older resident confined to bed, has emphysema and is receiving oxygen therapy. On entering the resident's room, the nurse notices flames coming from a garbage can. The nurse's *initial* response should be to:

① Push the fire alarm in the hall

② Alert the house supervisor immediately

③ Remove the resident and turn off the oxygen

④ Use the water pitcher to pour water in the garbage can

108. A resident refuses stool softener because the resident states that it is not needed. The nurse's *best* response is:

① "The physician has ordered this medication; you really need it."

② "You have the right to refuse this. I will respect your right."

③ "Let me give you this medicine now and in a while I will call your physician to see if we can hold it in the future."

④ "You do not have to take this medicine, but let me explain what this medication is for."

109. A resident has recently moved into a nursing home. A nurse learns that the resident is very "down" and feels worthless and unloved by the family. The family reports that the resident has made a previous suicidal gesture. Which is an *appropriate* nursing intervention at this time?

① The nurse should directly ask if the resident has thoughts or plans about committing suicide

② To prevent giving the resident ideas of self-harm, the nurse should avoid bringing up the subject of suicide

③ The nurse should indicate that others have felt the same way.

④ The nurse should outline some alternative measures to suicide during periods of depression

110. The physician orders promethazine (Phenergan) for a resident with nausea. The charting method for an injection of promethazine intramuscularly (IM) Z-track, would be which of the following?

① "Phenergan 50 mg IM given Z-track for complaint of nausea"

② "Phenergan 50 mg IM in the right dorsogluteal for complaint of nausea"

③ "Phenergan 50 mg IM given in the dorsogluteal Z-track for complaint of nausea"

④ "Phenergan 50 mg IM, Z-track in the right dorsogluteal for complaint of nausea"

111. The physiologic compensatory mechanism that is activated to counteract the effects of acid-base imbalance in a child with severe dehydration is:

① Profuse diaphoresis

② Renal retention of H+

③ Elevated temperature

④ Increased respirations

112. During the admission assessment, a resident with Alzheimer's disease tells the nurse, "You ask too many questions. Why can't you just leave me alone?" What is the *best* way for the nurse to respond?

① "These are important questions. We have to continue."

② "I know that you don't really feel that way."

③ "You sound upset. Would you like to rest for awhile?"

④ "You know your family wants you to cooperate."

113. Avoiding injury in the older adult involves:

① Eating low-energy food; daily outdoor exercise; keeping at least one room warm

② Using higher light intensity; avoiding objects on floor; avoiding use of blues and greens

③ Using direct lights, exposed light bulbs; using white surfaces

④ Keeping room temperature somewhat lower than usual; preparing signs with light backgrounds and dark lettering; daily contact with another person

114. The status of durable power of attorney that nursing home residents give to a person shall include but is not limited to:

① Selling his home, property, and other possessions that he has while he is alive, whether mentally competent or not

② Obtaining, inspecting, receiving, and disclosing medical records and information related to his physical/mental health history and medications

③ Giving the nursing home all his finances once he has passed away

④ Taking care of all his property, finances, and other responsibilities on his death

115. While working as a staff nurse on the same unit for 5 days, the nurse notices that several of the residents on the unit have developed urinary tract infections after being catheterized by the same nurse. The nurse should do which of the following to convey her concerns?

① Report the incident to the physician on the next rounds

② Confront the nurse and suggest that she has used an inappropriate technique

③ Follow the proper chain of command and report the incident so that Quality Assurance can follow up

④ Try to enter the room the next time this nurse performs a catheterization to observe her technique

116. A resident with chronic obstructive pulmonary disease (COPD) complains of a weight gain of 5 pounds in 1 week. The complication of COPD that may have precipitated this weight gain is:

① Polycythemia

② Cor pulmonale

③ Compensated acidosis

④ Left ventricular heart failure

117. A resident has a diagnosis of chronic brain syndrome, approaches the nurse's station and says to the nurse, "Could you please show me where I can get the bus home to Poughkeepsie?" Which response by the nurse would be most therapeutic?

① "Go straight down the hall and turn right."

② "Do you have money for the bus?"

③ "The last bus to Poughkeepsie left 10 minutes ago; you'll have to come back tomorrow."

④ "You don't live in Poughkeepsie anymore, Mr. Z. You live here with us in New City."

118. When setting limits on a resident's behavior, the nurse must identify the consequences to the resident should he exceed the established limits. The nurse knows that the *most appropriate* time to establish consequences is:
① Just before the anticipated behavior
② After the resident has exceeded the set limits
③ At the time the limits are set
④ When the staff can no longer tolerate the resident's behavior

119. A 70-year-old resident has been in a nursing home for several years because of increasing disability from rheumatoid arthritis. The main nursing intervention is:
① Ensuring complete bed rest with range-of-motion exercises
② Limiting activities because they tire her
③ Keeping the joints immobilized
④ Preventing contractures and maintaining range-of-motion in all joints

120. An appropriate nursing goal for a resident who is in the terminal stages of an illness should be:
① Assisting the resident through each stage of the death and dying process
② Reassuring the resident that he or she has nothing to fear in death
③ Secluding the resident from others
④ Engaging the resident in future planning

121. The physician tells the resident that an above-the-knee amputation (AKA) is necessary. After the physician leaves the resident's room, the resident turns her head away from the nurse and begins to cry. The nurse would:
① Leave the room quietly and allow her to cry without embarrassment
② Stay and encourage her to talk about post-operative coughing and deep breathing
③ Leave the room and call a family member to come to the hospital to console her
④ Stay with her while quietly holding her hand

122. After 1 month in a nursing home a Jewish resident says she misses lighting her candles on Friday night (Shabbas licht). The nurse's *best* response would be:
① "I'll ask the charge nurse if we can arrange that for you."

② "Candles do have a peaceful effect."
③ "Habits are hard to break."
④ "The fire department will not allow it."

123. In planning nursing care for a resident receiving warfarin (Coumadin), the nurse must be aware that the antidote for warfarin is:
① Protamine sulfate
② Vitamin K
③ Folic acid
④ Calcium gluconate

124. The mental process most sensitive to deterioration with aging seems to be:
① Judgment
② Creativity
③ Intelligence
④ Short-term memory

125. Several evenings before a resident's death, she confides to the nurse, "I just keep on hoping that someone will find a cure for this so I can continue to raise my family." What should be an appropriate response by the nurse?
① "I'll keep praying for you. There must be a cure somewhere."
② "I'll try to do everything I can to help you and keep you comfortable."
③ "I just read an article in a nursing journal about all the work being done at another hospital. I'll see what I can find out."
④ "Try to have more peace of mind with what you have accomplished."

126. Which of these may indicate that death is approaching?
① Decreased body temperature
② Deep, slow respirations
③ Dry, cool skin
④ Dull, glazed eyes

127. The nurse would be aware that a resident with chronic renal failure recognizes an adequate source of high biological value protein when the food the resident selected from the menu was:
① Apple juice
② Raw carrots
③ Cottage cheese
④ Whole wheat bread

128. A 3-year-old with acute asthma is short of breath, the respirations are 56, the pulse is 102, and there is a nonproductive cough. The nurse would expect the child's blood gas values to indicate a:
① pH of 7.32

② PO$_2$ of 95 mm Hg
③ HCO$_3$ of 26 mEq/L
④ PCO$_2$ of 40 mm Hg

129. Which of the following is a right of a resident in a nursing home?
① Taking any medications they feel they need
② Refusing treatment ordered by the physician
③ Making as much noise as they want
④ Demanding their meals at the times they prefer

130. The nurse is providing a sitz bath for a resident. The nurse knows to establish the temperature of the water at:
① 75° F to 80° F (23.8° C to 26.6° C)
② 85° F to 90° F (29.4° C to 32.2° C)
③ 100° F to 105° F (37.7° C to 40.5° C)
④ 120° F to 125° F (48.8° C to 51.6° C)

131. In planning for a resident's wound care, what important nursing measures should the nurse consider *first*?
① Preparing supplies
② Checking drainage tubes
③ Giving assistance to resident's needs
④ Reducing the transfer of microorganisms

132. What should the nurse do to meet an alert resident's right for informed consent?
① Close the door and pull the curtain.
② Explain what is being done and why.
③ Prevent a resident from leaving the facility.
④ Get all consents in writing.

133. To evaluate nursing care you must determine if:
① All assigned nursing measures were completed
② Goals are being accomplished
③ Resident feels better
④ Resident is happy with the quality of care

134. The son of a delirious resident states, "I feel so helpless. I just don't know what to do." Which of the following is the *best* way to help the resident's son deal with the resident's illness?
① Reassure him that the resident will be fine in a few days
② Suggest that he not visit the resident until there is improvement
③ Role model how best to interact with the resident
④ Refer him to the physician to answer his concerns

135. A Catholic resident tells the nurse that before getting ill, she used to go to Mass and receive communion every morning. The nurse should:
① Have the priest come and give her last rites.
② Assign her to a room with another Catholic resident.
③ Arrange for her to receive communion daily.
④ Tell the resident the name of the nearest Catholic church.

136. In planning care for an infant with human immunodeficiency virus (HIV), it is most important for the nurse to:
① Wash hands frequently
② Notify the Centers for Disease Control and Prevention
③ Implement universal precaution protocol
④ Wear mask, gown, and gloves at all times

137. A resident with tuberculosis requires a sputum specimen for acid-fast bacillus. The *most appropriate* nursing intervention for sputum collection is:
① Encourage the resident to do abdominal breathing while coughing
② Cleanse the resident's mouth with hydrogen peroxide before taking the specimen
③ Instruct the resident to take a deep breath and cough from the diaphragm
④ Keep the resident in a semi-Fowler's position while obtaining the specimen

138. For a resident with gout, which of the following drugs would most likely be on the drug profile?
① Allopurinol
② Corticosteroids
③ Acetaminophen
④ Estrogen replacement

139. A resident tells the nurse that he is having trouble breathing. The nurse should take which of these actions *first*?
① Determine the pulse rate
② Report this to the team leader
③ Elevate the head of the bed to high-Fowler's position
④ Instruct the resident to breathe deeply

140. The dietary practice that will help a resident reduce the dietary intake of sodium is:
① Increasing the use of dairy products
② Using an artificial sweetener in coffee
③ Avoiding the use of carbonated beverages

④ Using catsup for cooking and flavoring foods

141. During the evening shift, a resident asks the nurse for assistance with writing a living will. The nurse recognizes which of the following as the primary purpose of a living will?

① It provides that the family may make all decisions regarding the resident's health care when the resident is no longer able to decide for himself or herself

② It provides for the distribution of all the resident's material possessions

③ It states exactly what measures are to be taken to save the resident's life

④ It provides that extraordinary measures not be taken to save a resident's life if he or she becomes terminally ill

142. When providing nursing care for older adults in institutions, which of the following is a major consideration?

① Providing personal hygiene

② Eliminating all resident responsibilities

③ Fostering social privacy

④ Making decisions for the resident

143. A resident requires a tracheotomy. Which of the following procedures should be carried out by the nurse when suctioning secretions in the client?

① Oxygenate, suction for 30 seconds, oxygenate

② Oxygenate, suction for 15 seconds, cough and deep-breath

③ Oxygenate, suction for 10 seconds, oxygenate

④ Oxygenate, suction for 25 seconds, allow to rest

144. Chlorothiazide (Diuril) is given to expel fluid from the body and prevent pulmonary edema. When evaluating resident response to the drug, the nurse should also observe for:

① Hematuria

② Nausea and vomiting

③ Diarrhea

④ Muscular weakness and cramping

145. Chest pain is a common symptom in a resident with pneumonia, usually occurring on the affected side. When it does occur, the nurse should encourage the resident to:

① Breathe deeply to relieve the pain

② Lie on the affected side to cough

③ Cough frequently

④ Lie on the unaffected side to cough

146. A resident with spinal cord injury has a sudden extreme elevation in blood pressure, a throbbing headache, nasal stuffiness, sweating and flushing, and chills and pallor. These symptoms indicate:

① Urinary tract infection

② Autonomic dysreflexia

③ Transient ischemic attack

④ Septicemia

147. A resident has been pacing up and down the corridor for several hours. The nurse observes the resident yelling, "Get out of my way, moron." The *most appropriate* nursing response should be to tell the resident:

① That his behavior is unacceptable and will not be tolerated

② That, if he does not "cool it," he'll be put in seclusion

③ That if he does not stop bothering the other residents, his afternoon privileges will be taken away

④ To come to the medication room for his Ativan

148. The health care team includes:

① The physician and nurse

② The resident and his family

③ Social workers and physical therapists

④ All of the above

149. Chloral hydrate (Noctec) was ordered for an 83-year-old resident in a nursing home. In planning care for the resident, the nurse must know that chloral hydrate is a(n):

① Sedative

② Antiepileptic

③ Antidepressant

④ Tranquilizer

150. At a staff meeting the question of a staff nurse returning to work after a drug rehabilitation program is discussed. The nursing supervisor helps the staff to decide that the best way to handle the nurse's return would be to:

① Offer the nurse support in a direct straightforward manner

② Avoid mentioning the problem unless the nurse brings up the topic

③ Assign another staff member to keep the nurse under close observation

④ Make certain the nurse is assigned to administer only nonnarcotic medications

Answers and Rationales for Comprehensive Examination

1. **4** Residents with depression are difficult to relate to because of their feelings of hopelessness and apathy. The lack of success by the nursing assistants may lead to withdrawal or feelings of anger toward the resident.
   1 Residents with depression are not necessarily lazy.
   2 Poor personal grooming may be a factor; however, this can be easily managed.
   3 Residents with depression are typically dependent on others.

2. **3** This does not take away the resident's only way of coping, and it permits future movement through the grieving process when the resident is ready.
   1 The resident's denial should be neither supported nor taken away; encouraging denial is a form of false reassurance.
   2 This is false reassurance.
   4 The resident must not be abandoned; the nurse's presence is a form of emotional support.

3. **4** Unless the tray was also contaminated, the drape can be replaced easily, and the tray can still be used.
   1 Sterile trays are quite expensive and unless contaminated, the tray should be saved.
   2 This is unsafe and could result in contamination to the resident.
   3 The physician should be informed of the contamination, but starting over may not be necessary; see rationale for answer 4.

4. **3** The resident is still denying the illness and has not resolved the basic problem that led to the alcoholism.
   1 This is incorrect because the resident is still denying the illness; willpower alone will not keep the resident away from alcohol.
   2 This may be true, but it does not ensure compliance or successful rehabilitation.

4 This is not helpful unless the basis of the conflicts and the resident's role in resolving them are understood by the resident.

5. **2** Lethargy leading to coma develops because of metabolic acidosis (ketoacidosis).
   1 This is not a symptom of ketoacidosis.
   3 This may be a symptom of hypoglycemia, not ketoacidosis.
   4 This is not a symptom of ketoacidosis.

6. **3** Decreased metabolism and excretion of drugs occur in the aged; therefore it is prudent to give smaller doses, farther apart.
   1 Smaller dosages may not achieve a desired effect, and because metabolism is decreased in older adults, there is a risk for accumulation if doses are given too close together.
   2 Larger dosages closer together are never given, as metabolism and excretion are decreased in the normal aging process.
   4 Larger dosages could potentially lead to toxicity because metabolism and excretion are slowed in the aged.

7. **1** Theophylline (Theo-Dur) relaxes smooth muscle in the bronchi so that ventilation becomes easier.
   2 This is not an action of this medication.
   3 This is not an action of this medication.
   4 This is not an action of this medication.

8. **1** Shearing force occurs when two surfaces move against each other; when the bed is at an angle greater than 30 degrees, the torso tends to slide and cause this phenomenon.
   2 This would raise the head of the bed too high to prevent the resident from sliding in bed.
   3 This would raise the head of the bed too high to prevent the resident from sliding in bed.
   4 This would raise the head of the bed too high to prevent the resident from sliding in bed.

9. **2** Hearing impairment common with advancing age.
   1 Personality and reality contact alterations.
   3 Loss of visual accommodation in advancing age.
   4 Cognitive dysfunction characterized by disorientation and confabulation.

10. **4** This drug relaxes the respiratory muscles; it inhibits transmission of nerve impulses by binding with cholinergic receptor sites and antagonizing the action of acetylcholine; the resident will die without mechanical ventilation.
   1 This is not the priority.
   2 This is not the priority.
   3 This is not the priority.

11. **2** Rechecking assures equipment is functioning, and reporting to the immediate supervisor (charge nurse) brings prompt attention to the changes because these changes indicate increased intracranial pressure.
   1 Delay of reporting could have serious consequences, and therefore it is not correct procedure.
   3 Delay of reporting could have serious consequences, and therefore it is not correct procedure.
   4 These changes are significant and need to be reported.

12. **4** Most seizure disorders can be controlled partially or completely by anticonvulsants. These drugs also act to raise the seizure threshold. The choice of medication depends on the type of seizures.
   1 Digitalis preparations and atropine are examples. They are used to slow and strengthen the heartbeat and increase the heart rate.
   2 Anticonvulsants are central nervous system (CNS) depressants.
   3 Antispasmodics are used to treat muscle spasms and are not anticonvulsants.

13. **2** Listening allows the resident to express feelings more freely and fully and encourages the resident to work through those feelings.
   1 This response ignores the resident's need to express his or her feelings to the nurse.
   3 This response ignores the resident's need to express his or her feelings to the nurse.
   4 This insensitivity ignores the resident's feelings and blocks communication.

14. **1** Chest tubes are inserted between the ribs into the pleural space to allow drainage of secretions, blood, and air.
   2 The negative pressure within the thoracic cavity is restored when the lung is expanded.
   3 Atmospheric pressure rushing into the thoracic cavity causes the lung to collapse.
   4 The thoracic cavity pressure is normally negative as opposed to the atmospheric pressure. The pressure is not equal.

15. **1** This provides for systemic monitoring of fluid intake and output.
   2 This is indicative, but daily weights are needed for closer monitoring.
   3 Activity is not a factor in fluid balance.
   4 Activity is not a factor in fluid balance.

16. **2** This is necessary to prevent flooding of the trachea with fluid; some systems have receptacles attached to the tubing to collect the fluid, and others have to be temporarily disconnected while emptying the fluid.
   1 This circumstance does not require assistance from a respiratory therapist.
   3 This is unsafe; humidity is necessary to preserve moisture of the respiratory tract and liquefy secretions.
   4 The amount of condensation is irrelevant in terms of recording the intake and output.

17. **3** Kyphosis alters the center of gravity, which contributes to alterations in balance and gait.
   1 Decreased endurance and fatigue should not change the center of gravity or alter the gait; a lack of stamina by itself should not cause falls.
   2 Age is incidental; one should not accept falls as an inescapable aspect of aging.
   4 Although kyphosis alters the line of vision downward, this by itself would not cause increased falls.

18. **4** This is a miotic that constricts the pupil, permitting fluid drainage, which reduces intraocular pressure.
   1 This is a topical anesthetic; it will not reduce the increased intraocular pressure associated with glaucoma.
   2 This is contraindicated; this dilates the pupil and paralyzes ciliary muscles.
   3 This is contraindicated; this is a mydriatic that dilates the pupil, obstructing drainage, which increases intraocular pressure.

19. **3** The orthopneic position lowers the diaphragm and provides for maximum thoracic expansion.
   1 This would not facilitate thoracic expansion because it still permits abdominal organs to press against the diaphragm.
   2 This would not facilitate thoracic expansion because it still permits abdominal organs to press against the diaphragm.
   4 Although this could help, it would not be as beneficial as the orthopneic position.

20. **3** Tachycardia and palpitations, not bradycardia, occur.
    1 Nausea may occur; it reflects a central emetic reaction to levodopa.
    2 Anorexia may occur; decreased appetite results because of nausea and vomiting.
    4 Changes in affect, mood, and behavior are related to toxic effects of the drug.

21. **3** Massage increases circulation to the affected area, thereby supplying nutrients to promote tissue health.
    1 Alcohol causes drying, and rubbing the area may promote tissue destruction.
    2 A semi-Fowler's position would cause direct pressure to the coccyx region.
    4 Heating increases vasodilation; this measure is suggested when dealing with an open wound.

22. **1** Surgical asepsis means that the defined area will contain no microorganisms.
    2 This would be true of isolation procedures.
    3 This would apply to isolation and medical asepsis.
    4 This would apply to medical asepsis.

23. **1** These are common side effects of cholinergic drugs, although increased peristalsis occurs more frequently than does an increase in urination.
    2, 3, 4 See rationale for answer 1; only part of each of these responses is correct, which makes the response totally incorrect.

24. **3** Giving aspirin will reduce inflammation and decrease pain and stiffness in the morning.
    1 A warm bath would relax muscles and decrease pain and stiffness. A cool bath is contraindicated.
    2 This type of exercise is too strenuous for rheumatoid arthritis.
    4 This type of exercise is too strenuous for rheumatoid arthritis.

25. **4** Can increase intraocular pressure as a result of the mydriatic effect of the drug.
    1 Especially in the geriatric resident with a history of urinary retention.
    2 Not usually a contraindication.
    3 Because the heart rate may be increased, careful consideration must be given before these drugs are given to such residents.

26. **1** The licensed practical nurse or licensed vocational nurse works under the direction of a physician and registered nurse. Bedside nursing interventions appropriate to the terminally ill are provided.
    2 This is the responsibility of the primary nurse who is usually a licensed registered nurse. The primary nurse evaluates the resident's response to treatment and is an advocate between resident, family, physician, and an interdisciplinary team.
    3 The hospice volunteer usually assumes these duties. The volunteer has completed volunteer training of at least 24 hours and continues support throughout the bereavement period.
    4 These functions are through the primary pastor who supports the resident and family in coping with their fears and uncertainties.

27. **2** Dysphagia is defined as difficulty in swallowing. If the resident has lost the gag reflex, he may easily aspirate oral fluids.
    1,3 The resident has difficulty swallowing. not in communicating (aphasia).
    4 Means of assessing the gag reflex.

28. **3** This nonjudgmentally points out the resident's behavior.
    1 This is too confrontational; resident may not be able to answer the question.
    2 This is too confrontational and an assumption by the nurse.
    4 This is too judgmental, an assumption, and a stereotypical response.

29. **3** Small doses of these drugs can cause toxic levels; gentamicin sulfate is an aminoglycoside and is considered a potent bactericidal antibiotic reserved for life-threatening infections; theophylline is the prototype of the xanthine derivatives used in the treatment of emphysema and other COPDS.
    1,2 Three of the four drugs listed in these responses are classified as antibiotics and do not require routine monitoring of drug level; aspirin is an antiinflammatory agent also not indicative of monitoring drug levels.
    4 Residents receiving Demerol or morphine sulfate necessitate observation of vital signs but routine monitoring of drug levels is not necessary.

30. **3** Expressive aphasia results from damage to Broca's speech area. The resident understands what is said to him and knows the words he wishes to say, but he cannot form the words verbally. Many times he may still be able to write words.
    1,2 One or both of these actions will not facilitate communication efforts and will usually increase resident frustration over his or her inability to communicate.
    4 Safety is not an issue and unnecessary items do not hamper communication ability provided the resident is given the appropriate items with which to communicate.

31. **2** Bacteria are spread by contaminated stool; thus to protect others, isolation procedures must be initiated immediately on admission.
   1 This is part of the initial assessment and would have been accomplished before admission.
   3 Although this will be done, the priority is to establish appropriate isolation precautions.
   4 Although this will be done, the priority is to establish appropriate isolation precautions.

32. **1** Lack of motivation is the most serious impediment to successful continuous ambulatory peritoneal dialysis (CAPD); CAPD may be contraindicated for some residents such as those who are blind or have a colostomy, a psychosis, or PVD.
   2 This is not a contraindication if the resident is receiving medical supervision.
   3 This is not a contraindication if the resident is receiving medical supervision.
   4 This is not a contraindication if the resident is receiving medical supervision.

33. **1** The use of direct eye contact is one of the characteristics of attentive listening, conveying an attitude of caring and interest.
   2 The overuse of personal experiences focuses on the nurse and not the resident.
   3 The misuse of social graces implies that the nurse is not attentively listening.
   4 Providing privacy is an appropriate action to the situation; however, the use of direct eye contact best indicates that the nurse is interested in what the resident is saying.

34. **3** Nothing is achieved if the equipment is working and the resident is not responding.
   1 This is presumptive; the data base is incomplete for the assessment that surgery is necessary.
   2 Endotracheal intubation does not permit verbal communication.
   4 This is important but not the priority.

35. **1** Seizures for whatever reason are a major nursing concern and occur whenever there is damage to the motor centers of the brain.
   2 Muscle tone can either be increased or decreased, depending on the nature and distribution of neuromuscular dysfunction.
   3 Muscle tone can either be increased or decreased, depending on the nature and distribution of neuromuscular dysfunction.
   4 While sensory impairments, hearing loss, and/or abnormalities of vision are important, they are not life-threatening.

36. **3** This is the saftest since this position prevents aspiration of saliva and vomitus.
   1, 2, 4 These positions (prone) are not appropriate for an unconscious resident because of the

possibility of aspirating saliva or vomitus; changing position (turning from side to side) every 2 hours along with proper skin care are also recommended nursing interventions.

37. **1** Never use a suppository directly from a refrigerator, because cold causes constriction.
   2 Lubrication ensures easy, painless insertion.
   3 Ineffective when inserted into a bolus of stool.
   4 Glycerin suppositories are inserted after 20 minutes if resident has not had a bowel movement.

38. **4** The port on the drainage tubing is specifically designed for obtaining specimens.
   1 Attaching a new drainage bag requires opening the closed system, which is to be avoided.
   2 This would require opening the closed system, which is to be avoided.
   3 On most catheters, inserting a needle would leave a hole, which would then leak urine.

39. **3** MDS clearly identifies areas that need to be addressed in planning resident care.
   1 This is not true. It is a valuable tool in planning care.
   2 This is incorrect. It is comprehensive information pertinent to the resident as a total person and his needs.
   4 This is not necessarily true. Some states have been given permission to use an alternate version.

40. **2** The use of reassuring clichés is a barrier to therapeutic communication because these responses tend to convey to the resident that the nurse feels the resident is worrying needlessly or that the nurse does not understand the problem.
   1 The nontherapeutic technique of disagreeing with the resident implies that what the resident said is not acceptable. Disagreeing may serve to threaten the resident.
   3 By belittling the resident's feelings, the nurse devalues them by implying they are commonplace and insignificant. Belittling serves to lower the resident's self-esteem.
   4 The technique of giving approval creates a block by shifting the focus to the nurse's values. The nurse now becomes judgmental.

41. **4** Safety is the priority during the seizure.
   1 It would be unsafe to leave the child having the seizure.
   2 Attempting to open clenched jaws could result in injury to the child's teeth and jaw.
   3 This may cause airway occlusion by forcing the neck onto the chin; a small flat blanket is more effective.

42. **3** To prevent possible obstruction as a result of thickening and expansion of the drug.

   1,2 Administration of this type of laxative is not limited to any specific time.

   4 This type of laxative is bland and not affected by digestive juices therefore giving with an antacid is not necessary.

43. **3** The nurse should encourage daily exercise as tolerated to prevent pneumonia and to maintain joint mobility. Encourage participation in previous work, as well as social and diversional activities to avoid social withdrawal.

   1 Many residents with Parkinson's disease live for years.

   2 At this time there is no known way to stop progression of this disease.

   4 There is no known cure at this time.

44. **4** RAPs are a tool that identifies problems and specific interventions to address in care plans.

   1 This is untrue because it is a valuable tool in planning care and possible changes as needs change.

   2 This is incorrect because this tool generates comprehensive information pertinent to the resident as a total person and his needs.

   3 This is incorrect because this tool provides the specific care needs.

45. **4** The action of Micronase is to stimulate the pancreas to produce more insulin and to increase the sensitivity of insulin receptors on the cell.

   1 Oral hypoglycemics are not insulin and cannot replace it.

   2 Oral hypoglycemics have no digestive action.

   3 Oral hypoglycemics have no effect on weight.

46. **4** Increased pulmonary pressure occurs with fluid buildup in the lungs (pulmonary edema).

   1 Fatigue does occur, but it is not a significant indication of complications.

   2 Restlessness may occur without indicating a major problem.

   3 This is not indicative of the diagnosis.

47. **1** Increased weight in childhood and middle age predisposes a person to the disorder; high salt intake also increases the risk.

   2 Not totally correct response, although smoking is considered a risk factor.

   3 Not totally correct response, although age is considered a risk factor.

   4 Not totally correct response, although age is considered a risk factor.

48. **4** Sublingual nitroglycerin should be taken at the *earliest* sign of chest discomfort. The resident should sit down, place one tablet under the tongue, and allow it to dissolve.

   1 A resident may be taught to dissolve one tablet under the tongue 5 minutes before participat-

ing in an activity that the resident knows causes chest discomfort. However, taking the medication at the *earliest* sign of chest discomfort is the most appropriate resident response in the beginning stage of resident teaching.

   2 Sublingual nitroglycerin is for use when chest discomfort occurs.

   3 Sublingual nitroglycerin is for use when chest discomfort occurs.

49. **4** Increased rate and depth of breathing result in excessive elimination of CO_2 and respiratory alkalosis results.

   1 Hypoxia is associated with respiratory acidosis, not respiratory alkalosis which is related to hyperventilation.

   2 With hyperventilation, CO_2 levels will be decreased (hypocapnia), not elevated.

   3 This results from excess hydrogen ions caused by a metabolic problem, not a respiratory problem.

50. **1** The U.S. Congress sought federal approval to ensure quality of care.

   2 This is incorrect because this requirement is for both Medicare and Medicaid.

   3 This is incorrect because this requirement is for both Medicare and Medicaid.

   4 This is incorrect because this requirement is for both Medicare and Medicaid.

51. **4** The smooth muscle relaxant action causes dilation of the coronary arteries, and this action provides blood and oxygen to the heart muscle.

   1 Has no effect on the pumping mechanism.

   2 Has no effect on cardiac output.

   3 Dilates the arteries.

52. **2** Dosage individualized according to blood coagulation tests; the therapeutic aim is to produce prolongation of the prothrombin time within 1.3 to 1.5 times the control.

   1 Fibrinogen is a plasma protein essential to the blood-clotting process.

   3 The time required for blood to stop flowing from a tiny wound; prolonged bleeding times are most often the result of uremia, a disorder of platelet function or the ingestion of aspirin.

   4 Process of blood returning to a portion of the capillary system after being interrupted briefly; when cardiac output is reduced and digital perfusion is poor, then capillary refill is slow.

53. **1** Attentive listening promotes emotional well-being.

   2 This measure does not necessarily promote emotional well-being.

   3 This procedure may only be promoting physical well-being.

4 The promotion of emotional well-being usually implies some contact between the resident and the nurse; avoidance behavior may not necessarily do this.

54. **3** The causative factor of stress is considered with rest and privacy for toileting.
   1 Rest is needed, but privacy for toileting is an important factor.
   2 Restrictions may be needed to decrease stress and provide rest that is needed.
   4 This does not allow for rest and privacy in toileting.

55. **4** There is an obstruction or cutting off of the blood supply to the coronary artery or its branches.
   1 This is not related to the situation.
   2 This is not related to the situation.
   3 The coronary arteries can become occluded by a thrombus or emboli.

56. **3** Recovery from aphasia is a continuous process; the amount of recovery cannot be predicted.
   1 This response abdicates the nurse's responsibility; the physician cannot predict return of function.
   2 This gives false reassurance; it may take a year or longer or may never return.
   4 This gives false reassurance; it may take a year or longer or may never return.

57. **2** Obtain bowel history; assess evacuation pattern; plan program; implement program; evaluate program.
   1 Part of assessment is obtaining a bowel history.
   3 Follow steps of the nursing process.
   4 Follow steps of the nursing process.

58. **3** This follows universal precaution guidelines to decrease the possibility of needlestick injury.
   1 This action is a violation of the Centers for Disease Control and Prevention (CDC) guidelines for universal precautions.
   2 This maneuver is in violation of CDC standards and has been linked to an increased incidence of needlestick injury.
   4 This action is not recommended and is not regarded as safe practice.

59. **2** Of the four choices, this is the most important safety measure.
   1 To maintain the bed in low position is appropriate, but it is not the highest priority in this situation.
   3 Removing the pillow may be warranted; however, it is more a comfort measure than a safety measure.
   4 This is an important factor in safety principles, but it is not the highest priority in this situation.

60. **3** Decreases physiologic manifestations.
   1 Signs of anxiety.
   2 Paradoxical reaction.
   4 Signs of anxiety.

61. **3** Intermittent claudication is the pain that occurs during exercise because of a lack of O_2 to muscles in the involved extremities.
   1 It is the exercise, not the lack of it, that precipitates the pain.
   2 This is related to a venous problem, not an arterial one.
   4 This is related to a venous problem, not an arterial one.

62. **3** This pause allows added time for gaseous exchange at the alveolar capillary beds.
   1 Inhalation should be through the nose to moisten, filter, and warm the air.
   2 This decreases the effectiveness of respirations.
   4 The expiratory phase should be lengthened, and exhalation should be through pursed lips.

63. **1** Eating small meals will decrease the amount of O_2 necessary for digestion at any one time.
   2 Lying down increases intraabdominal pressure, pushing a full stomach against the diaphragm and limiting respiratory excursion.
   3 While fluids do help liquefy secretions, they should not be encouraged in a resident with right ventricular heart failure.
   4 Protein maintains or increases hydrostatic pressure; it does not decrease it.

64. **4** Immobility promotes urinary stasis, lending itself to stone formation.
   1 Increased fluid intake would decrease the formation of urinary stones.
   2 Fat and protein metabolites are not known to be associated with urinary calculi.
   3 Exercise may decrease stone formation, but it is not a significant preventive measure.

65. **3** Relieving the resident's anxiety helps to reduce the stress that may bring on further anginal episodes.
   1 Although this is important, relieving anxiety may reduce the need for vasodilators. Assuring the resident that the medication will be given promptly is a means of relieving anxiety.
   2 This should not be a primary goal, but it is included as follow-up instructions.
   4 Monitoring the weight is not necessary unless edema is present. This might indicate further problems.

66. **2** The nurse lets the resident express all feelings and gives the resident reassurance.
   1 This is not the best time to teach the resident.
   3 The resident is concerned about his or her condition and needs to be reassured.
   4 By avoiding the subject, the nurse might think that the nurse does not care.

67. **3** The test consists of the tubercle bacillus extract being injected intradermally in the inner aspect of the upper arm; 48 hours is the amount of time needed for the extract to permeate the system.
   1 This is too short of a period.
   2 This is too short of a period.
   4 This is too long of a period for the extract to take effect.

68. **3** Placing the walker flat on the floor provides stability; putting weight on the walker equalizes weight bearing on the upper and lower extremities.
   1 This is unsafe; this places the walker too far in front of the resident for safe transfer of body weight.
   2 It is not possible to move the walker and have it bear weight at the same time; the walker should be flat on the ground when stepping forward.
   4 This is unsafe; all four points of the walker should be flat on the ground when the resident is stepping forward.

69. **3** This includes the resident in the problem-solving process.
   1 This does not include the resident in the problem-solving process; more data should be obtained from the resident before deciding on an intervention, which may or may not be appropriate.
   2 This does not include the resident in the problem-solving process; more data should be obtained from the resident before deciding on an intervention, which may or may not be appropriate.
   4 This does not include the resident in the problem-solving process; more data should be obtained from the resident before deciding on an intervention, which may or may not be appropriate.

70. **2** Urinary tract infections affect the genitourinary tract and interfere with the voluntary control of micturition.
   1 This is a neurologic, not a genitourinary, factor.
   3 These are iatrogenic factors.
   4 This is an environmental factor.

71. **1** Can produce drug-diet interactions due to high content of tryamine.

2, 3,4 These foods do not contain a high content of tryamine and may be safely consumed by residents taking MAO inhibitor drugs.

72. **3** Respiratory compensation to acidosis involves increased CO_2 elimination through hyperventilation, with a resulting increase in pH to normal limits.
   1 Hypoventilation would not increase expiration of CO_2 with the ultimate increase in pH.
   2 If the resident is hypoventilating, blood H+ ions would increase because of CO_2 retention; pH would decrease.
   4 With hyperventilation there would be an increase in CO_2 elimination, not a decrease; the pH would increase, not decrease.

73. **2** Immediate defibrillation is the first choice to correct ventricular fibrillation.
   1 From a cardiac perspective, atropine's main action is to increase the heart rate; therefore it would be contraindicated in the treatment of ventricular fibrillation.
   3 Endotracheal intubation does not affect the electrical activity of the heart; however, the situation may warrant intubation once the fibrillatory state is corrected.
   4 Cardioversion is used for terminating rapid, less lethal dysrhythmia, not ventricular fibrillation.

74. **2** Oxygen is necessary for the production of fire.
   1 Oxygen does not burn itself; it supports combustion.
   3 This is irrelevant to the need for safety precautions.
   4 This is irrelevant to the need for safety precautions.

75. **4** Insulin in tablet form would be inactivated by gastric juices; insulin given by injection bypasses the destructive gastric juices.
   1 Oral insulin would be inactivated in the stomach; oral hypoglycemics contain substances such as sulfonylurea that stimulate beta cells to produce insulin.
   2 This is incorrect information for a resident who is currently insulin-dependent; this provides false reassurance.
   3 This does not answer the resident's question; insulin is administered IV or subcutaneously and the route depends on the resident's needs.

76. **4** The warning feelings some people experience are odd sensations such as unpleasant odors, spots before their eyes, flashing lights, vertigo, tingling, or numbness.
   1 This occurs during the recovery stage, in the postictal period. During this time there are common complaints of headaches and muscle aches.

2 This is sometimes reported postictally.

3 Hallucinations are not reported in most seizure activities.

77. **3** Could lead to adverse reactions; if the heart rate is 60 bpms or below the normal action of the drug would cause a further lowering of the heart rate.

　1 The average systolic blood pressure is 120 mm Hg.

　2 Digitalis is a cardiotonic and has two main actions: (1) increasing of strength of the heart muscle contraction and (2) slowing of the heart rate.

　4 These symptoms may or may not be related to the resident's condition; proper assessment and reporting of the resident's condition may be warranted.

78. **2** This allows the resident input into decisions about his or her care.

　1 This does not allow for the resident's individual needs.

　3 This is not an important factor at this time.

　4 The resident is the primary focus at this point.

79. **2** This type pacemaker synchronizes impulses to the atria and ventricles to more closely simulate the normal action of the heart; it may be a fixed-rate or, most usually, a demand mode pacemaker and may stimulate the atria, the ventricles, or both.

　1 The physiologic pacemaker stimulates both the atria and ventricles to contract.

　3 It affects the electrical conduction system of the heart, not the anatomic structures.

　4 It will increase the heart beat to a more normal rate.

80. **2** High biologic value (HBV) protein contains essential amino acids needed by the body for tissue building and repair.

　1 A high-caloric diet would provide for weight gain.

　3 Low biologic value (LBV) proteins avoid the accumulation of urea in the body.

　4 This is not the purpose of high biologic value proteins; sodium restrictions would decrease blood pressure.

81. **4** This action assesses the arterial blood flow to both legs; Doppler pressure measurements can also be implemented.

　1 There is a need to increase the collateral circulation to the leg; elevation is not recommended.

　2 Blood work will not directly provide this information.

3 Movement is needed to increase the collateral circulation to the leg.

82. **2** Angina pectoris usually occurs during exertion and usually subsides with rest and vasodilators.

　1 This is typical of pain with a myocardial infarction.

　3 Although this may be present with angina, it is typical of pain with a myocardial infarction. The key is to distinguish between the two conditions.

　4 Radiating pain is typical for both angina and myocardial infarction; however, this kind of pain seems more common with angina.

83. **4** This statement reflects on the resident's feelings, allowing for open communication.

　1 This is giving advice, closing communication between nurse and resident.

　2 Silence would not be an appropriate method of fostering communication at this time.

　3 Commenting on how everyone else feels does not help the way the resident feels; this blocks communication.

84. **4** Although other selections may be true, this selection enables the nurse to design a plan that will ultimately promote the change to a healthful behavior.

　1 This fact could be incorporated in the resident teaching; however, it is not the prime consideration in promoting healthy behaviors.

　2 This is inappropriate because it challenges the resident's sense of being and does not promote a therapeutic relationship.

　3 This fact should be included in promoting healthful behaviors, but it is not the correct answer given the other selections.

85. **4** Restrained residents should have a method for calling for help in the absence of a staff member.

　1 Unsafe; no method has been provided for the resident to call for help.

　2 This should be done every 2 hours, not 3 hours; this does not focus on the right to call for help.

　3 While this may support social friendships, it does not provide for safety as roommates are not responsible for one another.

86. **4** Immediate action is required for choking.

　1 Situation is an emergency—this is not relevant emergency action.

　2 Situation is an emergency—this is not relevant emergency action.

　3 Situation is an emergency—this is not relevant emergency action.

87. **1** Changing damp gowns and bedding prevents the child from chilling.
    2 This does not directly aid in promoting safety or comfort.
    3 The child needs freedom to move in the crib.
    4 The child should be positioned for maximum lung expansion, for example in high-Fowler's position.
88. **2** Essential to know that tube is in stomach and not in the lungs.
    1 Improper placement of the tube.
    3,4 Medication administered through an NG tube is usually in liquid form; if tablets are used they must be crushed and mixed with 30 ml of water before administering through the NG tube.
89. **3** Studies and evidence do not support this idea; creativity and intelligence do not change with age.
    1 This statement is true.
    2 This statement is true, although elderly people generally do not limit their ability to manage their households.
    4 The majority of older adults have at least one weekly contact with family and a network of friends.
90. **4** This is actual and factual data that does not imply the nurse's opinion or dissatisfaction.
    1 This is labeling the resident instead of describing what was measurable about his or her behavior.
    2 Although it is important to note in the chart, this is too vague as written.
    3 The first part is an opinion and labels the resident.
91. **4** The supine position with the head elevated 30 degrees allows for proper drainage of cerebral edema and will help reduce intracranial pressure (ICP).
    1 This will not help reduce ICP.
    2 This will not help reduce ICP.
    3 This will increase ICP.
92. **2** Frequent turning decreases the incidence of complications, provides good circulation, and maintains good skin integrity.
    1 Referring to an adjustment period produces anxiety and fear.
    3 The resident may experience phantom pain.
    4 This increases the incidence of complications, poor circulation, and poor skin integrity.
93. **1** Exercise causes muscle contractions, which require an increase in arterial circulation to supply oxygen and nutrients for energy being expended.

2 This is important for the person with diabetes, but it does not improve arterial blood flow.
    3 This would reduce arterial blood flow; the legs should be kept dependent.
    4 Hot water is contraindicated because it can burn the skin and/or cause drying; also, individuals with peripheral vascular disease have an altered perception of temperature.
94. **2** Flight of ideas refers to scattered thoughts, as evidenced by illogical connections made during verbalizations.
    1 Confusion is usually a matter of being disoriented as to time, place, or person.
    3 Delusions are fixed false beliefs.
    4 Hallucinations are the perceptions of sensory stimuli when no external objects are present.
95. **2** Body fluid that is lost normally is not replaced by intake of food and fluids.
    1 Edema, not dehydration, occurs.
    3 Uremia, not dehydration, occurs.
    4 Incontinence, not necessarily dehydration, occurs.
96. **3** Keeping the skin clean and dry aids in the prevention of infection.
    1 The child's position should be changed often to avoid constant pressure to one area as well as severe itching.
    2 To reduce itching and subsequent scratching a minimum amount of clothing is recommended.
    4 Warm, moist dressings would increase the itching; cool moist dressings should be used.
97. **2** This allows for drainage of secretions, blood and air through gravity.
    1 This is contraindicated because the drainage would flow back into the thoracic cavity, causing further complications.
    3 This is contraindicated because drainage would reenter the pleural space.
    4 The level is of primary importance to prevent complications and respiratory distress.
98. **1** This response presents reality, acknowledges the resident's statement, and casts doubt on the resident's altered thought process, all of which are therapeutic.
    2 This challenges the resident's thought process, which the resident may be compelled to defend; therefore, this would be nontherapeutic.
    3 This challenges the resident's thought process, which the resident may be compelled to defend; therefore this would be nontherapeutic.
    4 This reinforces the resident's hallucination and is thus nontherapeutic.

99. **4** According to state nurse practice acts, the nurse who draws up the medication is responsible for giving the drug.
 1 Not a responsible action for this situation.
 2 Not a responsible action for this situation.
 3 Not a responsible action for this situation.
100. **2** A portable chest x-ray examination should be done in the room to prevent disease transmission to others in the hospital.
 1 Because the resident is coughing frequently, the mask is needed; disease transmission during a trip to the radiology department is high.
 3 The infection control nurse could be contacted, but she will probably suggest either notifying the physician or a portable chest x-ray examination, as in the rationale for answer 2.
 4 Although the technicians should be protected, the risk of contamination during a trip to the radiology department is high.
101. **2** Any resident who has been sedated, or who is not fully conscious, may not sign the consent for a surgical procedure.
 1 Many residents face contradictory feelings regarding their impending surgery, but their consent is legal unless they withdraw the consent.
 3 A second opinion is not required for a consent to be legal.
 4 A complete history and physical are needed before surgery, but they do not affect the legality of consent.
102. **1** This indicates decrease in myocardium contraction and buildup of fluid in the lungs.
 2 This is not indicative of holding the medication.
 3 This is a positive sign that is sought.
 4 This is not indicative of a problem by itself.
103. **3** Family processes, altered, is the nursing diagnosis that is evident in the family's behavior. Assistance with coping behaviors can be facilitated by the nurse.
 1 When a nursing diagnosis is written, the relational statement should be something that the nurse can change. This is not true in this statement.
 2 The nurse cannot change or cure the resident's illness.
 4 Inappropriate nursing diagnosis; this is not evident.
104. **3** All medication orders in question should be clarified with the physician as soon as possible, especially orders that need to be given immediately.

1 The practical/vocational nurse does not have the authority to prescribe and therefore may not independently alter a physician's order.
 2 If the medication is out of the therapeutic dose range, the nurse is responsible to ensure the safety of the resident by clarifying the order and not giving a potentially dangerous dosage.
 4 Holding a "now" order of medication until the physician makes rounds may have deleterious effects on the resident and is personal nursing judgment.
105. **4** Respiratory isolation prevents transmission of disease through air droplets. A gown would usually not be required.
 1 The glass thermometer should be left in the room to prevent its use by any other resident.
 2 Hands should be washed before caring for any resident.
 3 A mask is always worn while caring for any resident in respiratory isolation.
106. **2** There is a lack of neural control of individual muscle fibers, resulting in a characteristic mask-like facies.
 1 This is unrelated to Parkinson's disease; this is often associated with a CVA.
 3 Movement usually abolishes tremors, which are known as nonintention tremors.
 4 This does not occur; both arms fall rigidly to the sides and do not swing with a normal rhythm when walking.
107. **3** The nurse's initial concern is the resident. To control the environment, the nurse should remove him from the room and have the oxygen discontinued.
 1 The fire alarm may not be necessary at this time. The nurse should further assess the situation.
 2 The supervisor should be notified, but only after the resident is safely out of the room.
 4 This is an acceptable response but only after the resident is safe.
108. **4** Resident's may refuse medication, but nurses who are responsible for the resident's safety, the plan of care, and the legal status of a nursing license will provide and document the teaching provided to the resident regarding the actions of the drug and reasons for its use.
 1 The response discounts the resident's rights to participate in and decline treatment if desired.
 2 This answer is true, but it is less complete than answer 4.
 3 This response does not allow the resident to make the decision now; it is bargaining with the resident to avoid a problem.

109. **1** This response is appropriate to clarify the situation and assess the potential for violence. The nurse should ask, "Are you thinking of hurting yourself now?" If the answer is yes, the nurse should ask, "How are you going to hurt yourself?" Following a response, the nurse should ask, "Can you agree not to hurt yourself for (a specific period) without talking with me first?" If the resident will not commit to not acting, the nurse should stay with her while appropriate alternative care is sought.
   2 Avoiding the subject is unwise; it is best to investigate.
   3 It is not necessary to describe other residents who have had similar feelings.
   4 It is premature to outline alternative measures.

110. **4** The amount, route, place and reason are all listed in this description.
   1 Although the description of the discomfort is good, the notes do not state where it was given.
   2 This charting does not indicate that the injection was given Z-track.
   3 This charting does not designate on which side the injection was given.

111. **4** In metabolic acidosis the lungs try to compensate by blowing off excess carbonic acid in the form of carbon dioxide.
   1 This is a compensatory mechanism to reduce fever by evaporation.
   2 This indicates renal compensation for alkalosis.
   3 This is not an adaptation to metabolic acidosis; fever with dehydration results from inadequate fluid for perspiration and cooling.

112. **3** This acknowledges that the resident is probably tired and may be frightened as a result of his mental deficits. It gives him the opportunity to feel some control in the process of being evaluated and makes the nurse an ally, not an enemy.
   1 This is true, but there is nothing to be gained and it needlessly aggravates the resident to continue to question him when he is obviously unwilling to continue at this time.
   2 There is no reason to doubt the truth of what the resident says he is feeling. Doubting him may make him angry and argumentative.
   4 This might also be true, but his family's wishes are not the priority at this time.

113. **2** Blues and greens are not seen clearly by older adults. Avoiding objects on the floor prevents falls, and using higher-intensity light assists in better vision as the size of the pupil decreases and is less responsive to light.
   1 High-energy food is necessary because aging affects taste, digestion, and metabolism. Because an older adult may not be aware of extreme loss of body heat, measures to prevent hypothermia include keeping room temperatures slightly higher than usual and staying indoors as much as possible on windy, wet, and cold days.
   3 Because of changes in visual acuity and problems with color interpretation, light intensity, and depth perception is aided by avoiding direct lights and white surfaces that produce glare; exposed bulbs can result in burns because of slower response time and reduced ability to feel pain.
   4 Slightly higher-than-normal room temperature prevents hypothermia; signs should have dark backgrounds and light lettering to be more easily seen; daily contact with another person helps in avoiding isolation.

114. **2** These are all aspects related to his physical and mental health while a resident is in the nursing home.
   1 This does not have to do with personal finances.
   3 This does not have to do with responsibilities after death.
   4 This does not have to do with responsibilities after death.

115. **3** It is important for the nurse to always follow facility policy and procedure for reporting errors or omissions. The Quality Assurance committee should be made aware of such incidents to determine if a problem does exist.
   1 The physician is not next in authority on the unit and would probably defer to the supervising nurse.
   2 Confrontation is not the responsibility of the staff nurse; it could result in unpleasant working conditions.
   4 Unnecessary and inappropriate; follow facility policy and procedure.

116. **2** An initial symptom of right ventricular heart failure because of COPD (cor pulmonale) is sudden weight gain.
   1 This is associated with polycythemia vera, not COPD.
   3 A sudden weight gain is not associated with this condition.
   4 Right, not left, ventricular heart failure occurs with COPD.

117. **4** Reality orientation—only response that does not reinforce confusion and disorientation.
   1 Reinforces disorientation and confusion.

2 Reinforces disorientation and confusion.

3 Reinforces disorientation and confusion.

118. **3** Realistic consequences should always be addressed at the time limits are set. It is important that the resident know what consequences have been established so he has the opportunity to discuss his reactions and feelings.

    1 As a motivation to change his behavior, the resident should know the consequences at the time the limit is set.

    2 Again, consequences should be preestablished to be consistently enforced by all staff members.

    4 Manipulative resident behavior can be quite frustrating to staff members. Manipulative behaviors should be immediately identified, and consequences enforced to motivate the resident to change his behavior.

119. **4** Active/passive exercising allows continued movement of the joints to prevent complications and assists in reducing pain.

    1 Bed rest limits activity and contributes to complications even with range-of-motion exercises.

    2 Balanced, rather than limited, activity with rest is needed to prevent complications even if it does tire the resident.

    3 Immobility leads to joint damage and deformity.

120. **1** This is an appropriate goal.

    2 False reassurance is not helpful.

    3 Secluding the resident is not helpful.

    4 Future planning may only depress the resident more.

121. **4** Crying is normal and residents need to vent their grief. Holding her hand is a nonverbal means of communicating understanding and empathy.

    1 The resident needs to know that you are there for her; leaving is an inappropriate nursing action.

    2 Stay, but does talk about postoperative care; she is not ready to hear that, she is still unaccepting of what her physician has just told her.

    3 The resident needs someone with her now for support; calling her husband at this moment is not priority unless the resident requests you do so.

122. **1** The performance of religious rituals, if done safely, should be supported because they meet spiritual and emotional needs.

    2 This does not recognize the religious importance of the candles and does not help the resident meet the need to perform this religious act.

    3 This denies the resident's feelings and ignores the religious importance of lighting the candles.

    4 Untrue; if performed safely, it can be done.

123. **2** Vitamin K is the antidote for an overdose of warfarin (Coumadin).

    1 This is an antidote for heparin.

    3 This is not an antidote for warfarin.

    4 This is not an antidote for warfarin.

124. **4** In older adults, there is a progressive atrophy of the convolutions with a decrease in the blood flow to the brain, which may produce a tendency to become forgetful, a reduction in short-term memory, and susceptibility to personality changes.

    1 People with a normal aging process show little or no change in their judgment.

    2 Creativity is not affected by aging; many people remain creative until very late in life.

    3 There is little or no intellectual deterioration; intelligence scores show no decline up to the age of 75 to 80.

125. **2** This is the recommended statement by E. Kubler-Ross. It is important for the resident to know that the nurse will try to help the resident. This response does not negate the resident's sense of hope.

    1 This relates a false sense of hope.

    3 This relates a false sense of hope and gives the resident a sense of doubt about the adequateness of her health-care providers.

    4 This does not recognize the resident's concerns or feelings.

126. **4** Common indication.

    1 Body temperature is often elevated.

    2 Respirations are often rapid and shallow.

    3 Skin is often cool and clammy.

127. **3** One cup of cottage cheese is approximately 225 calories, 27 g of protein, 9 g of fat, 30 mg of cholesterol, and 6 g of carbohydrate; proteins of high biologic value (HBV) contain optimal levels of the amino acids essential for life.

    1 Apple juice is a source of vitamin C, not protein.

    2 Raw carrots are a carbohydrate source and contain beta carotene.

    4 Whole wheat bread is a source of carbohydrates and fiber.

128. **1** This is below the normal range of 7.35 to 7.45; hypoxia causes hypercapnia, resulting in a fall in the pH.

    2 This is within the normal limits of 80 to 100 mm Hg.

    3 This is within the normal limits of 21 to 28 mEq/L.

    4 This is within the normal limits of 35 to 45 mm Hg.

129. **2** The resident has a right to refuse treatment; the physician must inform the resident of the risks involved with no treatment.
    1 If done safely, self-administration of medications is allowed; however, medications must be ordered by the doctor.
    3 Residents do not have a right to disturb the quality of life of other residents.
    4 This is not practical; meals are usually scheduled during traditional mealtimes.

130. **3** 100° F (37.7° C) to 105° F (40.5° C) is warm to the body.
    1 This option is cooler than body temperature and will defeat the goal of warmth to the perineum.
    2 This option is cooler than body temperature and will defeat the goal of warmth to the perineum.
    4 This temperature is hot enough to endanger skin integrity.

131. **4** Residents are often immunosuppressed and have decreased resistance; strict asepsis is needed to minimize exposure to microorganisms.
    1 Preparing supplies is important, but most important is to prevent contamination of supplies.
    2 Drainage tubes will be checked as part of the assessment, but reducing the spread of microorganisms takes priority.
    3 Giving assistance to resident's needs will be done, but most important in planning wound care is to avoid a wound infection.

132. **2** Informed consent means the resident knows what and why something is going to be done as well as who is going to do it.
    1 These actions support privacy, not informed consent.
    3 This violates informed consent; an alert resident has the right to leave a facility.
    4 Consents may be written or verbal; a verbal consent can be a gesture such as shaking the head yes or lifting up to get on a bedpan; legal written consents are obtained by the nurse.

133. **2** Goals/objectives are the expected results of nursing actions.
    1 Nursing measures other than those assigned are often necessary to meet resident needs.
    3 In many situations, nurses provide excellent care, yet the resident may not feel better.
    4 At times, good nursing care may not make the resident happy.

134. **3** Role modeling by the nurse is the best way to teach the resident how to maximize strengths and cope with deficits until there is improvement.

1 This gives false reassurance; it may take much longer and there is no way to predict how much the resident will recover.
2 This would deprive the resident of the comfort of his visits and denies him the opportunity to monitor progress.
4 This will not necessarily answer his questions any more completely or give him any more reassurance than talking with the nurse.

135. **3** Communion can be brought daily to the resident by a priest or lay minister of the Catholic church.
    1 This ignores the resident's need to go to Mass and receive communion daily.
    2 Unnecessary; the resident's spiritual needs must be met.
    4 The resident may not be able to follow through with this information; the nurse should communicate with the church to have someone visit the resident.

136. **3** Implementation of the universal precaution protocol is recommended in all health-care facilities when dealing with residents with HIV or AIDS.
    1 Although this is still a procedure in the nursery, universal precautions are being used in health-care facilities when caring for residents with HIV or AIDS. In fact, regardless of whether an infant or its mother is tested for the virus, most health-care facilities recommend that nurses wear gloves during initial care of the newborn.
    2 It is not the responsibility of the nurse to report to the CDC; the nurse is responsible to his or her supervisor, whose duty it is to report such cases.
    4 The mask, gown, and gloves at all times are not really necessary because most residents with HIV are not necessarily ill with the signs and symptoms of active AIDS. Use of masks, gowns, and gloves is for the resident whose immune system places him at risk.

137. **3** Coughing from the diaphragm will generate sputum as deeply as possible from the respiratory tract.
    1 Abdominal breathing is too shallow to encourage the expectoration of sputum.
    2 This will destroy bacteria that are an important part of the specimen.
    4 A high-Fowler's position is preferable to encourage the expectoration of sputum.

138. **1** Allopurinol inhibits the formation of uric acid.
    2 Corticosteroids are antiinflammatory agents and would be used in treatment of lupus erythematosus.
    3 Acetaminophen (Tylenol) is an analgesic.
    4 Estrogen replacement is recommended for osteoporosis.

139. **3** Elevating the head of the bed to high-Fowler's position would be the first nursing action for a resident who is experiencing dyspnea.

    1,2 Elevating the head of the bed will facilitate breathing; checking pulse and reporting to the team leader are secondary to assuring airway patency.

    4 Airway patency is priority, then pulse check and reporting; telling the resident to breath deeply may or may not be appropriate, depending on the reason for the dyspnea.

140. **3** Carbonated beverages are generally high in sodium and should be avoided.

    1 Many of these products contain sodium.

    2 This product may contain sodium.

    4 This product may contain sodium.

141. **4** A living will allows the resident to decide that extraordinary measures not be taken.

    1 The intent of a living will is to allow the resident, not the family, to decide what measures will be taken.

    2 This is a legal (probated) will; it does not take the place of a living will.

    3 A living will states what should not be done in the event of a terminal illness.

142. **1** The major need is personal and body functioning.

    2 This is an inappropriate response; they need to have a purpose in life.

    3 Isolation with only some group contact is unacceptable. It causes a mere state of existence rather than as full a life as possible.

    4 This is an unacceptable approach. These residents should be involved in making as many decisions as possible to maintain a sense of self-worth.

143. **3** When suctioning a resident, it is important to give oxygen before and after because suctioning removes oxygen as well as secretions. The length of time to suction would be 10 to 15 seconds. At least 5 minutes should elapse between each suctioning.

    1 Thirty seconds is too long; this would remove oxygen from the system.

    2 Coughing and deep breathing should not be performed as part of the suctioning procedure. Oxygenation is the last step.

    4 Twenty-five seconds is too long and would remove oxygen from the system. The last step is to oxygenate.

144. **4** These symptoms indicate a decrease in potassium, a side effect of too much fluid loss.

    1 Hematuria is not a side effect of this medication.

    2 These are side effects that bear watching, but they are not significant.

    3 Diarrhea by itself is not indicative of a problem.

145. **2** Lying on the affected side helps to splint the chest and assist in coughing.

    1 Because it is painful to breathe, the resident will avoid deep-breathing.

    3 Coughing increases the pain if there is no chest support.

    4 In this position the resident will be unable to give support to the affected side. This will not help the amount of pain the resident is experiencing.

146. **2** Autonomic dysreflexia may occur in 85% of all spinal cord-injured residents with lesions at T6 level or above.

    1 This symptom does not describe this condition.

    3 This symptom does not describe this condition.

    4 This symptom does not describe this condition.

147. **4** The pacing and the yelling indicate that the resident could benefit from PRN medication at this time before becoming more out of control.

    1 This has a threatening quality that is inappropriate.

    2 Residents should never be threatened.

    3 Residents should never be threatened.

148. **4** All are included for the reasons listed below.

    1 The physician and nurse coordinate the total care.

    2 The resident and his or her family are active participants and consumers of care.

    3 Total care involves all health providers and skills.

149. **1** This interferes with the transmission of impulses from the thalamus to the cortex of the brain, causing sedation.

    2 An antiepileptic (anticonvulsant) drug such as phenytoin (Dilantin) decreases convulsions/seizures.

    3 An antidepressant is a substance such as amitryptyline that decreases depression.

    4 A tranquilizer is a substance used to calm anxious or agitated people without decreasing consciousness.

150. **1** This allows the resident to use the staff as a support system and removes an opportunity to deny the problem.

    2 This supports and permits denial; both the resident and the staff know a problem exists, and the resident must admit it.

    3 This is a nonprofessional approach that would be nontherapeutic for the resident.

    4 This is a nonprofessional approach that would be nontherapeutic for the resident.

References/Bibliography

AJN/Mosby: *AJN/Mosby nursing boards review,* ed 9, St. Louis, 1994, Mosby.

AJN/Mosby: *The AJN/Mosby question and answer book,* ed 4, St. Louis, 1994, Mosby.

Babcock D and Miller M: *Client education: theory and practice,* St. Louis, 1994, Mosby.

Balzer-Riley J: *Communications in nursing: communicating assertively and responsibly in nursing, a guidebook,* ed 3, St. Louis, 1995, Mosby.

Barkauskas V et al.: *Health and physical assessment,* St. Louis, 1994, Mosby.

Bernhard LA and Walsh M: *Leadership: The key to the professionalization of nursing,* ed 3, St. Louis, 1995, Mosby.

Burke M and Walsh M: *Gerontological nursing: care of the frail elderly,* St. Louis, 1992, Mosby.

Castillo H: *The nurse assistant in long-term care: a rehabilitative approach,* St. Louis, 1992, Mosby.

Christ MA and Hohlack, FJ: *Gerontologic nursing:a study and learning tool,* 1988, Springhouse.

Christensen B and Kockrow: *Foundations of nursing,* ed 2, St. Louis, 1995, Mosby.

Christensen PJ and Kenney J: *Nursing process: applications of conceptual models,* ed 4, St. Louis, 1995, Mosby.

Edmunds M: *Introduction to clinical pharmacology,* ed 2, St. Louis, 1995, Mosby.

Eliopoulos, C: *Manual of gerontologic nursing,* St. Louis, 1995, Mosby.

Giger J and Davidhizar R: *Transcultural nursing: assessment and intervention,* ed 2, St. Louis, 1995, Mosby.

Green E and Karz J: *Clinical practice guidelines for the adult patient,* St. Louis, 1994, Mosby

Hermey C: *Quick reference for IV therapy,* St. Louis, 1995, Mosby.

Hoeman S: *Rehabilitation nursing: process and application,* ed 2, St. Louis, 1995, Mosby.

Hogstel M: *Clinical manual of gerontological nursing,* St. Louis, 1992, Mosby.

Husted G and Husted J: *Ethical decision making in nursing,* ed 2, St. Louis, 1995, Mosby.

Ingalls AJ and Salerno MC: *Study guide to accompany the 8th edition of Ingalls and Salerno's maternal and child health nursing,* ed 6, St. Louis, 1995, Mosby.

Iyer P and Camp N: *Nursing documentation: a nursing process approach,* ed 2, St. Louis, 1995, Mosby.

Jaffe M: *Geriatric nutrition and diet,* ed 2, St. Louis, 1995, Mosby.

Kelly K and Mass M: *Managing nursing care: promise and pitfalls* (SONA, Vol 5), St. Louis, 1993, Mosby.

Kelly KJ: *Nursing staff development: current competence, future focus,* Philadelphia, 1992, Lippincott Co.

Laraia MT and Stuart: *Quick psychopharmacology reference,* ed 2, St. Louis, 1995, Mosby.

Lewis S and Collier I: *Medical-surgical nursing: assessment and management of clinical problems,* St. Louis, 1992, Mosby.

Marquis B and Huston C: *Leadership roles and management functions in nursing: theory and application,* Philadelphia, 1992, J.B. Lippincott Co.

McKenry L and Salerno E: *Mosby's pharmacology in nursing,* ed 19, St. Louis, 1995, Mosby.

Myers J: *Quick medication administration reference,* ed 2, St. Louis, 1995, Mosby.

Perry A and Potter P: *Clinical nursing skills and techniques,* ed 3, St. Louis, 1994, Mosby.

NGNA: *NGNA Core curriculum for gerontological nurses and associates,* St. Louis, 1995, Mosby.

Phipps W et al.: *Medical-surgical nursing: concepts and clinical practice,* ed 5, St. Louis, 1995, Mosby.

Potter P: *Pocket guide to health assessment,* ed 3, St. Louis, 1994, Mosby.

Potter P and Perry A: *Basic nursing: theory and practice,* ed 3, St. Louis, 1994, Mosby.

Redman B: *The process of patient education,* ed 7, St. Louis, 1993, Mosby.

Rubin IL and Crocker AC: *Developmental disabilities: delivery of medical care for children and adults,* Philadelphia, 1989, Lea and Febiger.

Saxton D: *Mosby's comprehensive review of nursing,* ed 14, St. Louis, 1993, Mosby.

Saxton D et al: *Mosby's review questions for NCLEX-RN,* ed 2, St. Louis, 1995, Mosby.

Seidel H et al.: *Mosby's guide to physical examination,* ed 3, St. Louis, 1995, Mosby.

Sorrentino SA and Hogan J: *Mosby's textbook for LTC assistants,* ed 2, St. Louis, 1994, Mosby.

Soule B et al.: *Infection and nursing practice, prevention and control,* St. Louis, 1995, Mosby.

Stuart G and Sundeen: *Principles and practice of psychiatric nursing,* ed 5, St. Louis, 1995, Mosby.

Suddarth DS: *The Lippincott manual of nursing practice,* Philadelphia, 1991, JB Lippincott Co.

Swearingen P: *Manual of medical-surgical nursing care: nursing interventions and collaborative management,* ed 3, St. Louis, 1994, Mosby.

Umiker W: *Management skills for the new health Care supervisor,* Rockville, Md., 1988, Aspen Publishers.

Vitale B and Nugent P: *Long term care: test-taking review for nurse aides and assistants,* St. Louis, 1990, Mosby.

Watt-Watson J and Donovan M: *Pain management: nursing perspective,* St. Louis, 1992, Mosby.

Williams SR: *Essentials of nutrition and diet therapy,* ed 6, St. Louis, 1994, Mosby.

Williams SR: *Nutrition and diet therapy,* ed 7, St. Louis, 1994, Mosby.

Wold G: *Basic Geriatric nursing,* St. Louis, 1993, Mosby.

Wong D: *Whaley and Wong's nursing care of infants and children,* ed 5, St. Louis, 1995, Mosby.

Yannes-Eyles M: *Mosby's comprehensive review of practical nursing,* ed 11, St. Louis, 1994, Mosby.

Yannes-Eyles M: *Mosby's Q&A for NCLEX-PN,* St. Louis, 1994, Mosby.

Index